Yes/No Medical Spanish

Comprehensive Handbook of Clinical Spanish

Yes/No Medical Spanish

Comprehensive Handbook of Clinical Spanish

Tina M. Kaufman, PhD, PA-C
Physician Assistant III
Parkland Memorial Hospital
Dallas, Texas

Ticiano Alegre, MD
Faculty
North Lake College
Irving, Texas

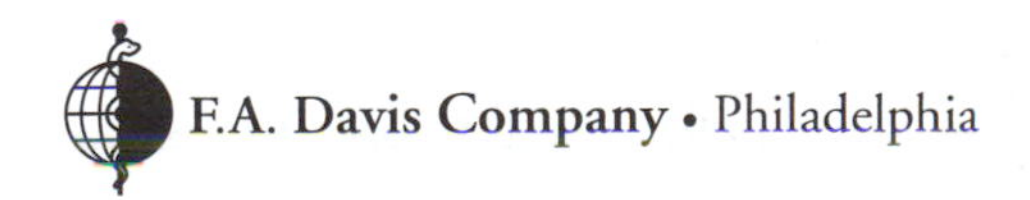

F.A. Davis Company
1915 Arch Street
Philadelphia, PA 19103
www.fadavis.com

Printed in the United States of America

Last digit indicates print number: 10 9 8 7 6 5 4 3 2 1

Senior Acquisitions Editor: Andy McPhee
Developmental Editor: Robyn Alvarez
Manager of Content Development: George W. Lang
Art and Design Manager: Carolyn O'Brien

Library of Congress Cataloging-in-Publication Data

Kaufman, Tina M.
Yes/no medical Spanish : a comprehensive handbook of clinical Spanish /
Tina M. Kaufman, Ticiano Alegre.
p. ; cm.
Includes index.
English and Spanish.
ISBN-13: 978-0-8036-2124-4
ISBN-10: 0-8036-2124-8
1. Spanish language—Conversation and phrase books (for medical personnel) I. Alegre, Ticiano. II. Title.
[DNLM: 1. Medical History Taking—Phrases—English. 2. Medical History Taking—Phrases—Spanish. 3. Physical Examination—Phrases—English. 4. Physical Examination—Phrases—Spanish. 5. Physician-Patient Relations—Phrases—English. 6. Physician-Patient Relations—Phrases—Spanish. W 15 K21y 2010]
PC4120.M3K33 2010
468.3'42102461—dc22

2009034330

"It is because the body is a machine that education is possible. Education is the formation of habits, a superinducing of an artificial organisation upon the natural organisation of the body."

—*Thomas Henry Huxley*
(19th-century English physician)

Foreword

The social and cultural diversity of our society is nowhere more evident than in health care practice. Because illness beliefs and behavior are so influenced by culture, and because establishing a trust relationship with patients is so important for effective treatment, today's student clinicians must acquire the knowledge, skills, and attitudes needed to understand and respond effectively to their patients' cultural differences. In recent years such cultural competence has become a byword in health care education.

However, the most obvious and fundamental barrier to communication is lack of a common language. In the metropolitan area where I practice, dozens of languages are spoken by people from several continents, but the Latino community is by far the largest, constituting nearly 15% of our patient population. While many of these patients are bilingual, many others are not, especially the elderly and those who have arrived recently in the United States. How can we provide optimal medical care for these patients? The best approach, of course, would be to train a sufficient number of thoroughly bilingual clinicians. Failing that, we are obligated to ensure that our clinics and hospitals provide the services of professional Spanish translators.

Nonetheless, situations commonly arise when non-Spanish speaking health care professionals must assess and treat patients who speak no English or whose English is rudimentary. Such patients may sometimes be accompanied by family members willing to translate, but communication via relatives can present privacy problems and may not always be reliable. Moreover, professional translators may be a scarce resource, often unavailable in triage situations and urgent care. Clinicians are then faced with a dilemma. How might they perform a targeted patient assessment, given the lack of a common language?

This is where a book like Kaufman and Alegre's *Yes/No Medical Spanish* provides an invaluable service. By presenting basic Spanish words, phrases, and questions related to symptoms of illness and other aspects of the clinical examination, the text allows the learner to accomplish much more than might appear at first glance. First, of course, the language tools, in conjunction with nonverbal communication, will allow the learner to accomplish the basic task of clinical assessment. In addition, the learner's willingness to communicate in Spanish, even if carried out in a rudimentary fashion, will help generate a trusting relationship. Patients and their families almost always appreciate attempts to "reach out" to them in their own language. Finally, the discipline of learning and using these basic tools will likely help students develop confidence not only in their ability to manage the difficult situation at hand, but also in a capacity to learn the language in greater depth. Clinical practice provides a great venue for doing so. With sufficient practice, what began as a series of yes/no questions, might eventually lead to the satisfying accomplishment of true clinician–patient conversation in Spanish.

—Jack Coulehan, MD, MPH
Professor Emeritus
Stony Brook University School of Medicine

Reviewers

Paul Arnstein, RN, PhD, FNP
Associate Professor
Community Health Nursing
Boston College
Chestnut Hill, MA

Hannah Kathleen Bomar, PA-S
Physician Assistant Student
Baylor College of Medicine
Allied Health Department
Houston, TX

Anna M. Choo, JD, MD
Resident Physician
Emory University
Physical Medicine and Rehabilitation
Atlanta, GA

Yovana Coupey
Medical Spanish Program Coordinator
Albert Einstein College of Medicine
Bronx, NY

Katherine M. Erdman, MPAS, PA-C
Assistant Director
Physician Assistant Program
Baylor College of Medicine
School of Allied Health Sciences
Houston, TX

Alejandro Garcia-Lemos, MA
General Manager
Comunicar Language and Consulting Services
Spanish Translation and Interpretation
Columbia, SC

Michele Iannuzzi Sucich, MD
Family Practitioner and Geriatrician
Private Practice
Poughkeepsie, NY

Ashlee Elizabeth Jontz, RN, BSN
Staff Nurse/Adult Nurse Practitioner Student
Good Samaritan Hospital
Arizona State University
Chandler, AZ

Naghmeh Khodai, MD
Resident Physician
Rush Medical Center
OB/Gynecology Department
Chicago, IL

V. Maloof, MD
Phlebotomy Program Director
Griffin Technical College
Griffin, GA

John Tobias Musser, MD
Physician
Emory University
Physical Medicine and Rehabilitation
Atlanta, GA

Maurizio Najt
Medical Spanish Instructor
Albert Einstein School of Medicine
Bronx, NY

Diane E. Nuñez, MS, ANP-C, BC
Clinical Associate Professor
Arizona State University
College of Nursing and Healthcare Innovation
Phoenix, AZ

Megan Spears, RN, BSN
NP student
Arizona State University
Chandler, AZ

Daniel Wood, MPAS, PA-C
Clinical Assistant Professor
University of Texas Health Science Center at San Antonio
Physician Assistant Studies
San Antonio, TX

Erica Young, PA-C
Medical Department
University of Texas Medical Branch
Houston, TX

Acknowledgments

I wish to gratefully acknowledge all the people whose support, assistance, and encouragement went into the making of this book. I would like to express my gratitude first and foremost to my co-author Ticiano Alegre, my teacher, colleague, and friend.

My appreciation and thanks go out to *all* the incredible people at F.A. Davis who worked so hard on making this book a reality, and more specifically to the following: Yvonne Gillam, who helped create the podcasts; George Lang, whose support and encouragement were unlimited; Andy McPhee, who decided to take a chance on the concept (and us!); and Robyn Alvarez, for her painstaking work on editing the manuscript and really helping us put it all together and make it look like a book. I really cannot thank them enough. And I cannot forget to thank all my Spanish-speaking patients who, over the years, have been gracious and good humored in allowing me to "practice" on them. And last, I owe a special thanks to Sandi, as always, for her input, advice, patience, and support. She is the best!

—Tina M. Kaufman, PhD, PA-C

What can I say, what can I say. Many years ago I was studying for a midterm. It was late, I was tired, and I could not get a clear thought on what I was reading. I was thinking about someone, I was thinking about something, I was just thinking about everything. I kept asking myself questions about why and when and what. I remembered not coming up with any adequate answers. During a break, as I was heading out of the bathroom, I remembered looking into the mirror and at that instance I realized many things. I was very thankful to God, I was very thankful to my mother, I was very thankful to those who always support me and love me. Without them nothing could have been possible, nothing is currently possible, and nothing will be possible nor have meaning. Therefore, my love, my mind, and my ink goes to them, but especially to my patient wife and my inquisitive son, because they allow me to do what I do.

—Ticiano Alegre, MD

Contents

Yes/No Medical Spanish

Comprehensive Handbook of Clinical Spanish

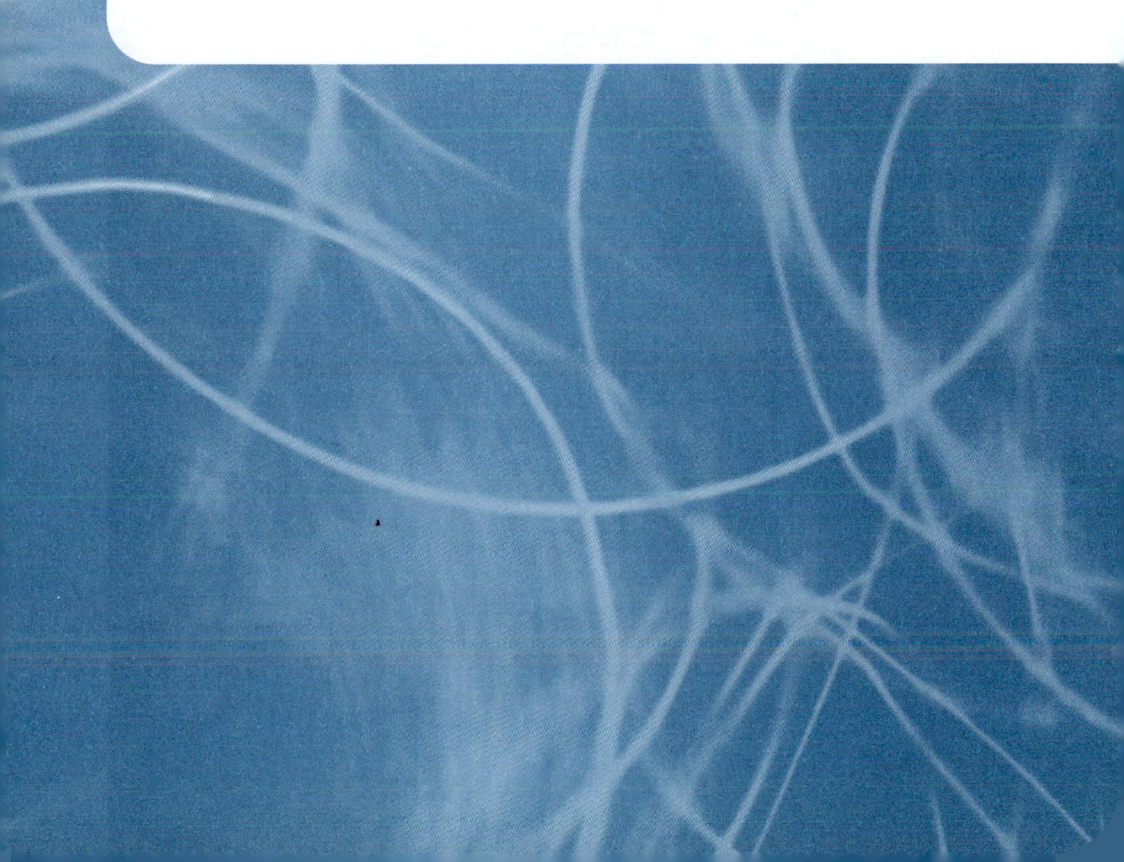

Chapter 1

Breaking Down Language Barriers

According to the U.S. Census Bureau, as of mid-2007, Latinos make up over 15% of the U.S. population, and remain not only the country's largest minority group, but also the fastest growing, with a 29% increase between 2000 and 2007.[1] Many Latinos are limited in English language proficiency, with a limited ability to read, write, speak, or understand English. In fact, according to a 2000 U.S. Census Survey, 45% of all Spanish speakers self-reported that they spoke English "not well" or "not at all."[2]

These language barriers in the Latino population may adversely affect their use of health care services. It is well documented that Latinos as a group, and Spanish-speaking individuals specifically, often experience a lower quality if health care in the United States compared to English-speaking individuals.

---

[1]Annual Estimates of the Population by Sex, Race, and Hispanic Origin for the United States: April 1, 2000 to July 1, 2007 (NC-EST2007-03) http://www.census.gov/popest/national/asrh/NC-EST2007-srh .html. Accessed 1/20/09.

[2] Language Use and English-Speaking Ability: 2000. US Census Bureau. http://www.census.gov/ prod/2003pubs/c2kbr-29.pdf. Accessed 1/20/09.

Studies show that Spanish-speaking patients experience longer wait times, less help from office staff, and difficulties with provider communication.[3,4] Without interpreter or translator services, these language barriers and cultural differences can lead to a reluctance to seek medical care, resulting in suboptimal health care overall.

In order for clinicians to provide quality health care to Spanish-speaking patients, they must be able to communicate effectively. To care for the increasing Spanish-speaking patient populations across the country, there is a strong push in all healthcare areas to create a more ethnically diverse nursing work force. In addition, healthcare employers in hospitals and clinics are making extra efforts and providing incentives to recruit bilingual nurses and clinicians.

While there is a growing trend in the United States among health professions' training programs to provide medical Spanish, it still remains the exception rather than a required component of the curriculum. Among the U.S. Physician Assistant programs surveyed in 2005, only 31% offered any type of medical Spanish training, with only 12.9% of those as a formal class.[5]

The idea for this book came during a night course in medical Spanish, when we—the teacher (a physician educator) and the student (a clinically practicing physician assistant)—realized a need for a new approach to a handbook of clinical medical Spanish. It was obvious early on in the course that, to communicate effectively with Spanish-speaking patients, a non-Spanish-speaking clinician would need more expertise than a semester of night courses could provide. As a non-Spanish-speaking clinician, the challenge is not in learning how to ask questions in Spanish; rather the more daunting task is comprehension of the verbal reply in Spanish. Medical Spanish textbooks currently available are designed to teach open-ended questions. While open-ended questions are considered optimal for obtaining medical histories, they are impractical if the history taker is not fluent in the language. The reply is frequently lost in translation, if not misunderstood altogether.

Dissatisfied with the currently available medical Spanish textbooks, we designed this book to provide the reader with specific sets of directed questions intended to elicit specific medical histories in an organized, algorithmic fashion. Avoiding the open-ended format wherever possible, the

---

[3] Fiscella K, Franks P, Doescher MP, Saver BG. Disparities in health care by race, ethnicity, and language among the insured: findings from a national sample. *Med Care.* 2002;40(1):52–59.

[4] Woloshin S, Schwartz LM, Katz SJ, Welch HG. Is language a barrier to the use of preventive services. *J Gen Intern Med.* 1997;12(8):472–477.

[5] Gonzalez CM, Parma LA. Medical Spanish and physician assistant education; Usage, barriers and need. *Perspect Physician Assistant Educ.* 2005;16(1):18–20.

questions are designed in a progressive, history-specific format to elicit either a yes or no answer. Of course, not all questions are amenable to a yes/no format; in these instances, the answers may require a simple day or date or number as an answer.

We do not intend for this book to replace an interpreter; however, in busy private practice or more rural areas, interpreters may not be readily available. This book strives to bridge the gap between those providers whose understanding of Spanish is little to none, and the Spanish-speaking patient. The contents of this book may be used in a variety of clinical settings: the routine outpatient office visit, the emergency room, or inpatient hospital environment. The book is clearly geared toward health care providers such as physicians, physician assistants, nurse practitioners, and nurses. However, many others in the health care field will find this book useful, including medical assistants, receptionists, and front-end office staff.

The chapters of this book are separated into sections that are easily referenced for either inpatient or outpatient encounters. When a patient is admitted to the hospital and a comprehensive history is required, there are sections for adult, obstetric, and pediatric patients.

There are several chapters for the outpatient encounter. There is a chapter that specifically addresses active medical conditions for which the patient needs ongoing follow up, such as diabetes or hypertension, as well as a chapter with commonly encountered symptoms for which the patient may present for more urgent or emergent care, such as chest pain, dyspnea, ear ache, or back pain.

Unique in other ways, this book offers information for both nurses and providers to instruct patients on such topics as nutrition, exercise, and diabetes care, and screening questions on dementia, depression, domestic violence, and alcohol abuse.

One of the more unique aspects of this book is its usefulness as a teaching resource for the student in health care. The organizational structure of the questions are designed not only to elicit specific histories, but may be used by the student as a reference for learning medical history taking. Students often use acronyms to memorize the components of taking a history of present illness, and in this book we teach the acronym OLD CARTS, as well as the key history components required for proper reimbursement. Additionally, Chapter 7, "Comprehensive Adult History," and Chapter 8, "Review of Systems" follow the standard format and order taught in most medical history textbooks.

In this age of ever-increasing demands on the clinician's time, we intend for you to use this book as a quick reference without requiring any background knowledge in the Spanish language. While patients usually are quite forgiving if pronunciation is not exact, in some instances the meaning of the word changes with incorrect pronunciation. We have included sections to teach basic pronunciation and grammar to enhance provider-patient communication. Because words and phrases with similar meanings often vary depending on the region or culture, alternate words or phrases are set in bold for easy reference throughout the text to denote regional variations.

Finally, there are two bonus features available to the reader: Podcasts are available for download on DavisPlus (http://davisplus.fadavis.com) to assist the reader with language skills such as pronunciation, verb conjugation, everyday phrases, and a typical patient encounter; and patient education handouts are available in both Spanish and English for download.

The unique features of this book—the yes/no format; the organization; the inpatient, emergency and ambulatory care clinical scenarios; and a focus on cultural competency, patient education, and prevention—will make *Yes/No Medical Spanish: A Comprehensive Handbook of Clinical Spanish* the most invaluable reference on the market. We sincerely hope that you find this book an important resource in your health care endeavors and that it helps us all improve the quality of health care for Spanish-speaking patients.

Chapter 2

Pronunciation and Grammar

This chapter was designed for the health care workers' (HCW) need for simple and to-the-point grammar. Here you will find useful information about how to pronounce the Spanish alphabet, as well as how to understand some of the simplest grammar concepts of the language. This chapter will provide particular conjugations as well as information about basic mechanics of the Spanish language.

Pronunciation

The Alphabet

Letter	Pronunciation	Letter	Pronunciation
a	*ah*	n	*eneh*
b	*beh*	ñ	*en-yeh*
c	*seh*	o	*oh(au)*
ch	*che*	p	*peh*
d	*deh*	q	*ku*
e	*eh*	r	*ere*
f	*eh-feh*	s	*ese*
g	*heh*	t	*teh*
h	*ah-che*	u	*oo*
i	*ee*	v	*veh*
j	*houtah*	w	*doble veh*
k	*kah*	x	*eh-kees*
l	*ele*	y	*ee-griegah*
ll	*eh-yeh*	z	*zeh-ta*
m	*emeh*		

Vowels

Vowel	Pronunciation	English Examples	Spanish Examples
A	*ah*	father	paso, arte, alma
E	*eh*	met	peso, estilo
I and Y	*ee*	machine and corky	piso, Díos, Ynez
O	*oh*	sold, note	pozo, olmo
oo (rare) is pronounced as a long O			
U	*oo*	like oo in moon and moot	puso, unido *(never like U in mute)*
		between G and E or I, it is not pronounced, as in guest, guide	guerrilla

Consonants

There are a number of hard and soft sounding consonants based on vowel combinations that are easy to confuse while speaking.

Consonant/consonant-vowel combination	Hard or Soft	Pronunciation
j	hard	*h*
ba; ca	hard	*bah; cah*
be; ce	soft	*beh; seh*
bi; ci	soft	*bee; see*
bo; co	hard	*boh; ko*
bu; cu	hard	*boo; coo*

There are also a number of rules that determine the way certain consonants are pronounced.

Consonant	English Examples	Spanish Examples
C plus A, O, U or a consonant	Like hard C in cat, copy, and cooper	cama, como, cura, cual, clamor, acción
C plus E or I	Like soft C in certain	centro, cero, hacer, decir
CH	Like ch in church	chocolate, leche, churro
G plus A, O, U or a consonant	Like hard G in gate	García, golfo, gusano, amigo, gracias (The G in the gua combination is pronounced so softly by some that it sounds almost like *wah*, as in *Guadalupe*, *guayabera*)
G plus E or I	like hard H in hag, hog, hug	gente, ingeniero, gitano, agitar
H	not pronounced, as in heir	hijo, hotel, herencia, humano
J	like hard H in hot, harp	José, Jesús, Guadalajara
LL	Y sound, as in yes	calle, llano, llave
Ñ	like NI in onion and NY in canyon	cañon, España, tamaño

Consonant combination/consonant-vowel	Hard or Soft	Pronunciation
QU	like K in kite and QU in quay	querida, quetzal, Quito
S	like SS in miss	mesa, Jesús, rosa, asistir
X before a consonant	like English S	extraño
	like English X, as in exit	Éxito
Z	like SS in kiss	zona, zapato, mestizo

The remaining consonants are pronounced approximately as they are in English.

Syllable Stresses

The following are general rules for the placement of stress (Donde va la fuerza de pronunciacion):

1. 9Words ending in a vowel, N, or S are stressed on the next-to-last syllable.
2. Words ending in all other letters are stressed on the last syllable.
3. Words that do not follow these first two rules carry written accent marks.
4. Capital letters often are not marked with a written accent.

Grammar

Nouns

As in English, a noun is the part of speech used for people, places, objects, and conditions.

They are either masculine or feminine.

Rule	Spanish Example	English Translation
Most nouns that end in *–o* are masculine.	**el carro**	the car
Most nouns that end in *–a* are feminine.	**la puerta**	the door

Grammar (cont)

Rule	Spanish Example	English Translation
Exceptions:		
Some feminine nouns end in *–o.*	**la mano**	the hand
Some masculine nouns end in *–a.*	**el problema**	the problem
Nouns ending in *–ción, –sión, –dad, –tad, –tud, lud,* and *–umbre* are generally feminine.	**la** canción **la** televisión **la** calidad **la** amistad **la** salud **la** multitud **la** lumbre	the song the television the quality the friendship the health the multitude the fire

There are a number of rules for making nouns plural in Spanish. Some are similar to English rules and some are quite different.

Rule	Spanish Example	English Translation
For a noun that ends in a vowel, add *–s.*	el chequ**e** becomes los cheque**s**	the checks
For a noun that ends in a consonant, add *–es.*	el guardia**n** becomes los guardian**es**	the guardians
For a noun that ends in *–z,* change the **z** to a **c** and add *–es.*	el albatro**z** becomes los albatro**ces**	the albatrosses
A noun that ends in *–es* will remain the same (only the article **el** or **la** changes to **los** or **las** to indicate plural).	**El** martes becomes **los** martes	Tuesdays

Articles

Articles are a part of speech used to modify nouns and to specify their application. They agree in gender and number with the nouns they modify.

Spanish uses four **definite articles:** *el, la, los,* and *las*. The correct choice depends on the gender and number of the noun being modified. All of these words translate to the English *the*. Use the following rules to determine which to use:

Rule	Spanish Example	English Translation
Proper noun that is modified by an adjective	**El** estudioso niño	the boy who studies very much
Weight or measure	**La** carne de cerdo está a tres dolares **la** libra	Pork is going for three dollars a pound.
Names of some cities, countries, and continents	**La** China, **Los** Estados Europeos, **La** Paz, **La** America Central	China, European Union, La Paz (capital of Boliva), Central America
Name of a subject	Me gusta **la** geometría.	I like geometry.
Noun in apposition with a pronoun	Nosotros **los** irlandeses	We, the Irish
With nouns listed in a series	Pongo **el** plátano, **el** melón y **la** naranja en la canasta.	I put the banana, the watermelon, and the orange in the basket.
Intangible concept	**La** pena es **la** hermana de **la** experiencia.	Sorrow is the sister of experience.
Infinitives used as nouns	**El** cantar es divertido.	Singing is fun.
Titles, ranks, and professions	**El** Capitán Ramirez está aquí.	Captain Ramirez is here.
Days of the week	De vez en cuando vamos a la ciudad **los** domingos.	Occasionally we go to the city on Sundays.

Articles (cont)

Rule	Spanish Example	English Translation
Seasons	En **el** verano hace mucho calor.	In the summer it is very hot.
Showing possession	**Los** zapatos de José están en el cuarto de María.	Jose's shoes are in Maria's room.
Telling time	Son **las** dos.	It's two o'clock.

Indefinite articles also vary according to gender and number. In Spanish, the indefinite articles are *un/una*, which translate to *a/an*, and *unos/unas*, which translates to *some*.

Rule	Spanish Example	English Translation
Indefinite articles go *before* the noun		
Masculine		
Singular: **Un**	**un** libro	a book
	un techo	a roof
	un zapato	a shoe
	un pelo	a hair
	un periódico	a newspaper
Plural: **Unos**	**unos** archivos	some records
	unos peines	some combs
	unos cuartos	some rooms
Feminine		
Singular: **Una**	**una** pluma	a pen/feather
	una camisa	a shirt/blouse
	una libreta	a notebook
	una lámpara	a lamp
Plural: **Unas**	**unas** camas	some beds
	unas almohadas	some pillows
	unas sabanas	some bed sheets

Pronouns

A pronoun is a functional word that is used in place of a noun or noun phrase. The following table shows the **personal pronouns** and their English translations.

Spanish	English
yo	I
tú	you (familiar)
él	he
ella	she
usted	you (formal)
nosotros	we
ellos	they (masculine)
ellas	they (feminine)
ustedes	you (formal)

There are other types of pronouns as well that we use in other situations. **Reflexive pronouns** are used whenever the subject of a verb is also its object. Reflexive pronouns are used when the subject of a sentence is acting on itself.

Spanish Pronoun	English Translation	Spanish Example	English Translation
Me	myself	Me visto.	I'm dressing myself.
Te (informal)	yourself	¿Te vistes?	Can you dress yourself?
Se	himself, herself, itself, themselves, yourself (formal), yourselves (formal), each other	Tina se quiere.	Tina loves herself.
Nos	ourselves, each other	Nos aceptamos.	We accept ourselves. or We accept each other.

Interrogative pronouns are those we use to ask questions.

Spanish	English
¿Quién? ¿Quiénes?	Who? Whom?
¿Qué?	What?
¿Cuál? ¿Cuáles?	What? Which?
¿Cuánto? ¿Cuánta?	How much?
¿Cuántos? ¿Cuántas?	How many?

Possessive pronouns indicate ownership. In Spanish, possessive pronouns vary according to the gender of the noun they replace.

Singular (masc/fem)	Plural (masc/fem)	English Translation
el mío, la mía	los míos, las mías	mine
el tuyo, la tuya	los tuyos, las tuyas	yours (familiar singular)
el suyo, la suya	los suyos, las suyas	yours (his, hers, its)
el nuestro, la nuestra	los nuestros, las nuestras	ours
el suyo, la suya	los suyos, las suyas	yours (formal)/theirs

Demonstrative pronouns indicate specific nouns. As with other pronouns, they vary by gender and number.

Masculine	Feminine	Neutral	English Translation
este	esta	esto	this one (over here)
estos	estas		these (over here)
ese	esa	eso	that one (over there, closer)
esos	esas		those (over there, closer)
aquel	aquella	aquello	that one (over there, farther)
aquellos	aquellas		those (over there, farther)

Objects of Prepositions

When the pronoun is acting as the object of the preposition, a different set of pronouns is used. Use the object of preposition pronoun to replace the noun that comes right after the preposition.

Subject Pronouns	Object of Preposition Pronouns	Spanish Example	English Translation
yo	mí	Sandi conversa **de mí**.	Sandi talks **about me**.
tú	ti	Sandi conversa **de ti**.	Sandi talks **about you** [singular informal].
él	él	Sandi conversa **de él**.	Sandi talks **about him**.
ella	ella	Sandi conversa **de ella**.	Sandi talks **about her**.
usted	usted	Sandi conversa **de usted**.	Sandi talks **about you** [singular formal].
nosotros/as	nosotros/as	Sandi conversa **de nosotros**.	Sandi talks **about us**.
vosotros/as	vosotros/as	Sandi conversa **de vosotros**.	Sandi talks **about you** [plural informal].
ellos/as	ellos/as	Sandi conversa **de ellos**.	Sandi talks **about them**.
ustedes	ustedes	Sandi conversa **de ustedes**.	Sandi talks **about you** [plural formal].

These rules govern the use of objects of prepositions.

Rule	Spanish Example	English Translation
Whenever the object of preposition **mí** follows the preposition **con**, the two words combine to form **conmigo**.	¿Quieres venir **conmigo**?	Do you want to come **with me**?
Whenever the object of preposition **ti** follows the preposition **con**, the two words combine to form **contigo**.	No quiero nada **contigo**.	I don't want anything to do **with you**.

Adverbs

Adverbs modify verbs, adjectives, and other adverbs.

Rule	Adjective	Feminine Singular Form	Adverb
Most Spanish adverbs are formed by adding *–mente* to the feminine singular form of the adjective. This ending corresponds to *–ly* in English.	brusco (rough) inteligente (intelligent) fácil (easy)	brusca (rough) inteligente (intelligent) fácil (easy)	brusca**mente** (roughly) inteligente**mente** (intelligently) fácil**mente** (easily)
Another way to form an adverb is to use the preposition **con** and the singular form of the noun.	bondadoso (kind)	bondadosa (kind)	bondadosamente (kindly) or con bondad (with kindness)

Adverbs cont.

Rule	Adjective	Feminine Singular Form	Adverb
An adverb can go before the adjective it modifies but usually follows the verb it modifies			La crema es **muy** sabrosa (the cream is **very** delicious).

There are three types or classes of adverbs:

Type	Rule	Spanish Example	English Translation
Equality	Use **tan** followed by an adjective, or use an adverb and add **como** and **tanto**.	José es **tan** alto **como** Pedro.	Joseph is **as** tall **as** Peter.
		Tengo **tanto(s)** caballos **como** ustedes.	I have **as many** horses **as** you guys.
Inequality	Place **mas** or **menos** before and **que** after the adjective, adverb or the noun	Juan es **más** musculoso **que** Roberto.	John is **more** muscular **than** Bob.
		María es **menos** sensitiva **que** Patricia.	Mary is **less** sensitive **than** Patricia.
Superlatives	Place a definite article and **mas** or **menos** in front of the adjective	Kurt es el muchacho **más/menos** delgado de la clase.	Kurt is the **thinnest/least thin** boy in the class.
		Bob es el **más/menos** bravo de la escuadra.	Bob is the **bravest/least brave** of the squadron.

Adjectives

Adjectives are a part of speech that modifies a noun, usually describing it or making its meaning more specific.

Rule	Spanish Example	English Translation
Most feminine adjectives end in –*a*.	bonita	beautiful
Most masculine adjectives end in –*o*.	guapo	handsome
They must agree with the gender and number of the nouns they modify.	Los **niños** son **inteligentes**.	The children are intelligent.
They are made plural the same way as nouns.	Los **caballos** son **veloces**.	The horses are speedy.
Those ending in –*án* and –*ón* are made feminine by adding –*a* and *dropping* the accent.	La mula es muy **haragana**.	The mule is very sluggish.
A nationality ending in a consonant is converted to feminine by adding –a and *dropping* the accent.	Japones→ Japones**a**	Japanese
Adjectives ending in –dor are converted to feminine by adding –*a*.	trabajador→ trabajador**a**	hard-working

There are a number of different types of adjectives. **Possessive adjectives** indicate ownership.

Masculine	English Translation	Feminine	English Translation
mi libro	**my** book	**mi** mano	**my** hand
mis libros	**my** books	**mis** manos	**my** hands
tu libro	**your** book (familiar singular)	**tu** mano	**your** hand (familiar singular)
tus libros	**your** (familiar plural) books	**tus** manos	**your** hands (familiar plural)
su libro	**his** book; **her** book; **your** (formal) book; **their** book	**su** mano	**your** hand; **her** hand; **your** (formal) hand; **their** hand
sus libros	**his** books; **her** books	**sus** manos	**his** hands; **her** hands; **your** (formal) hands; **their** hands
nuestro libro	**our** book	**nuestra** mano	**our** hand
nuestros libros	**our** books	**nuestras** manos	**our** hands

Demonstrative adjectives specify particular nouns.

Masculine	Feminine	English Translation
este	esta	**this** one
estos	estas	**these**
ese	esa	**that** one (closer)
esos	esas	**those**
aquel	aquella	**that** one (farther)
aquellos	aquellas	**those** (farther)

Skin Cancer

Actinic Keratoses

- A precursor to squamous cell carcinoma that appears as a scaly, erythematous patch, and is evidence of significant sun damage to the skin.
- Usually present on sun-exposed skin (face, ears, hands, arms) along with other signs of sun damage, such as thickened, yellowish skin.
- Treatment: Eliminate by liquid nitrogen, trichloroacetic acid, topical cream, chemical peels, or laser. Confirm diagnosis before treatment.

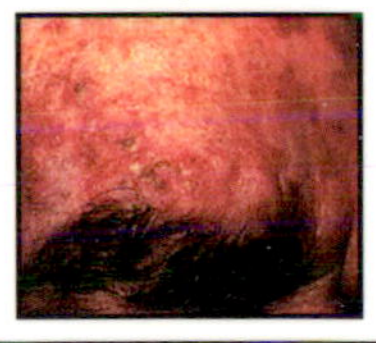
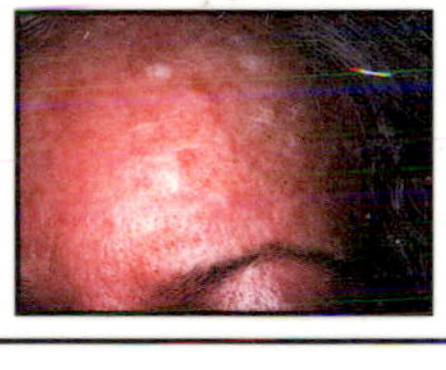
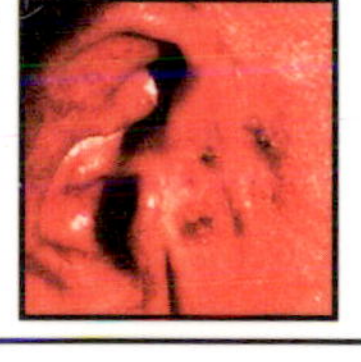

Basal Cell Carcinoma

- Usually appears as a pink, pearly, translucent papule with prominent telangiectasia that may ulcerate in the center.
- Usually present on sun-exposed skin, particularly the head and neck.
- Diagnosis: Perform a punch biopsy to remove lesion for clinical diagnosis.

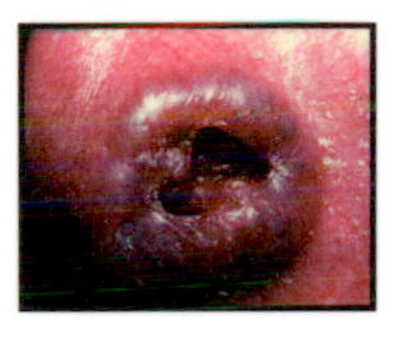
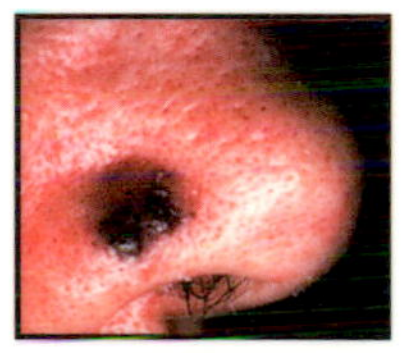
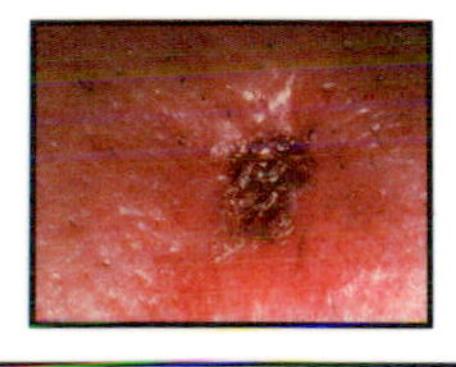

Squamous Cell Carcinoma

- Usually appears as a red nodule with a central crust.
- Usually present on sun-exposed skin (face, lip, ear, neck, hands, arms) or can develop on traumatized or chronically inflamed skin (e.g., burn scars, ulcers, or radiodermatitis sites).
- Diagnosis: Perform a punch biopsy to remove lesion for clinical diagnosis.

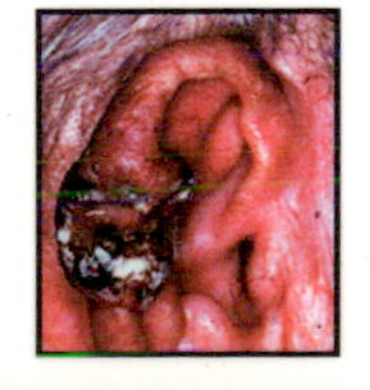
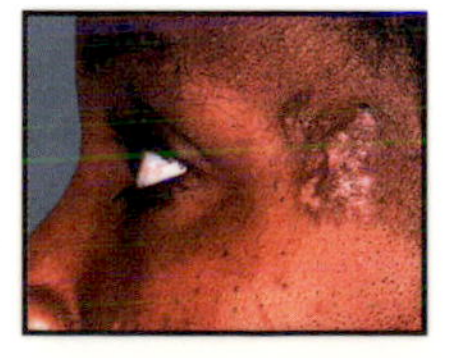
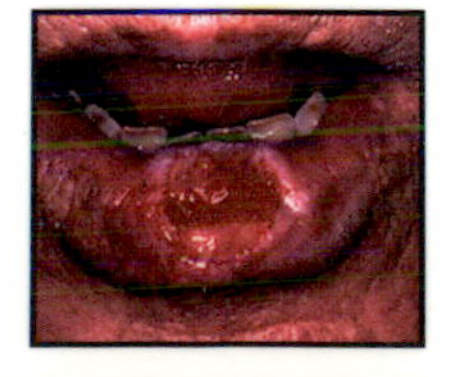

Malignant Melanoma

Asymmetry

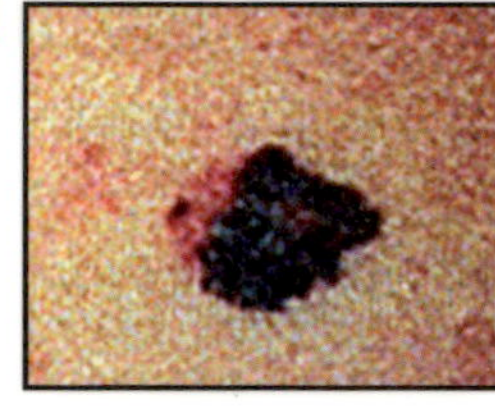

Border

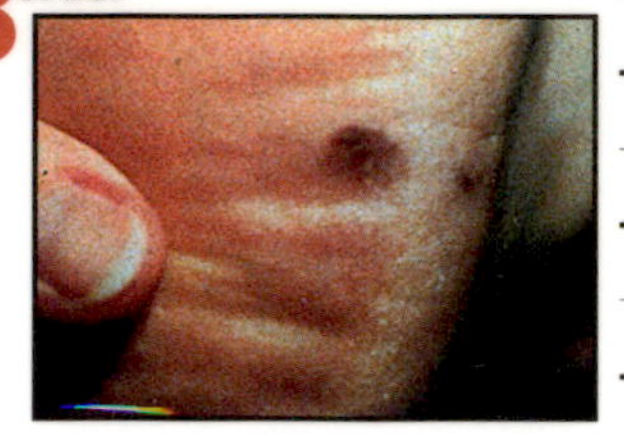

Color

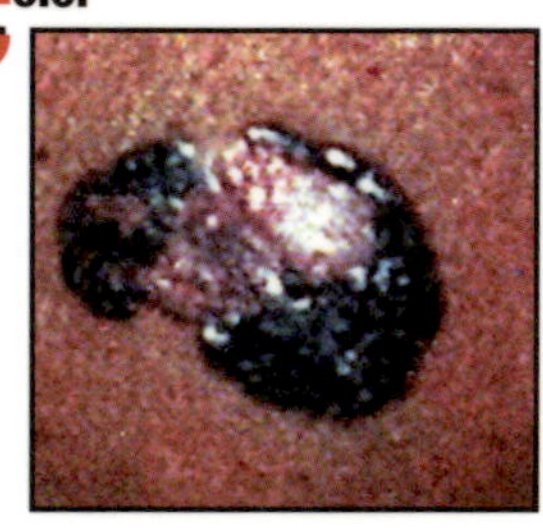

Diameter

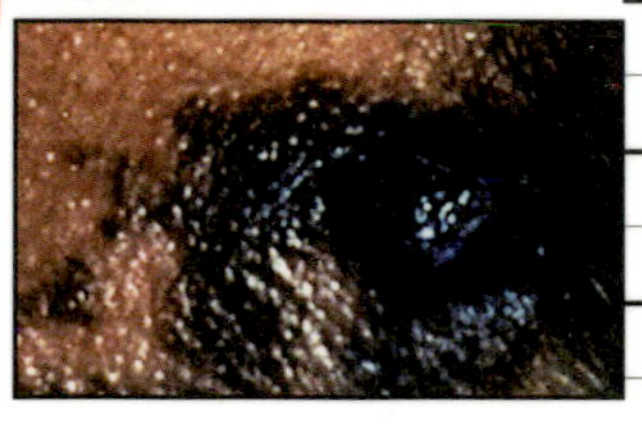

1cm 2cm 3cm 4cm 5cm 6cm 7cm 8cm 9cm 10cm 11cm

Malignant Melanoma

- Appears as a lesion that is asymmetrical, has notched or poorly defined borders, varies in color (tan, brown, black, blue, red, or white areas in any combination), and often is larger than 6 mm in diameter.
- Usually present on areas covered by clothing. In women, about 50 percent of melanomas are found on the lower extremities, mostly the legs; in men, 50 percent occur on the trunk and 24 percent on the head and neck.
- Diagnosis: Perform excisional or incisional biopsy for lesions suspected of being melanoma.

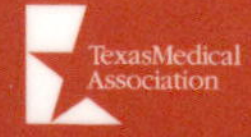

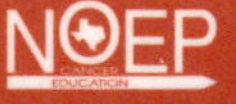

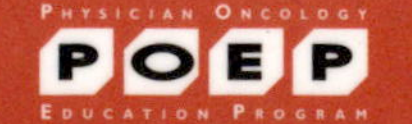

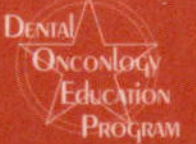

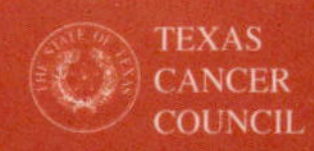

Limiting adjectives go before the noun.

Type	Spanish Example	English Translation
Demonstratives	**esta** libreta	**this** notebook
	estos pacientes	**these** patients
Possessives	**mis** guantes	**my** gloves
	tu archivo	**your** file
Indefinite articles	**unas** mesas	**some** tables
	un periódico	**a** newspaper
Cardinal numbers	**ocho** doctores	**eight** doctors
	tres cuchillos	**three** knives
Ordinal numbers	el **tercer** piso	the **third** floor
	el **primer*** piso	the **first** floor

*In some instances the adjective will lose the "o" ending before a masculine singular noun. In this case we do **not** say **el primero piso** but **primer piso**. Another example is **algun perro** (some dog)—we do **not** say **alguno perro**.

Descriptive adjectives follow two rules:

Rule	Spanish Example	English Translation
They follow the nouns they modify.	el perro **grande**	the **big** dog
	la rosa **roja**	the **red** rose
When they are not adding a particular characteristic or emphasis and are associated with the noun, they will go before the noun (this type of adjective is used often in poetry).	la **roja** rosa de la India	the Indian **red** rose
	el **blanco** cielo de invierno	the **white** sky of winter

Verbs

Verbs express action, a state of being, or the relationship between the subject and object in a sentence. In Spanish, they are categorized according to infinitive endings: *–ar*, *–er*, and *–ir*. If the verb agrees with the formula below, it is considered a regular verb. If it does not, then it is considered an irregular verb.

The following is an example of how we would conjugate the verb *to cook* in English in the first person in the various tenses:

Tense	Example
Present	I **cook** on Sunday all day.
Imperfect	I **was cooking** on Sunday all day.
Preterit	I **cooked** on Sunday all day.
Future	I **will cook** on Sunday all day.
Conditional	I **would have** cooked on Sunday all day . . .
Present Subjunctive (represents the things we recommend or wish we or someone else would do but haven't actually done yet)	I **hope to cook** all day on Sunday.
Imperfect Subjunctive (If this were to happen . . .)	**If I were to cook** on Sunday all day . . .

Follow the rules in the charts below for the various conjugations. For regular verbs using the ending *–ar*, as in *cocinar* (to cook):

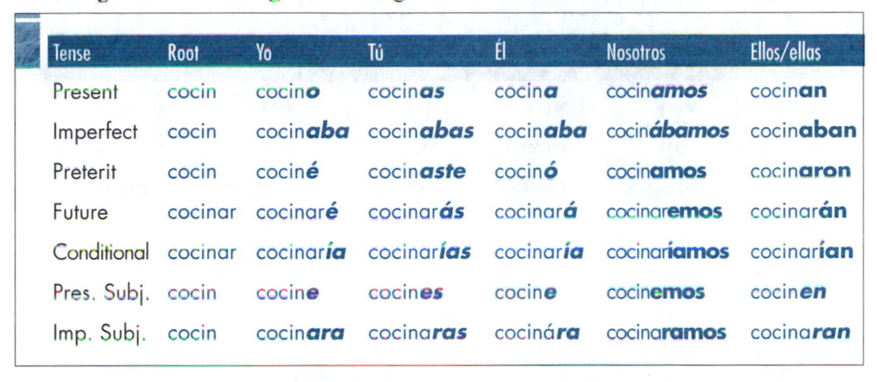

Tense	Root	Yo	Tú	Él	Nosotros	Ellos/ellas
Present	cocin	cocino	cocinas	cocina	cocinamos	cocinan
Imperfect	cocin	cocinaba	cocinabas	cocinaba	cocinábamos	cocinaban
Preterit	cocin	cociné	cocinaste	cocinó	cocinamos	cocinaron
Future	cocinar	cocinaré	cocinarás	cocinará	cocinaremos	cocinarán
Conditional	cocinar	cocinaría	cocinarías	cocinaría	cocinaríamos	cocinarían
Pres. Subj.	cocin	cocine	cocines	cocine	cocinemos	cocinen
Imp. Subj.	cocin	cocinara	cocinaras	cocinára	cocinaramos	cocinaran

For regular verbs using the ending *–er*, as in *correr* (to run):

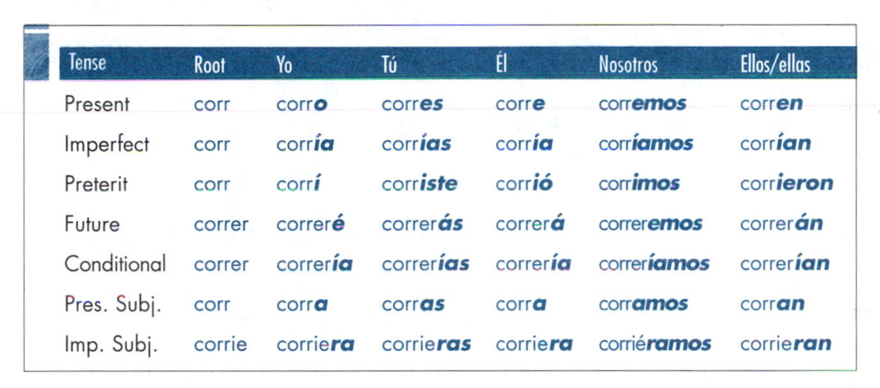

Tense	Root	Yo	Tú	Él	Nosotros	Ellos/ellas
Present	corr	corro	corres	corre	corremos	corren
Imperfect	corr	corría	corrías	corría	corríamos	corrían
Preterit	corr	corrí	corriste	corrió	corrimos	corrieron
Future	correr	correré	correrás	correrá	correremos	correrán
Conditional	correr	correría	correrías	correría	correríamos	correrían
Pres. Subj.	corr	corra	corras	corra	corramos	corran
Imp. Subj.	corrie	corriera	corrieras	corriera	corriéramos	corrieran

For regular verbs using the ending *–ir*, as in *escribir* (to write):

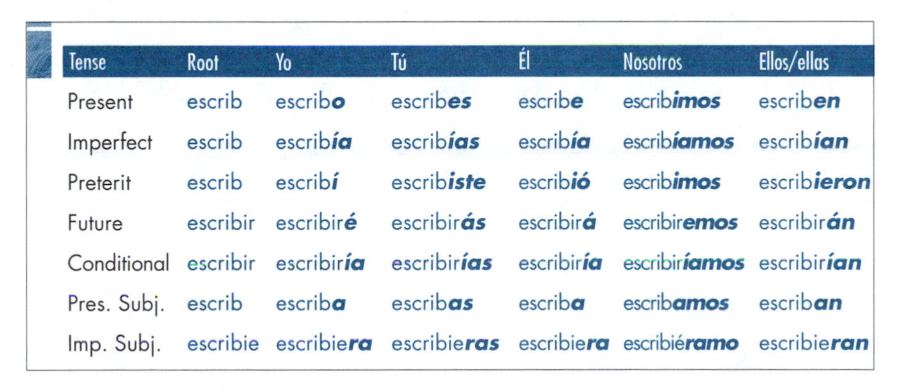

Tense	Root	Yo	Tú	Él	Nosotros	Ellos/ellas
Present	escrib	escribo	escribes	escribe	escribimos	escriben
Imperfect	escrib	escribía	escribías	escribía	escribíamos	escribían
Preterit	escrib	escribí	escribiste	escribió	escribimos	escribieron
Future	escribir	escribiré	escribirás	escribirá	escribiremos	escribirán
Conditional	escribir	escribiría	escribirías	escribiría	escribiríamos	escribirían
Pres. Subj.	escrib	escriba	escribas	escriba	escribamos	escriban
Imp. Subj.	escribie	escribiera	escribieras	escribiera	escribiéramo	escribieran

The following table lists the most common **irregular verbs** and their conjugations in the present tense.

	Yo	Tú	Él	Nosotros	Ellos/Ellas
Ir (to go)	**voy**	**vas**	**va**	**vamos**	**van**
Ser (to be)	s**oy**	**eres**	**es**	s**omos**	s**on**
Tener (to have)	**tengo**	**tienes**	**tiene**	**tenemos**	**tienen**
Venir (to come)	ven**go**	v**ie**nes	v**ie**ne	ven**imos**	v**ie**nen
Dar (to give)	d**oy**	d**as**	d**a**	d**amos**	d**an**
Decir (to tell/say)	d**igo**	d**i**ces	d**i**ce	dec**imos**/	d**icen**
Estar (to be)	est**oy**	est**ás**	est**á**	est**amos**	est**án**
Haber (to have)	**he**	**has**	**ha**	**hemos**	**han**

To conjugate more than one verb in a sentence, use the following rules:

1. Verbs separated by the conjunction y (and): Conjugate both verbs when y separates the verbs: **Yo corro y juego**. (I run and play.)
2. Verbs separated by the conjunction **pero** (but): You do *not* need to conjugate both verbs since the conjunction **pero** is separating two sentences: **Me gusta correr pero brincar no me gusta mucho**. (I like to run, but I do not like to jump so much.)
3. Two verbs in a row: Conjugate the first verb and leave the second verb in the infinitive form: **Usted necesita beber leche**. (You need to drink milk.)

Mood

Each verb has various moods (sometimes called the mode). They indicate the attitude of the speaker about the factuality or likelihood of what is expressed. Each mood has three non-finite forms:

1. An **infinitive**, ending in –ar, –er, and –ir
2. A **gerund**, which has several different forms; see "The English *–ing*" below
3. A **past participle**, formed by dropping the infinitive ending (–ar, –er, –ir) and adding –ado (for –ar *verbs*) or –ido (for –er and –ir verbs). For example, caminar: camin– + –ado → caminado

The **indicative mood** is used in typical speech when making statements. The indicative is the most common of moods and is used in expressing facts and actual situations. It indicates action, process, or identity as taking place in reality. For example:

Como (I eat, I am eating)
He comido (I have eaten)
Estoy comiendo (I am eating)
He estado comiendo (I have been eating)

The **subjunctive** mood is used to discuss potential, hypothetical, possible, or desirable events, or events portrayed subjectively. It indicates action, process, or identity as dependent on the speaker's reaction to it. To conjugate the present subjunctive, drop the –o from the first person of the present indicative and add the subjunctive endings as seen below:

	–ar verbs: caminar	*–er* verbs: correr	*–ir* verbs: vivir
yo	cami**ne**	corr**a**	viv**a**
tú	camin**es**	corr**as**	viv**as**
él/ella	camin**e**	corr**a**	viv**a**
usted	camin**e**	corr**a**	viv**a**
ustedes	camin**en**	corr**an**	viv**an**
nosotros	camin**emos**	corr**amos**	viv**amos**
ellos/ellas	camin**en**	corr**an**	viv**an**

The **conditional mood** ("would") creates situations that can be characterized by "if this, then that." For example:

Si fuera doctor, diagnosticar su problema **sería** [from the infinitive ser] fácil.

If I **were** a doctor, diagnosing you **would** be easy.

To conjugate the conditional mood, add –ía to the root for most conjugations:

	Bailar	Comer	Vivir
yo	bailar**ía**	comer**ía**	vivir**ía**
tú	bailar**ías**	comer**ías**	vivir**ías**
él/ella	bailar**ía**	comer**ía**	vivir**ía**
usted	bailar**ía**	comer**ía**	vivir**ía**
ustedes	bailar**ían**	comer**ían**	vivir**ían**
nosotros	bailar**íamos**	comer**íamos**	vivir**íamos**
ellos/ellas	bailar**ían**	comer**ían**	vivir**ían**

The **imperative mood** expresses commands. The imperative mood has only one tense: the present tense. To form the present tense of the imperative mood, we need to take the regular infinitive verbs (*–ar*, *–er*, *–ir*) and conjugate them in the present indicative, then replace *–er* and *–ir* with *–e* or *–ar* with *–a*. For example:

Infinitive	Conjugation	Translation	Imperative	Translation
Comer	Yo como.	I eat.	¡Com**e**!	Eat!
Escribir	Yo escribo.	I write.	¡Escrib**e**!	Write!
Hablar	Yo hablo.	I speak.	¡Habl**a**!	Speak!

The English –ing

A gerund is a verb that ends in -ing and functions or is used as a noun; gerunds can be subjects, subject complements, direct objects, indirect objects, and objects of prepositions. To form the gerund of regular verbs in Spanish, drop the infinitive ending (–ar, –er, –ir) and add –ando to the stem of –ar verbs and **–iendo** to the stem of –er and –ir verbs.

The gerund is a form of the verb that always ends in **–ndo** in Spanish, for example: escribiendo (writing), corriendo (running), masticando (chewing).

Form	Example	English Translation
verb (most commonly is used in the progressive form)	Roman está **caminando** toda la casa.	Roman is **walking** all over the house.
adjective	Anne Marie está **cocinando** una cena deliciosa.	Anne Marie is cooking a very delicious dinner.
noun	Ticiano y Anne Marie están delgados por que están **comiendo** menos durante la cena.	Ticiano and Anne Marie are thinner because they are **eating** less during dinner.
adverb	Sandi estaba **bailando** toda la noche.	Sandi was **dancing** all night long.

The Famous Ser and Estar

Ser and estar are two of the most common verbs used in Spanish, and they can be used as classic grammar tools. The following table shows the uses of ser:

Rule	Spanish Example	English Translation
Describes characteristics of a/an		
object	Mi libro **es** verde.	My book **is** green.
animal	Mi caballo **es** blanco.	My horse **is** white.
person	Mi amigo **es** alto.	My friend **is** tall.
Deals with		
origin	Yo **soy de** Puerto Rico.	I **am from** Puerto Rico.
material	El lápiz **es de** madera.	The pencil **is made of** wood.
ownership (when followed by the preposition **de**)	El reloj **es de** mi tío.	The watch **belongs to** my uncle.
time	¿Qué hora **es**?	What time **is** it?
dates	¿Qué día **es**?	What day **is** it?

The following table shows the uses of estar:

Rule	Spanish Example	English Translation
Indicates location	San Jose **está** en Costa Rica	San Jose **is** in Costa Rica
Indicates state or condition	Él **está** enfermo.	He **is** sick.
	Él **está** hecho pedazos.	He **is** [or **feels**] worthless/demoralized.
	Él **está** muerto.	He **is** dead.

Chapter 3

Vocabulary

This section encompasses a compilation of reference words most often used in the health care system. They will be greatly useful in many instances when or where the health care worker needs a particular word or phrase to fully translate a complicated concept.

This section will also be an extra aid in various scenarios where prior chapters might not contain the necessary words for which the health care worker is looking.

Despite every attempt to format questions in a yes/no format, certain questions will arise that necessitate qualitative, quantitative or time-dependent answers. This chapter includes a wealth of useful words and phrases that will assist the provider in navigating questions involving numbers, days, colors, anatomy, etc.

While it is possible to flip to this chapter when necessary, it is probably not the most time-efficient method for the busy health care provider. Memorizing some common numbers, days, time-related words, and simple interrogatives in the beginning will greatly assist the provider with many of the clinical questions in later chapters.

Basic Phrases

Introductory Phrases	Frases Preliminares
Hello, my name is . . .	Hola, me llamo . . . Hola, **mi nombre es** . . .
I am . . .	Yo soy un/una . . .
a physician assistant/nurse practitioner.	asistente de doctor/enfermera profesional. asistente de doctor/**enfermera especializada**.
the nurse for Dr. _____.	la enfermera del Doctor ____.
the medical assistant.	el asistente de médico.
the radiology technician.	el tecnólogo radiológico.
the receptionist.	la recepcionista.
the office manager.	la gerente de oficina.
the lab technician.	el técnico de laboratorios.
Do you speak English?	¿Habla usted inglés?
How may I help you?	¿Como lo puedo ayudar?
Repeat please.	¿Repita por favor?
Slowly, please.	Despacio, por favor.
I do not understand.	No entiendo
Do you understand?	¿Usted entiende?
Say yes, no, or I don't know.	Diga si, no o no se.
Good morning/afternoon/evening.	Buenos días/buenas tardes/buenas noches.

Basic Phrases

I speak very little Spanish.	Yo hablo un poco de español. Yo hablo un **poquito** de español.
I do not speak Spanish.	Yo no hablo español.
Do you speak English?	¿Usted habla Inglés?
Is there someone with you that speaks English?	¿Hay alguien con usted que habla Inglés?
Please use English as much as possible.	Por favor use Inglés lo más posible. Por favor **hable** Inglés lo más posible.
I am learning to speak Spanish.	Yo estoy aprendiendo español.
How do you say ___ in Spanish?	¿Como se dice ___ en español?
I am going to get someone that speaks Spanish.	Voy a buscar a alguien que habla español.
What is your name?	¿Cuál es su nombre? **¿Como se llama?**
Pleased to meet you.	Gusto en conocerle. **Mucho gusto** en conocerle.
Thank you.	Gracias
You are welcome.	De nada.

Simple Interrogatives

how	cómo
which	cuál
which (plural)	cuáles
when	cuándo
how much	cuánto/a
how many	cuántos/as
where	dónde
why	por qué
for what reason	para qué
what	qué
who	quién
who (plural)	quiénes
whom, to whom	a quiénes

Basic Phrases

Directions

above	arriba
around	alrededor
around the corner	a la vuelta
backward	hacia atrás
behind	detrás de
below	debajo de
come in	pase **pásele**
Continue straight along the hall.	Siga derecho por el pasillo.
down	abajo
elevator	elevador
escalators	escaleras
face down	boca abajo
face up	boca arriba
floor	piso
forward	adelante
Go down to the third floor.	Baje al tercer piso.
Go there.	Vaya allí.
Go up the elevator to the fifth floor.	Suba por el elevador al quinto piso.
Go up the stairs.	Suba por los escalones.
Go up to the first floor.	Suba al primer piso.
here	aquí
in front	al frente
inside	adentro
is over there (further/closer)	está allá/allí
near	cerca
next to	al lado
on the other side of the hall	en la otro lado del pasillo
on top of	encima de
on your left side	sobre el lado izquierdo
on your right side	sobre el lado derecho
outside	afuera
over here (in this area)	acá
Please follow me.	Por favor sígame.

Basic Phrases

stairs	los escalones
straight	derecho
that one (farther from the listener)	aquel
there (in sight)	allí
there (further)	allá
this one (closer to the speaker)	éste/ésta
that one (closer to the listener)	ése
through the door	por la puerta
to the left	a la izquierda
to the rear	al fondo allá atrás
to the right	a la derecha
toward	hacia
up	arriba

In the Hospital

basement	sótano
business office	oficina de comercio oficina de **negocios**
cafeteria	cafetería
cardiac rehabilitation	rehabilitación cardiaca
cardiology	cardiología
cardiovascular lab (testing)	laboratorio cardiovascular (para pruebas)
central supply	área de suplido central **cuarto de suministro** central **cuarto de surtido** central **cuarto de provisiones** central
chapel	capilla (feminine) gremio (masculine)
chaplain	capellán
clinic	la clínica
counseling	consejero
dermatology	dermatología
dialysis	diálisis
emergency room	sala de emergencia
endocrinology	endocrinología

Basic Phrases	*Frases Básicas*
family medicine	medicina de familia
gastroenterology	gastroenterología
gift shop	tienda de regalos
ground floor	planta baja
gynecology	ginecología
hospital	hospital
hydrotherapy	hidroterapia *hidropatía*
infectious disease	enfermedades infecciosas
internal medicine	medicina interna
labor and delivery	sala de parto **labor y expulsión**
laboratory	laboratorio
lobby	sala de espera
medical records	archivos médicos
nephrology (renal)	nefrología
neurology	neurología
neurosurgery	neurocirugía
newborn nursery	unidad de recién nacidos **enfermería** de recién nacidos
obstetrics	obstetricia
occupational therapy	terapia ocupacional
oncology	oncología
operating room	sala de operaciones
ophthalmology	oftalmología
oromaxillofacial surgery (dental)	cirugía oromaxilofacial
orthopedics	ortopedia
orthotics	relacionado con aparatos ortopédicos
otolaryngology (ear, nose and throat)	otorolaringologo (oído, nariz y garganta)
parking	estacionamiento
pediatrics	pediatría
pharmacy	farmacia
physical medicine and rehabilitation	rehabilitación y medicina física
physical therapy	fisioterapia

Basic Phrases

plastic surgery	cirugía plástica
prosthetics	protética
psychiatry	psiquiatría
psychology	psicología
pulmonary lab	laboratorio pulmonar
pulmonology	pulmonologia
radiology	radiología
recovery room	sala de recuperación *cuarto de recuperación*
registration	registración
respiratory therapy	terapia respiratoria
rheumatology	reumatología
room	sala
speech therapy	foniatría
social work	asistencia social
social worker	trabajador/a social **asistente social** **visitador/a social**
surgery	cirugía
thoracic surgery	cirugía torácica
urology	urología
vascular surgery	cirugía vascular
waiting room	sala de espera

Relationships

wife	esposa
husband	esposo
partner/lover	compañero/a
friend	amigo/a
fiancé	novio de compromiso
boyfriend	novio
girlfriend	novia
mother	madre

Basic Phrases

father	padre
stepmother	madrastra
stepfather	padrastro
stepdaughter	hijastra
stepson	hijastro
parents	los padres
sister	hermana
brother	hermano
daughter	hija
son	hijo
child	niño
children	niños
baby	bebe
grandmother maternal grandmother paternal grandmother	abuela abuela materna abuela paterna
grandfather	abuelo
grandparents	abuelos
grandchildren	nietos
grandson	nieto
granddaughter	nieta
aunt	tía
uncle	tío
niece	sobrina
nephew	sobrino
godfather	padrino
godmother	madrina
goddaughter	ahijada
godson	ahijado
cousin	primo
mother-in-law	suegra
father-in-law	suegro
sister-in-law	cuñada
brother-in-law	cuñado

Basic Phrases

family	familia
relative	pariente
neighbor	vecino
roommate	compañero de cuarto
single	soltero/a
married	casado/a
separated	separado/a
divorced	divorciado/a
widowed	viudo/a

Colors

black	negro
blue	azul
brown	café **marrón**
clear	claro
gold	dorado
gray	gris
green	verde
orange	anaranjado, naranja
pink	rosado
red	rojo
white	blanco
yellow	amarillo

Numbers, Time, and Distance

Numbers

1	uno
2	dos
3	tres
4	cuatro
5	cinco
6	seis
7	siete
8	ocho
9	nueve
10	diez
11	once
12	doce
13	trece
14	catorce
15	quince
16	dieciséis
17	diecisiete
18	dieciocho
19	diecinueve
20	veinte
21	veinte y uno
22	veinte y dos
23	veinte y tres
24	veinte y cuatro
25	veinte y cinco
26	veinte y seis
27	veinte y siete
28	veinte y ocho
29	veinte y nueve
30	treinta
31	treinta y uno
32	treinta y dos

Numbers, Time, and Distance

40	cuarenta
50	cincuenta
60	sesenta
70	setenta
80	ochenta
90	noventa
100	cien
101	ciento uno
102	ciento dos
110	ciento diez
120	ciento veinte
200	doscientos
201	doscientos uno
220	doscientos veinte
500	quinientos
700	setecientos
900	novecientos
1000	mil
10,000	diez mil
1,000,000	un millón
half	medio/a
quarter	cuarto
double	doble

Ordinal

first	primero
second	segundo
third	tercero
fourth	cuarto
fifth	quinto
sixth	sexto
seventh	séptimo
eighth	octavo
ninth	noveno
tenth	décimo

Numbers, Time, and Distance

eleventh	undécimo
twelfth	dos decimo
thirteenth	tres décimo
fourteenth	cuatro decimo
twentieth	vigésimo
1/4	un cuarto
1/3	un tercio
1/2	un medio
2/3	dos tercios
3/4	tres cuartos

Time

second	segundo
minute	minuto
hour	la hora
yesterday	ayer
today	hoy
tomorrow	mañana
the day after tomorrow	pasado mañana
the day before yesterday	antes de ayer
last night	anoche
tonight	esta noche
the night before last	antenoche
now	ahora
What time is it?	¿Qué hora es?
It is 1:00 [for 1:00 only].	Es la una.
It is 12:00 [for 2:00–12:00 only].	Son las doce.
3:15	tres y cuarto **tres y quince**
3:30	tres y media **tres y treinta**
3:35	cuatro menos veinticinco
3:45	cuatro menos cuarto **cuatro menos quince**

Numbers, Time, and Distance

At what hour?	¿A qué hora?
At 1:00.	A la una.
At [2:00–12:00].	A las [dos-doce].
early	temprano
late	tarde
earlier	más temprano
later	tarde
early in the morning	temprano por la mañana
in the morning (no specific time)	por la mañana
in the daytime	durante el día
at noon	al mediodía
at midnight	a la medianoche
at bedtime	al acostarse
at night	por la noche
before	antes
after	después
every day	todos los días
every other day	cada dos días
weekly	semanalmente
weekend	fin de semana
monthly	al mes
yearly	anual
every hour	cada hora
at the same hour	a la misma hora
at intervals	de vez en cuando

Dates

day	día
week	semana
month	mes
year	año

Days of the Week

Sunday	domingo
Monday	lunes
Tuesday	martes

Numbers, Time, and Distance

Wednesday	miércoles
Thursday	jueves
Friday	viernes
Saturday	sábado
on Monday	el lunes
on Mondays	los lunes

Months

January	enero
February	febrero
March	marzo
April	abril
May	mayo
June	junio
July	julio
August	agosto
September	septiembre
October	octubre
November	noviembre
December	diciembre
on March 1	en marzo primero
on April 31	en abril treinta y uno

Recent Years

1998	noventa y ocho
1999	noventa y nueve
2000	dos mil
2001	dos mil uno
2002	dos mil dos
2003	dos mil tres
2004	dos mil cuatro
2005	dos mil cinco
2006	dos mil seis
2007	dos mil siete
2008	dos mil ocho
2009	dos mil nueve

Numbers, Time, and Distance

2010	dos mil diez
2011	dos mil once
2012	dos mil doce

Distance

inch(es)	pulgada(s)
foot/feet	pie/pies
mile(s)	milla(s)
block(s)	bloque(s) **manzana(s)** **cuadra(s)**
centimeter(s)	centimetro(s)
meter(s)	metro(s)

Health Care

Anatomy

abdomen	el abdomen
ankle	el tobillo
appendix	la apéndice
arm	el brazo
artery	la arteria
back	la espalda
bladder	la vejiga
blood	la sangre
bones	los huesos
bowel	el vientre
brain	el cerebro
breast	el seno
buttocks	las nalgas
cervix	el cuello de matriz
cheek	la mejilla
chest	el pecho
ears	los oídos

Health Care

elbow	el codo
esophagus	el esófago
eye	el ojo
face	la cara
finger	el dedo de la mano
foot	el pie
gallbladder	la vesícula
gums	las encías
hand	la mano
head	la cabeza
heart	el corazón
heel	el talón
hip	la cadera
intestines	los intestinos
jaw	la mandíbula
kidney	el riñón
knee	la rodilla
leg	la pierna
ligament	el ligamento
lip	el labio
liver	el hígado
lungs	los pulmones
mouth	la boca
muscles	los músculos
neck	el cuello
nerves	los nervios
nose	la nariz
ovary	el ovario
pancreas	el páncreas
penis	el pene
perineum	el perineo
prostate	la próstata
rectal area	la sección rectal la parte rectal
ribs	las costillas

Health Care

shin	la espinilla
shoulder	el hombro
shoulder blades	el omóplato **las paletillas**
side	el lado **la canilla**
skin	la piel
skull	el cráneo
spine	la espina dorsal
spleen	el bazo
stomach	el estómago **la barriga**
teeth	los dientes
temples	las sienes
tendon	el tendón
testicles	los testículos
thigh	el muslo
throat	la garganta
thumb	el dedo pulgar
thyroid	las tiroides
toe	el dedo del pie
tongue	la lengua
trachea	la tráquea
uterus	el útero
vagina	la vagina
vein	la vena
vulva	la vulva
waist	la cintura
wrist	la muñeca

Health Care

Nutrition

Food	*Comida*
breakfast	el desayuno
lunch	el almuerzo
dinner	la comida **la cena**
snack	la merienda
low fat	poca grasa
low cholesterol	colesterol bajo
low salt	bajo en sal
liquid	liquido
baked	al horno
barbeque	barbacoa
boiled	hervido
broiled	asado a la parrilla
roasted	asado
grilled	a la parrilla **a la plancha**
fried	frito
breaded	empanado
canned	enlatado
cooked	cocinado
dried	seco
fresh	fresco
frozen	congelado **helado** **frisado**
raw	crudo
fats, oils	grasas, aceites
butter	mantequilla
shortening	manteca
lard	manteca
margarine	margarina
oil	aceite

Health Care

dairy	lácteo, relacionado con leche
	lechería
cheese	queso
cottage cheese	queso blanco grumoso
cream	crema
eggs	huevos
whites	la clara del huevo
yolk	yema
milk	leche
low fat	baja en grasa
skim	leche descremada
whole	leche entera
sour cream	crema agria
yogurt	yogurt
grains	granos
bread	pan
whole wheat	pan integral
whole grain	pan de trigo integral
white bread	pan de arina blanca
toast	tostado
cereals	cereales
oatmeal	avena
cream of wheat	crema de trigo
corn flakes	copos de maíz
bran flakes	copos de fibra
	copos de **salvados**
All Bran® cereal	solo fibra cereal
	toda fibra
crackers	galletas
pancakes	panqueques
	panqués
pasta	pasta
popcorn	palomitas de maíz

Health Care

rice	arroz
brown rice	arroz integral
meats/fish/poultry	carnes/pescado/aves
beef	carne de res
hamburger	hamburguesa
ribs	costillas
roast beef	rosbif
steak	bistec
chicken	pollo
breast	pechuga
leg	pierna
thigh	encuentro
wings	alas
white meat	carne blanca
dark meat	carne oscura
pork	puerco
bacon	tocino
chops	chuletas
ham	jamón
hot dog	perro caliente
loin	lomo
	solomillo
sausage	salchicha
	embutidos
	chorizo
goat	cabro
	cabrito
lamb	cordero
turkey	pavo
fish	pescado
anchovies	anchoa
catfish	bacalao
salmon	salmón
tuna	atún
white fish	atún blanco

Health Care

seafood	mariscos
shrimp	camarones
lobster	langosta
calories	calorías
diet	dieta
vegetables	vegetales
	viandas
asparagus	esparrago
beans	frijoles
broccoli	brécol
cabbage	repollo
carrots	zanahoria
cauliflower	coliflor
celery	apio
corn	maíz
cucumber	pepino
eggplant	berenjena
green beans	habichuelas verdes
	judías verdes
lettuce	lechuga
onion	cebolla
peas	guisante
potatoes	papas
baked	papas al horno
fried	papas fritas
mashed	pure de papas
salad	ensalada
spinach	espinaca
sweet potato	batata
	boniato
tomato	tomate
vinegar	vinagre

Health Care

fruits	frutas
apple	manzana
avocado	aguacates
banana	banana
	plátano
berries	bayas
	moras
cherries	cerezas
cranberries	arándanos
grapefruit	toronja
grapes	uvas
guava	guayaba
lemon	limón
lime	lima
melon	melón
mushroom	hongos
orange	naranja
peach	melocotón
pear	pera
pineapple	piña
plum	ciruela
prune	ciruela pasa
raisins	pasas
strawberry	fresas
watermelon	sandía
	melón
desserts	postres
cake	torta
	pastel
candy	dulces
cookies	galletas
ice cream	helado
pie	tarta
	pastel

Health Care

condiments	condimentos
chocolate	chocolate
garlic	ajo
herbs	hierbas
honey	miel
jam	mermelada
ketchup	salsa de tomate
mayonnaise	mayonesa
mustard	mostaza
peanut butter	mantequilla de maní
pepper	pimiento
salt	sal
spices	especias
sugar	azúcar

Beverages

alcohol	bebidas alcohólicas
beer	cerveza
gin	ginebra
liqueur	licor
rum	ron
scotch	Escocés
	whisky Escocés
vodka	vodka
whiskey	whisky
wine	vino
coffee	café
regular	regular
decaffeinated	descafeinado
instant	instantáneo
black	negro
with cream	con crema
no sugar	sin azúcar

Health Care

juice	jugo
apple	jugo de manzana
cranberry	arándano
grape	uva
grapefruit	toronja
guava	guayaba
lemonade	limonada
orange	jugo de naranja
prune	ciruela pasa
tomato	tomate
sodas	refrescos
diet sodas	refrescos de dieta
tea	té
water	agua

Medical Terminology

accommodations	alojamiento **plaza** **acomodaciones**
acne	acné
acute renal failure	fallo renal agudo
Adult Protective Services	Servicios de Protección de Adultos *Servicios de Protección para Adultos*
advocate	defensor **abogado** **partidario**
AIDS	SIDA (Síndrome de Inmunodeficiencia Adquirida)
alcoholic liver disease	enfermedad hepática por alcoholismo
allergic reaction	reacción alergica
amputation	amputación
anemia (low blood count)	anemia (conteo bajo de glóbulos rojos)
appendicitis (inflammation of the appendix)	apendicitis (inflamación de la apéndices)

Health Care

asthma	asma
atrial fibrillation (irregular heart beat)	fibrilación atrial (palpitación cardiaca *irregular/ latido cardiaco irregular)*
audiometry (hearing test)	audiometría (prueba de audición) *audiometría (**examen** de audición)*
bacterial infection	infección bacterial
behavioral counseling	consejería de comportamiento *consejería **para** comportamiento*
benign	benigno
bipolar disorder (manic depression)	desorden bipolar **desorden de bipolaridad**
bladder stones	piedras de vejiga
blind	ciego
bladder obstruction	obstrucción de vejiga *obstrucción **en la** vejiga*
blocked arteries	bloqueo arterial **arterias bloqueadas**
bony deformity	deformación ósea
bowel incontinence	incontinencia intestinal *incontinencia **rectal***
bowel obstruction	obstrucción abdominal
brain injury	trauma cerebral
brain tumor	tumor cerebral
broken bone	hueso roto *hueso **partido***
bronchitis	bronquitis
bunion	juanete
cancer	cancer
carpal tunnel syndrome (nerve in the wrist is squeezed)	syndrome de túnel carpiano
case manager	director del caso **jefe** del caso **encargado** del caso **gerente** del caso

Health Care

chemotherapy	quimo terapia
child advocate	defensor para niños **abogado de** niños **partidario de** niños
Child Protective Services	servicios de protección de niños
chlamydia	clamidia
chronic bronchitis	bronquitis crónica
chronic fatigue syndrome	síndrome de fatiga crónica
chronic renal failure	fallo crónico renal
cirrhosis (liver damage)	cirrosis (daño hepático)
cognitive defect	defecto cognoscitivo/de cognición
congestive heart failure	fallo cardiaco congestivo
counseling	orientación **consejería**
cystic fibrosis	fibrosis quística
deaf	sordo **sordera**
degenerative disc disease (degeneration of discs in the spine)	enfermedad degenerativa de los discos (degeneración de los discos vertebrales)
degenerative joint disease (arthritis)	enfermedad degenerativa de las articulaciones (artritis)
dementia	demencia
depression	depresión
developmental delay (developmental retardation)	retraso en el desarrollo (retraso en la edad evolutiva) retraso en el desarrollo (**retardación** en la edad evolutiva)
diabetes	diabetes
Down syndrome	síndrome de Down
eczema	eczema
emphysema	enfisema
endocarditis (infected heart valve)	endocarditis (infección de las valvulas cardiacas/del corazón.)
expected outcome	resultado esperado resultado **anticipado**

Health Care

farsighted or hyperopia (unable to see close objects)	hipermétrope (no puede ver objetos a corta distancia)
fatty liver (fat deposits in the liver)	hígado graso (depósitos de grasa en el hígado) hígado **adiposo**
fibromyalgia	fibromialgia
fungal infection	infección fungal
gallstones	piedras en la vesícula
gastroesophageal reflux (heartburn)	reflujo gatroesofágico (acidez gástrica de estomago) reflujo gatroesofágico (acidez **ardor** de estomago)
glaucoma (high pressure in the eyes)	glaucoma (alta presión en los ojos)
gonorrhea	gonorrea
hearing impaired	deficiencia auditiva **discapacidad auditiva** **defecto acústico**
heart defect	defecto cardiaco **defecto del corazón**
heart disease	enfermedad cardiaca enfermedad **del corazón**
heart murmur	soplo cardiaco soplo **en el corazón**
hepatitis	hepatitis
herpes	herpes
high blood pressure	presión sanguínea alta presión **arterial** alta **alta presión**
high cholesterol	colesterol elevado colesterol **alto**
HIV	(VIH) virus de inmunodeficiencia humana
hole in the heart	hueco cardiaco hueco **en el** corazón

Health Care

home health care	asistencia médica al hogar **ayuda salud** al hogar
hospice	centro de cuidados mínimos **centro de cuidados paliativos**
hyperthyroidism (too much thyroid hormone)	hipertiroidismo (alta cantidad de hormonas tiroideas)
hypothyroidism (not enough thyroid hormone)	hipotiroidismo (poca cantidad de hormonas tiroideas)
inflammatory bowel disease	enfermedad inflamatoria de los intestinos
irritable bowel disease	síndrome del intestino irritable
kidney stones	piedras renales
liver failure	fallo hepático
long term care	cuidado de larga duración
lymphedema (obstruction of the lymphatic fluid)	linfedema (obstrucción de los líquidos linfáticos)
malignant	maligno
meals on wheels	comidas gratis llevadas al hogar comidas **sin pago alguno** llevadas al hogar comidas **sin provecho económico** llevadas al hogar
medically necessary	medicament necesario
mental illness	enfermedad mental
multiple sclerosis	esclerosis múltiple
muscular dystrophy	distrofia muscular
myopia or nearsighted (unable to see objects far away)	miopía (no puede ver objetos a corta distancia) **corto de vista**
natural consequence	consecuencias naturales
nerve damage	daño en el nervio
neuropathy (nerve damage)	neuropatía (daño al nervio)
nursing home	centro de convalecencia **asilo de ancianos** **hogar de ancianos** **residencia de ancianos** **ancianato**

Health Care

osteoarthritis	osteoartritis
osteoporosis (weakening of your bones)	osteoporosis (debilidad ósea) osteoporosis (debilidad **de los huesos**)
outcome	resultados **consecuencias**
outpatient	paciente ambulatorio paciente **no hospitalizado** paciente **externo**
outpatient management	administración para el paciente ambulatorio **gerencia** para el paciente **no hospitalizado** **gerencia** para el paciente **externo**
pancreatitis	pancreatitis
paralyzed	paralizado
paraplegic	parapléjico
patient advocate	defensor al paciente **abogado** al paciente
pink eye	conjuntivitis contagiosa
pneumonia	neumonía
poliomyelitis	poliomielitis
prostatic hypertrophy (enlarged prostate)	hipertrofia prostática (próstata aumentada) hipertrofia prostática (próstata **grande**)
prosthesis	próstesis
prosthetic (artificial)	prostético (artificial)
psoriasis	soriasis
pulmonary edema (fluid in the lungs)	edema pulmonar (líquido en los pulmones)
pulmonary hypertension (high pressure in the lungs)	hipertensión pulmonar (alta presión en los pulmones)
quadriplegic	cuadripléjico
quality of life	calidad de vida
radiation therapy	terapia de radiación
Raynaud's disease	enfermedad de Raynaud

Health Care

rehabilitation hospital	rehabilitación hospitalaria
retinopathy (damage to the back of the eye)	retinopatía (daño en la parte de atrás del ojo) retinopatía (daño en la parte **inferior** del ojo)
rhabdomyolysis (muscle damage)	rabdomiolisis (daño muscular)
rheumatoid arthritis	artritis reumatoide
sarcoidosis	sarcoidosis
schizophrenia	esquizofrenia
sciatica (nerve irritation)	ciática (irritación al nervio/ciático)
side effect	efecto secundario
spina bifida	espina bífida
spinal cord injury	trauma en la columna vertebral trauma en la columna **espina dorsal**
spinal stenosis (narrow spinal canal compresses the spinal cord and nerves)	estenosis de la columna vertebral (el canal de la columna vertebral comprime la columna vertebral y los nervios espinales) estenosis de la **espina dorsal** (el **canal** de la **espina dorsal oprime** la **espina dorsal** y los nervios espinales)
sprain (of ligaments)	dislocación (de ligamentos) **torcedura** (de ligamentos)
stenosis (narrowing)	estenosis (angostamiento) estenosis (**estrechez**) estenosis (**encogimiento**)
stomach ulcers	ulceras estomacales
strain (of muscle)	distención (de músculo)
stroke	derrame **derrame cerebral (hemorrágico)** **infarto cerebral (isquémico)** **accidente cerebrovascular (ACV)**
syphilis	sífilis
systemic lupus erythematosis	lupus eritematoso sistémico
tendonitis (irritation of the tendon)	tendonitis (irritación del tendon)

Health Care

traumatic brain injury	lesión traumática cerebral
tuberculosis	tuberculosis
tumor	tumor
urinary incontinence	incontinencia urinaria
urinary obstruction	obstrucción urinaria
urinary retention	retención urinaria
viral infection	infección viral
warts	verrugas

Medical Occupations

anesthesiologist	anestesiólogo
chiropractor	quiropráctico
diabetic educator	educador diabético educador **de la diabetes**
dietician	dietista
dentist	dentista
doctor	doctor
gynecologist	ginecólogo
intern	internista
licensed practical nurse	enfermera practica autorizada enfermera practica **licenciada**
medical assistant	estudiante medico
medical student	estudiante de medicina
midwife	comadrona **partera** **matrona**
neurologist	neurólogo
nurse	enfermera
nurse anesthetist	enfermera anestesióloga enfermera **de anestesiología**
nurse practitioner	enfermera practica
nurse practitioner student	estudiante de enfermería practica
nursing student	estudiante de enfermería
obstetrician	obstetra
occupational therapist	terapista ocupacional

Health Care

ophthalmologist	oftalmólogo
paramedic	paramédico
pediatrician	pediatra
pharmacist	farmacéutico
physical medicine and rehabilitation	rehabilitación y medicina física
physical therapist	fisioterapia
physician assistant	asistente de médico
physician assistant student	estudiante de asistente médico
psychiatrist	psiquiatría
psychologist	psicólogo
radiologist	radiólogo
resident	residente
respiratory therapist	terapista respiratorio
speech therapist	foniatría
surgeon	cirujano
technologist	tecnólogo
urologist	urólogo
volunteer	voluntario

Medical Supplies

bed rails	barandillas de cama
bedside commode	tibor **retrete**
brace	abrazadera **suporte** **gancho**
cane	caña **bastón**
cast	molde **molde de yeso**
crutches	muletas

Health Care

diabetic supplies	suministros diabéticos
glucometer	glucómetro **medidor de azúcar en la sangre**
glucose test strips	tiras para la examinación de la glucosa
lancets (finger sticks)	lanceta **para pincharse el dedo** **para clavarse el dedo**
device that holds the finger sticks	dispositivos **aguantador de lancetas**
eggshell mattress	colchon en forma de cascara de huevos
electric wheelchair	silla de rueda eléctrica
hospital bed	cama de hospital
orthotic	aparato ortopédico
prosthesis	próstesis
prosthetic limb (artificial)	extremidad prostética (artificial)
rolling walker	andadera con ruedas
scooter	escúter **scooter** **motoneta** **patineta**
motorized scooter	escúter motorizado **scooter** motorizado **motoneta** motorizado **patineta** motorizado
shower chair	silla para la ducha **silla para sentarse en la ducha**
splint	tablilla
walker	andadera
wheelchair	silla de ruedas

Exercise Equipment

elliptical machine	máquina elíptica para hacer ejercicios
mini trampoline	mini-trampolín
rowing machine	máquina de remo para hacer ejercicio

Health Care

stair climber or step trainer	escladorea, escaladora de ejercicio,
stationary bicycle	bicicleta fija para hacer ejercicios
treadmill	rueda fija de andar para hacer ejercicios
weights	pesas
free weights	pesas libres
weight machines	máquinas de pesas para hacer ejercicios
upper body	cuerpo superior
lower body	cuerpo inferior
resistance bands	bandas de resistencias
exercise ball (inflatable)	bola inflable para hacer ejercicios

Special Procedures

arterial blood gases	gases de la sangre arterial
arteriogram	arteriograma
barium enema	enema de bario
barium swallow	tragar bario
biopsy	biopsia
bone	biopsia del hueso
bone marrow	médula ósea
breast	seno
liver	biopsia del hígado
lung	pulmones
kidney	riñones
muscle	biopsia del músculo
blood test	análisis de la sangre
bone density scan	gammagrafía ósea **estudio oseo por radionuclidos**
bronchoscopy	broncoscopia
catheterization	catéterilación
cardiac	cateterismo cardiaco
urethral	uretra
cauterization	cauterización
colonoscopy	colonoscopia
CT	tomografía computarizada

Health Care

culture	cultivo
nose	cultivo de la nariz
throat	cultivo de la garganta
urethral	uretra
urine	orine
vaginal	cultivo vaginal
cystoscopy	cistoscopia
echocardiogram	ecocardiograma
electrocardiogram	electrocardiograma
electroencephalogram	electroencefalograma
enema	enema
endoscopy	endoscopia
gastric lavage	lavado gastrico
Holter monitor	registro Holter **monitorización electrocardiografía ambulatoria**
incision and drainage	incisión y drenaje
joint aspiration	aspiración de coyuntura aspiración de **articulación**
joint injection	inyección de coyuntura inyección de **articulación**
laparoscopy	laparoscopia
lumbar puncture	punción lumbar
mammogram	mamograma
MRI	resonancia magnética
myelogram	mielograma
needle biopsy	biopsia con aguja biopsia **por** aguja
nerve conduction studies	estudios de conducción nerviosa
pacemaker	marcador de paso
intracardiac defibrillator	desfibrador intracardiaco
PAP smear	frotis Papanicolau **citología vaginal**
pelvic examination	examinación pélvica

Health Care

pregnancy test	prueba de embarazo
pulmonary function test (breathing test)	prueba de función pulmonar
rectal examination	examinación rectal
sigmoidoscopy	sigmoidoscopia
stool culture	cultura de heces fecales
stress test	examen de estrés
ultrasound	ultrasonido
upper GI series	series de placas esophagogastroduodenales
venogram	venograma
x-ray	radiografía **rayos X** **placas**

Legal/Disability Terminology

accident	accidente
appeal	apelación
appeal process	proceso de apelación
arbitration	arbitración
award	reconocimiento **premio**
case manager	director del caso **jefe** del caso **encargado** del caso **gerente** del caso
child advocate	defensor para niños **abogado de** niños **partidario de** niños
Child Protective Services	Servicios de Protección de Niños
chiropractor	quiropráctico
claim	demanda **reclamo**
court	corte
Department of Transportation	Departamento de Transportación

Health Care

Department of Vocational and Rehabilitation Services	Departamento de Servicios de Rehabilitación
deposition	deposición
disability	incapacidad **invalidez**
long term disability	incapacidad de larga duración **invalidez** de larga duración
partial disability	incapacidad parcial **invalidez** parcial
permanent disability	incapacidad permanente **invalidez permanente**
short term disability	incapacidad a corto plazo **invalidez a corto plazo**
temporary disability	incapacidad temporaria **invalidez temporaria**
total disability	incapacidad total **invalidez total**
disabled	descapacitado
guardian ad litem (guardian appointed for legal representation)	guardián designado (guardián decretado para representación legal) **tutor legal** (guardián **nominado** para representación legal) **tutor legal** (guardián **nombrado** para representación legal)
fraud	fraude
handicap	desventaja **impedimento** **retraso** **descapacidad**
handicap accessible	hándicap accesible hándicap posible
handicapped	hándicap **incapacitado** **impedido**

Health Care

handicapped license plate	matricula de hándicap **placa** de **incapacitado** **placa** de **impedido**
handicapped parking	estacionamiento de hándicap **parqueo** de **incapacitado** **aparcamiento** de **impedido**
handicapped placard	aviso de hándicap **letrero** de **incapacitado** **cartel** de **impedido** **plaqueta** de **impedido**
handi-ride	transportación publica para hándicap transportación **especial** para **incapacitado** transportación **especial** para **impedido**
hearing	audición
house arrest	arresto domiciliario
jail	cárcel
judge	juez
judgment	sentencia **dictar sentencia**
law	ley
lawsuit	demanda
lawyer	abogado
legal	legal
legal fees	honorarios legales **cargos** legales
liability	responsabilidad **deuda** **obligación legal**
light duty	trabajo ligero
litigation	litigación **demanda judicial** **pleito**
malpractice	negligencia **mal práctica**

Health Care

mobility impaired	movilidad discapacitada movilidad **deteriorada**
negligence	negligencia
parole	libertad balo palabra **libertad condicional** **libertad provisional**
parole officer	supervisor de la libertad condicional
pending	pendiente **en tramites** **por resolver**
prison	prisión **cárcel**
probation	período de prueba **período de libertad vigilada** **probación**
restricted duty	trabajo restringido
return to work	regreso al trabajo
review date	día de evaluación **día de revisión** **día de informe**
visually impaired	impedido visual **visualmente averiado** **ciego**
workers compensation	indemnización del trabajador
work restrictions	limitaciones en el trabajo **restricciones** en el trabajo
Have you filed a complaint?	¿Usted a presentado una queja? ¿Usted a presentado un **querella**? ¿Usted a presentado una **reclamo**?
Do you receive disability payments?	¿Recibe usted pagos por incapacidad?
Have you received disability in the past? How many years ago?	¿A usted recibido pagos por incapacidad en el pasado? ¿Cuántos años atrás?

Health Care

Do you have a handicapped license plate or placard?	¿Tiene usted una matricula o aviso de hándicap? ¿Tiene usted una **placa** o **letrero** de **incapacitado**? ¿Tiene usted una **placa** o **cartel** de **impedido**? ¿Tiene usted una **placa** o **plaqueta** de **impedido**?
Do you use handicapped parking?	¿Utiliza usted el estacionamiento para hándicap? ¿ **Usa** usted el estacionamiento para **incapacitado**? ¿ **Usa** usted el estacionamiento para **impedido**?
Have you filed a workers compensation claim?	¿A usted presentado un reclamo de indemnización del trabajador?
Have you filed a malpractice suit?	¿A usted presentado una demanda por negligencia? ¿A usted presentado una demanda **mal práctica**?
Is there a lawsuit pending concerning your accident/injury/illness?	¿Hay alguna demanda **pendiente** concerniente a su accidente/lesión/enfermedad? ¿Hay alguna demanda **pendiente** concerniente a su accidente/**herida**/enfermedad?
Do you have a lawyer?	¿Tiene usted un abogado?
Have you gone to court yet?	¿Fue usted ya a la corte?
Has the case been settled?	¿Ya su caso ha sido resuelto? ¿Ya su caso ha sido **establecido**?
Is this injury/illness part of a malpractice suit?	¿Esta lesión/enfermedad es parte del pleito por negligencia?
Is this injury/illness a workers compensation case?	¿Esta lesión/enfermedad es parte del caso de indemnización del trabajador?
Did this injury/accident happen while you were at work?	¿Esta lesión/enfermedad sucedió cuando usted estaba/se encontraba en su trabajo?

Health Care

Was this injury/illness related to your job?	¿Es esta lesión/enfermedad relacionada con su trabajo?
Have you ever had this same injury/illness before?	¿A usted tenido o padecido de esta lesión/enfermedad anteriomente?
How many months/years ago?	¿Cuántos meses/años atrás? ¿Cuántos meses/años **hace**?
Did the previous injury/ illness get better?	¿Su lesión/enfermedad previa mejoró?
Does your employer pay workers compensation benefits?	¿Su empresario paga de pagar indemnización para el trabajador? ¿Su **empleador se ocupa** de pagar indemnización para el trabajador? ¿Su **patrón se ocupa** de pagar indemnización para el trabajador?
Are you seeing another provider for your workers compensation injury/illness?	¿Esta usted viéndose con otro proveedor en referencia a su indemnización para el trabajador por su lesión/enfermedad?

Seasonal

Seasons

spring	primavera
summer	verano
autumn	otoño
winter	invierno

Weather

cold weather	clima frió
hot weather	clima caluroso
rain	lluvia
sleet	aguanieve
smog	niebla toxica
snow	nieve
sunny	soleado
windy	ventoso

Clothing/Accessories

belt	cinturón
blouse	blusa
bra	sujetadores **ajustadores** **bra**
bracelet	pulsera **brazalete**
clothes	ropa
coat	abrigo
dentures	dentaduras
diaper	pañal **pamper**
dress	vestido
earrings	aretes
glasses	lentes
gown	camisón **bata**
hat	sombrero
hose/stockings	medias
jacket	chaqueta **jacket**
jewelry	joyas
necklace	cadena
pants	pantalones
ring	sortija
robe	bata
shirt	camisa
shoes	zapatos
shorts	pantalones cortos **Bermudas**
skirt	faldas
socks	calcetines

Seasonal

sweater	suéter
underwear	ropa interior
watch	reloj
wig	peluca

Chapter 4

Meeting the Patient

This chapter includes the useful phrases one would use at the beginning of most medical encounters. From the time the patient presents to a health care facility, multiple people in various roles may interact with the patient at some point before the patient is actually seen by the health care provider. This section is designed for the front-end staff involved in a patient encounter. Triage questions will be particularly useful for nurses either in the emergency room setting or in an ambulatory urgent-care setting. Check-in and registration questions are somewhat self-explanatory and will likely be used by receptionists and business and financial office personnel. The section on vital signs, while consisting mostly of commands, will be most relevant to medical assistants, nurses, and, in some instances, even providers.

The section on medication history is critically important for any type of encounter. Not only will the front-end staff ask these questions, but the health care provider will also find these questions quite useful in most patient encounters. Verifying correct medication use will decrease the risk of many potential medical errors. And many Spanish-speaking patients, unless they are asked directly, are hesitant to volunteer that they are taking other non-prescribed medications, over-the counter or otherwise.

Triage

Please speak English as much as possible.	Por favor hable inglés lo más posible.
How old are you?	¿Qué edad usted tiene?
	¿**Cuántos años** tiene?
How are you feeling today?	¿Cómo se siente hoy?
Well?	¿Bien?
Sick?	¿Mal?
How do you feel now?	¿Cómo se siente ahora?
	¿Cómo se siente **ahorita**?
	¿Cómo se siente **en este momento**?
Well?	¿Bien?
Bad?	¿Mal?
Sick?	¿Enfermo?
Are you injured?	¿Está usted lastimado?
Were you in an accident?	¿Estuvo usted en un accidente?
In a car?	¿De carro?
	¿De **auto**?
	¿De **automóvil**?
	¿De **vehículo**?
In a bus?	¿De autobús?
	¿De **güagüa**?
In a train?	¿De tren?
Were you a pedestrian?	¿Usted era peaton?
How long ago did it happen (hours, days)?	¿Cuánto hace que ocurrió (horas, días)?
Show me where you were injured.	Enséñeme donde fue lastimado.
	Muéstreme donde fue lastimado.
Can you move it?	¿Puede mover la parte que fue lastimada?
Can you walk?	¿Puede caminar?

Triage

Did you hit your head?	¿Se dio usted en la cabeza?
	¿ **Se lastimó** usted en la cabeza?
Did you lose consciousness?	¿Perdió usted el conocimiento?
How many minutes were you unconscious?	¿Cuántos minutos estuvo usted sin conocimiento?
Was it witnessed?	¿Fue observado por alguien?
	¿Hubo algún testigo?
Are you sick?	¿Está usted enfermo?
Show me where you feel sick.	Enséñeme la parte la cual usted siente mal.
	Muéstreme la parte la cual usted siente mal.
Do you have pain?	¿Tiene dolor?
Are you pregnant?	¿Está usted embarazada?
	¿Está usted **encinta**?
What is the problem?	¿Cuál es el problema?
Can you show me what is wrong?	¿Puede usted enseñarme que es lo que está mal?
	¿Puede usted **mostrarme** que es lo que está mal?
How long ago did it start (minutes, hours, days, weeks, months)?	¿Cuánto hace que le empezó (minutos, horas, días, semanas, meses)?
Did it start suddenly?	¿Empezó de repente?
Did it start slowly?	¿Empezó despacio?
Is it constant?	¿Es constante?
Does it come and go?	¿Viene y se va?
Are you getting better?	¿Está usted mejorando?
Are you getting worse?	¿Está usted empeorando?
Have you had this problem before?	¿Ha tenido este problema antes?
Have you recently been around someone with these same symptoms?	¿Ha estado usted alrededor de alguien con estos síntomas ya mencionados?
Have you been around anyone who is sick?	¿Ha estado usted alrededor de alguien que está enfermo?

Triage

Are you taking any medicines for it?	¿Está usted tomando algún medicamento para esto? ¿Está usted tomando alguna **medicina** para esto?
Are they prescription?	¿Estos medicamentos son con receta? ¿Estas **medicinas** son **con prescripción**?
Over the counter?	¿Sin receta?
Do they make it better?	¿Lo/la mejoran?
Have you been in the hospital or ER lately?	¿Ha estado usted en el hospital o sala de emergencia recientamente?
For the same problem?	¿Por el mismo problema?
For a different problem?	¿Por otro problema diferente?
Do you have . . .	¿Tiene usted . . . ?

Refer to a dictionary or Past Medical History section under Chapter 7 for common disorders.

Have you ever had . . .	¿Ha tenido usted . . . ?

Check-in/Registration

Please speak English as much as possible.	Por favor hable inglés lo más posible.
Do you have an appointment?	¿Usted tiene una cita?
Who is your doctor/provider?	¿Quién es su doctor o proveedor médico?
What time is your appointment?	¿A qué hora es su cita médica?
What is your name?	¿Cuál es su nombre? **¿Cómo se llama?**
What is your last name?	¿Cuál es su apellido?
I'm sorry, but you are here on the wrong day.	Lo siento pero usted ha venido en el día equivocado.
I'm sorry, but the doctor/provider cannot see you today.	Lo siento pero el doctor/proveedor no lo podrá ver hoy.
We have to reschedule your appointment for another time.	Necesitamos darle otra cita para otro día.
Have you seen this doctor before?	¿Se ha visto usted antes con este doctor?

Check-in/Registration

Have you been seen in this clinic before?	¿Ha sido vista/o en esta clínica antes? ¿Ha sido vista/o en esta clínica **anteriormente?**
Have you seen a doctor about this problem before?	¿Ha visitado/**visto** usted anteriormente un(a) doctor(a) hacerca de este problema?
Are you being seen today for a new problem?	¿Lo están viendo hoy por un problema nuevo? ¿Lo están **ayudando** hoy por un problema nuevo?
Are you being seen today because you are sick?	¿Lo están viendo hoy por que está enfermo? ¿Lo están **ayudando** hoy por que **se encuentra** enfermo?
Please sign in and have a seat.	Por favor firme y siéntese. Por favor firme y **tome asiento**.
Do you have medical insurance?	¿Tiene usted seguro médico?
Do you have . . . *	¿Tiene usted . . .
Medicare?	Medicare? **seguro de salud para los jubilados en la seguridad social?**
Medicaid?	Medicaid? **Seguro médico para personas de bajos ingresos y recursos limitados?** **Ayuda médica federal y estatal?**
Medi-cal?	Medi-cal (ayuda médica estatal de California)?
Blue Cross/Blue Shield?	Cruz Azul?
Kaiser?	Kaiser?
Aetna?	Aetna?
Cigna?	Cigna?
United Health Care?	United Health Care (Ayuda de Salud Unida)?

Due to the many types of insurance plans available, you should use the original names whenever possible.

Check-in/Registration

Other insurance?	¿Otro tipo de seguro médico?
Please show me your insurance information.	Por favor enséñeme la información de su seguro médico. Por favor **muéstreme** la información de su seguro médico.
Is this a workers compensation case?	¿Este es un caso de compensación médica a través de su trabajo?
Do you have something with your address printed on it?	¿Tiene usted algún papel que contenga su dirección postal impresa?
Show me please.	Enséñeme por favor. **Muéstreme** por favor.
What is your address?	¿Cuál es su dirección? **¿Dónde vive?**
Is that an apartment?	¿Eso es un apartamento?
What is the apartment number?	¿Cuál es el número de su apartamento?
What city do you live in?	¿En qué ciudad usted vive?
What is your ZIP Code?	¿Cuál es su código postal?
Write your address.	Escriba su dirección.
What is your telephone number?	¿Cuál es su número teléfono?
What is your date of birth?	¿Cuál es su fecha de nacimiento? **¿Cuándo nació?**
Do you have something with your birthday printed on it?	¿Tiene usted algún papel que contenga su día de nacimiento impreso? ¿Tiene usted algún papel que contenga su **fecha de nacimiento impreso**?
Do you practice a specific religion?	¿Practica usted alguna religión en específico?
Are you Catholic?	¿Es usted católico?
Are you Protestant?	¿Es usted Protestante?
Are you Jewish?	¿Es usted Judío?
Are you Muslim?	¿Es usted musulmán?
Other?	¿Practica otro tipo de religión?

Check-in/Registration

What is your Social Security number?	¿Cuál es su número de seguro social?
Show me your card.	Enséñeme su tarjeta.
	Muéstreme su tarjeta.
Do you have a driver's license or identification card?	¿Tiene usted licencia de manejar u otra forma de identificación?
Do you have a utility bill in your name?	¿Tiene un recibo de sus utilidades (de agua o luz) en su nombre?
Do you work?	¿Usted trabaja?
Full time or part time?	¿Es usted un empleado a jornada completo o a jornada parcial?
	¿Es usted un empleado a **tiempo** completo a o **tiempo media**?
What is your employer's name?	¿Cuál es el nombre de su empleado?
	¿Cuál es el nombre de **su patrón**?
Address?	¿Su dirección?
Phone number?	¿Su número de teléfono?
What is your salary (more or less) per week or month?	¿Más o menos, cuál es su salario semanal o mensual?
Do you have a pay stub?	¿Tiene usted su talonario de pago?
	¿Tiene usted **recibos** de pago?
Do you receive disability or welfare payments?	¿Recibe usted pensión por invalidez o incapacidad/asistencia o bienestar social?
Are you an American citizen?	¿Es usted ciudadano Americano?
Do you have a visa?	¿Tiene usted visa?
Do you have a passport?	¿Tiene usted un pasaporte?
You need to go to the business office with your papers.	Usted necesita ir a la oficina de negocios con sus papeles.
Come back here to check in when you are done.	Regrese acá cuando usted esté listo para registrarse.
Whom do we contact in case of emergency?	¿A quién nosotros podemos llamar en caso de emergencia?
What is their address and phone number?	¿Cuál es la dirección y número de teléfono de estos?
Your co-pay for this visit is _____ dollars.	Su pago inicial por esta visita es _____ dólares.

Check-in/Registration

Will you be paying with cash, check, or credit card?	¿Usted va a pagar en efectivo/con cuenta de banco/con tarjeta de crédito? ¿Usted va a pagar en efectivo/ **con chequera**/con tarjeta de crédito?
Can you read English or Spanish?	¿Puede usted leer Ingles o Espanol?
Can you write in Engish or Spanish?	¿Puede usted escribir Inglés o Español?
Please fill out these forms.	Por favor llene estos papeles.
Please sign here.	Por favor firme aquí.
Please have a seat and wait for your name to be called.	Por favor siéntese y espere hasta que llamen su nombre.

Medications

Please speak English as much as possible.	Por favor hable inglés lo más posible.
Do you take any medicines?	¿Está usted tomando algún medicamento?
Did you bring your medicines?	¿Trajo sus medicamentos?
Let me see your medicines.	¿Déjeme ver sus medicamentos? ¿Déjeme ver sus **medicinas**?
How many times a day do you take this medicine?	¿Cuántas veces al día usted toma este medicamento? ¿Cuándo veces al día usted toma **esta medicina**?
Do you take this medicine . . .	¿Usted está tomando este medicamento . . . ¿Usted está tomando esta **medicina** . . .
in the morning?	en la mañana?
in the afternoon?	en la tarde?
in the evening?	al anochecer?
at noon?	al mediodía?
at bedtime?	antes de acostarse?
with meals?	con la comida?
before meals?	antes de comer?
after meals?	después de comer?

Medications

Do you know the names of the medicines?	¿Sabe usted el nombre de los medicamentos?
What is the name of the medicine?	¿Cuál es el nombre del medicamento?
	¿Cuál es el nombre **de la medicina**?
What is the dose in milligrams?	¿Cuál es la dosis en miligramos?
How many pills do you take each time/day?	¿Cuántas pastillas toma usted cada vez/por día?
Do you take any other medicines?	¿Está usted tomando algún otro medicamento?
	¿Está usted tomando alguna otra medicina?
Do you take any over-the-counter medicines like acetaminophen or aspirin?	¿Toma usted algún otro medicamento sin receta como acetaminofen o aspirina?
	¿Toma usted alguna otra **medicina** sin receta como acetaminofen o aspirina?
Do you take vitamins?	¿Toma usted vitaminas?
Do you know the names?	¿Sabe usted los nombres?
	¿Conoce usted los nombres?
Do you take herbal supplements?	¿Toma usted suplementos herbales?
Do you know the names?	¿Sabe usted los nombres?
	¿Conoce usted los nombres?
Are you allergic to any medicines?	¿Tiene usted alergia a algún medicamento?
	¿Tiene usted alergia a **alguna medicina**?
Which medicines?	¿Cuál medicamentos?
	¿Cuál **medicinas**?
Do you get a rash?	¿Le da a usted erupción?
	¿Le da a usted **salpullido**?
	¿Le da a usted **pintas rojas en su piel**?
Difficulty breathing or swallowing?	¿Dificultad al respirar o al tragar?
Swelling?	¿Hinchazón?
	¿Inflamación?

Medications

Have you had any bad reactions to any of your medicines?	¿Ha tenido usted alguna reacción adversa a alguno de sus medicamentos?
	¿Ha tenido usted alguna reacción **mala** a alguno de sus medicamentos?
	¿Ha tenido usted alguna reacción **dañina** a alguno de sus medicamentos?
	¿Ha tenido usted alguna reacción **no favorable** a alguna de **sus medicinas**?
Which medicine?	¿Cuál medicamento?
	¿Cuál **medicina**?
Did it give you a . . .	¿Le dio?. . .
rash?	erupciones?
	salpullido?
	pintas rojos en su piel?
swelling?	hinchazón?
cough?	tos?
headache?	dolor de cabeza?
muscle ache?	dolor muscular?
nausea?	nausea?
difficulty breathing?	dificultad al respirar?
excessive drowsiness?	somnolencia?
	modorra?
Did you take your medicines today?	¿Tomó usted sus medicamentos hoy?
Have you run out of any medicines?	¿Se le han acabaco algunas de sus medicamentos?
	¿Se le han **terminado** algunas de sus medicamentos?
	¿Se le han **agotado** algunas de sus **medicinas**?
How many days/weeks/months ago did you run out?	¿Cuántos días/semanas/meses hace que se les acabo los medicamentos?
Do you need refills?	¿Necesita repuestos para sus medicamentos?
	¿Necesita repuestos para **sus medicinas**?

Medications

Please bring all your medicines and supplements with you to each visit.	Por favor traiga todos sus medicamentos y suplementos con usted en su próxima visita. Por favor traiga **todas sus medicinas** y suplementos con usted en su próxima visita.

Vital Signs

Please speak English as much as possible.	Por favor hable inglés lo más posible.
Follow me.	Sígame.
Please sit down.	Por favor siéntese.
What is your telephone number?	¿Cuál es su número telefónico?
Are you allergic to any medicines? Which medicine?	¿Tiene usted alergia a algún medicamento? ¿Tiene usted alergia a **alguna medicina**? ¿Cuál medicamento? ¿Cuál **medicina**?
Do you get a rash?	¿Le da a usted erupción? ¿Le da a usted **salpullido**? ¿Le da a usted **pintas rojas en su piel**?
Difficulty breathing or swallowing?	¿Dificultad al respirar o al tragar?
Swelling?	¿Hinchazón? **¿Inflamación?**
Are you having pain today?	¿Tiene usted dolor hoy?
How bad is your pain? (One is almost no pain, and ten is you need to be in the ER.)	¿Qué tanto dolor tiene? (Uno es casi sin dolor, y diez es necesario ir a la sala de emergencia.)
Take off your coat.	Quítese su abrigo.
Lift up your sleeve.	Alce su manga.
Relax your arm and do not move.	Relaje su brazo y no se mueva.
Step on the scale please.	Párase en la balanza por favor. Párase en **la pesa** por favor.
How tall are you in feet?	¿Cuál es su estatura (en pies)? **¿Qué alto es usted** (en pies)?

Vital Signs

Please stand with your back against the wall.	Por favor párase con su espalda contra/**hacia** la pared.
Stand up straight.	Párese derecho.
Please come with me.	Por favor venga conmigo.
Please go to room number . . .	Por favor vaya al cuarto . . .
Please remove . . .	Por favor quítese . . .
your clothes from the waist up.	su ropa de la cintura para arriba.
all clothing and jewelry.	toda su ropa.
your clothes from the waist down.	su ropa de la cintura para abajo.
your pants.	sus pantalones.
your shirt.	su camisa.
your clothes except your underwear.	su ropa excepto su ropa interior.
your clothes including your underwear.	su ropa incluso su ropa interior.
Put on this gown.	Póngase esta bata.
Please remove your shoes and socks.	Por favor quítese sus zapatos y sus medias.
	Por favor quítese sus zapatos y sus **calzatines**.
The doctor/provider will be in to see you shortly.	El doctor/proveedor medico lo verá ya pronto.

Chapter 5

History of Present Illness for Common Symptoms

The history of present illness (HPI) is also called the primary history. It is a detailed set of questions designed to elaborate on the patient's chief complaint or presenting symptom. An accurate history is the first step in determining the etiology of the patient's concern. In fact, frequently, the diagnosis can be made simply on the history and physical examination.

There are several general questions that are applicable to most symptoms. Many acronyms have been proposed for memorizing the elements of the HPI. The one we include here is the OLD CARTS method:

Onset
Location
Duration
Characteristics
Aggravating factors
Relieving Factors
Treatments tried
Symptoms associated

Remember that an accurate history is not only important in determining the diagnosis, but is essential for proper reimbursement. The Centers for Medicare and Medicaid Services has defined criteria for what qualifies as a "reimbursable" HPI. A brief HPI includes one to three of the following, whereas an extended HPI must include four or more elements.

Timing **O**nset
Location
Duration
Quality (**C**haracteristics)
Severity (**C**haracteristics)
Context (**O**nset)
Modifying factors (**A**ggravating/**R**elieving factors)
Associated signs and symptoms (**S**ymptoms associated)

Included in this chapter are many of the acute symptoms most commonly encountered in clinical practice. The questions are designed to elicit a differential diagnosis for each complaint. Of course, not all the elements of the OLD CARTS questions can be applied to all symptoms; for example, insomnia has no location. But wherever possible, we attempted to incorporate as many questions as were appropriate to each symptom.

Abdominal Pain

Do you have abdominal pain?	¿Tiene usted dolor abdominal?
	¿Tiene usted dolor **de barriga**?
Show me where.	Enséñeme donde le duele.
	Muéstreme donde le duele.
How long ago did it start (hours, days, weeks, months)?	¿Cuándo fue que le empezó (horas, días, semanas, meses)?
Did it start suddenly?	¿Le empezó de repente?
Did it start slowly?	¿Le empezó despacio?
Is the pain constant?	¿El dolor es constante?
Does it come and go?	¿Viene y se va?
Is it getting worse?	¿El dolor se le está empeorando?
Slowly?	¿Despacio?
Rapidly?	¿Rápido?
Does it feel . . .	¿Se siente . . .
crampy?	con retorcijones?
achy	adolorido?
Does it feel like	¿Se siente . . .
burning?	ardiente?
stabbing?	punzante?
ripping?	rasgado?
tearing?	desgarrado?
Does the pain radiate . . .	¿El dolor se irradia . . .
	¿El dolor **se riega hacia otros lugares como** . . .
to your back?	hacia su espalda?
to your jaw?	hacia su quijada?
to your groin?	hacia su ingle?
to your shoulder?	hacia sus hombros?
to your arm?	hacia sus brazos?

Abdominal Pain

Do you have associated nausea or vomiting?	¿Tiene nausea o vómitos asociado con el dolor?
Do you vomit blood?	¿Está usted vomitando sangre?
Is it bloody?	¿Es sanguinolenta (el vomito contiene sangre)?
Does it look like coffee grinds?	¿El vómito se ve como café molido?
	¿El vómito **luce** como café molido?
Do you have fever?	¿Tiene usted fiebre?
Did you take your temperature with a thermometer?	¿Se tomó usted su temperatura con un termómetro?
What was it?	¿Cuál fue la temperatura?
Do you have diarrhea?	¿Tiene usted diarrea?
Do you have constipation?	¿Tiene usted constipación?
	¿Tiene usted **estreñimiento**?
Do you have blood in your stools?	¿Tiene usted sangre en sus heces?
	¿Tiene usted sangre en su **excreta**?
	¿Tiene usted sangre en su **excremento**?
Do you have black, sticky stools, like tar?	¿Son sus heces negras y pegajosas, como tar?
	¿Está su **excremento** negro y pegajoso, como **alquitrán**?
	¿Está su **excreta** negra y pegajosa, como **brea**?
Is your appetite normal?	¿Su apetito está normal?
Decreased?	¿Reducido?
	¿Bajo?
	¿Disminuido?
	¿Pobre?
Increased?	¿Aumentado?
Do you get the pain before meals?	¿Tiene usted dolor antes de comer?
With meals?	¿Al comer?
After meals?	¿Después de comer?

Abdominal Pain

Is the pain better with eating?	¿Su dolor se mejora al comer?
Worse?	¿Empeora?
No different?	¿Es igual?
When was your last period?	¿Cuándo fue su última menstruación?
	¿Cuándo fue su último **período**?
Does the pain start a few weeks after your period?	¿El dolor le empieza unas semanas después de su menstruación?
	¿El dolor le empieza unas semanas después de su **período**?

Anxiety

Do you have problems with anxiety or nervousness?	¿Tiene usted problemas de ansiedad o nerviosismo?
Do you feel anxious most days or just every once in a while?	¿Se siente usted nervioso(a) la mayoría de los días o de vez en cuando?
How long have you felt this way (days, weeks, months, years)?	¿Cuánto tiempo hace que usted se siente de esta manera (días, semanas, meses, años)?
	¿Cuánto tiempo hace que usted se siente de esta **forma** (días, semanas, meses, años)?
When you feel anxious, do you have associated chest pain?	¿Cuándo usted se siente ansioso/a también tiene dolor de pecho?
	¿Cuándo usted se siente ansioso/a también **le da** dolor de pecho?
Difficulty breathing?	¿Dificultad al respirar?
Dizziness?	¿Mareos?
Numbness?	¿Adormecimiento?
	¿Entumecimiento?
Tingling around the mouth?	¿Hormigueo alrededor de la boca?
Do you feel tired?	¿Se siente usted cansada?
Restless?	¿Inquieta?
	¿Impaciente?
Do you have difficulty sleeping or concentrating?	¿Tiene usted dificultad durmiendo o concentrándose?

Anxiety

Does it start suddenly? Gradually?	¿Le empieza de repente? ¿Gradualmente? **¿Despacio?**
Do you have sudden, brief attacks of intense anxiety or fright? Does it go away in a few minutes? Does something specific happen that causes the attacks?	¿Tiene usted breves ataques repentinos de ansiedad o miedo? ¿Tiene usted breves ataques **súbitos** de ansiedad o miedo? ¿Se le pasa en unos minutos? ¿Se le **van** en unos minutos? ¿Se le **desaparecen** en unos minutos? ¿Hay algo en específico que le ocurre a usted lo cual le causa estos ataques?
Do you have anxiety or fear when you are in enclosed places like elevators, tunnels, crowds?	¿Tiene usted ansiedad o miedo cuando usted está en lugares cerrados como elevadores, túneles, o muchedumbre? ¿Tiene usted ansiedad o miedo cuando usted está en lugares cerrados como elevadores, túneles, o con **mucha gente**?
Do you have anxiety when you are alone?	¿Tiene usted ansiedad cuando está solo/a?
Do specific things make you anxious, like heights, darkness, insects, needles?	¿Hay algunas cosas en específico que le dan ansiedad como alturas, oscuridad, insectos, agujas?
Have you ever been in a traumatic or life-threatening situation where you felt helpless?	¿Ha estado usted envuelto/a en una situación traumática la cual le amenazó su vida y se sintió indefenso/a? ¿Ha estado usted envuelto en una situación traumática o que le amenazó su vida en la cual se sentio **impotente**? ¿Ha estado usted envuelto/a en una situación traumática o que le amenazó su vida en la cual se sentio **que no pudo hacer nada**?
Have you ever been a victim of violence or sexual assault? Do you have frequent nightmares or flashbacks of the situation?	¿Ha sido usted la víctima de un acto violento o de un asalto sexual? ¿Tiene usted pesadillas frecuentes o escenas retrospectivas del incidente?

Anxiety

	¿Tiene usted pesadillas frecuentes de los **momentos en los cuales sucedió** el incidente?
Do you have intrusive thoughts that you can't stop thinking about?	¿Tiene usted pensamientos intrusos en los cuales no puede parar de pensar en ellos? ¿Tiene usted pensamientos **que le vienen a su cabeza** y que no puede parar de pensar en ellos?
Do you have certain behaviors that you feel you need to repeat, like washing your hands or checking things?	¿Tiene usted ciertos comportamientos que usted siente que tiene que repetirlos, como lavarse las manos o revisar algunas cosas? ¿Tiene usted ciertos comportamientos que usted siente que tiene que **hacerlos otra vez y otra vez** como lavarse las manos, o **inspeccionar** algunas cosas?
Do you feel depressed? Have you ever been treated for depression? What medication did you take? Did it help?	¿Se siente deprimido/a? ¿Ha sido usted alguna vez tratado(a) por depresión? ¿Qué medicamentos usted tomó o le fueron recetados? ¿Le ayudaron?
Have you ever taken medication for anxiety? What medication did you take? Did it help?	¿Ha usted alguna vez tomado medicamentos para la ansiedad? ¿Qué medicamentos usted usó/tomó? ¿Le ayudaron?

Chest Pain

Do you have chest pain? Are you having chest pain now? How long ago did it start (minutes, hours)?	¿Tiene usted dolor de pecho? ¿Tiene usted dolor de pecho en este momento? ¿Cuándo le empezo (minutos, horas)?

Chest Pain

Show me where the pain is.	Enséñeme donde le duele.
	Muéstreme donde le duele.
Is it getting better?	¿Se le está mejorando?
Worse?	¿Empeorando?
Have you had chest pain like this before?	¿Ha tenido usted anteriormente un dolor de pecho como este?
Are you getting chest pain more often or more severely recently?	¿Está usted teniendo últimamente dolor de pecho más a menudo?
	¿Más fuerte?
	¿Más severo?
How long have you been having chest pain (hours/days/weeks/months/years)?	¿Cuánto hace que usted está teniendo dolor de pecho (horas/días/semanas/años)?
How many times a day/week/month?	¿Cuántas veces al día/semana/mes?
Do you get it with activity?	¿El dolor le viene cuando usted esta activo(a)?
	¿El dolor le **empieza** cuando usted esta activo/a?
How much activity: walking one block?	¿Con cuánta actividad: caminando un bloque?
	¿Con cuánta actividad: caminando una **manzana**?
One mile?	¿Una milla?
kilometer	**¿Kilómetro?**
One flight of stairs?	¿Subiendo las escaleras solo una vez?
At rest?	¿Durante reposo?
	¿Sin actividad?
When you lie down?	¿Cuándo se acuesta?
Show me where the pain starts.	¿Enséñeme donde le empieza el dolor?
Does the pain stay there?	¿El dolor se le queda ahí?
	¿El dolor **no se le mueve**?
Does the pain radiate to the . . .	¿El dolor se le riega hacia . . . ?
arm?	¿el brazo?
back?	¿la espalda?
shoulder?	¿el hombro?
jaw?	¿la quijada?

Chest Pain

Show me where it goes.	Enséñeme adonde se le va. Enséñeme adonde se **le mueve**. **Muéstreme** para donde se **riega**.
How long does it last (seconds/minutes/hours)?	¿Cuánto tiempo le dura (segundos/minutos/horas)?
Does it feel . . . sharp? dull?	¿Lo siente . . . ? agudo? sordo? **mate**?
Does it feel like... squeezing? pressure? achy? tight? ripping? tearing? throbbing? burning?	¿Se siente como... apretado? con presión? adolorido? con poco movimiento? desgarrado? rasgado? pulsante? ardiente?
When you get the chest pain, do you have associated . . . nausea? vomiting? dizziness? fainting? excessive sweating? palpitations (heart racing or skipping beats)? anxiety?	¿Cuándo a usted le da el dolor de pecho, también tiene síntomas de . . . nausea? vómitos? mareo? desmayo? sudor excesivo? palpitaciones (siente que el corazón le corre o le salta latidos)? Ansioso/a?
Do you have difficulty breathing at rest? With activity?	¿Tiene usted dificultad respirando al descansar? Con actividad?
How many pillows do you use under your head when you sleep?	¿Cuántas almohadas usted utiliza debajo de su cabeza al dormir? ¿Cuántas almohadas usted **usa** debajo de su cabeza? ¿Cuántas almohadas usted se **pone** debajo de su cabeza?

Chest Pain

Can you breathe normally lying flat?	¿Puede usted respirar normalmente acostado?
Do you have difficulty breathing at night?	¿Tiene usted dificultad respirando por la noche, al dormir?
Do you have swelling in your legs?	¿Tiene usted hinchazón en sus piernas?
	¿Tiene usted **inflamación** en sus piernas?
For how many days, weeks, months?	¿Por cuantos días, semanas, meses?
Is it more or less than usual?	¿Es más o menos de lo usual?
	¿Es más o menos de lo **corriente**?
	¿Es más o menos de lo **normal**?
Do you have fever?	¿Tiene usted fiebre?
Do you have a cough?	¿Tiene usted tos?
Do you cough up blood?	¿Está usted tosiendo sangre?
Do you get heartburn or a bitter acid taste in your mouth?	¿Le da a usted ardor de estómago o siente un sabor acido-amargo en su boca con este dolor?
Does the pain get better with . . .	¿Se le mejora el dolor cuando . . . ?
rest?	descansa?
eating?	come?
sitting up?	Se sienta?
antacids?	Toma antiácidos?
Does it get worse with . . .	¿Se le empeora con . . . ?
activity?	actividad?
eating?	al comer?
lying down?	al acostarse?
coughing?	al toser?
breathing deeply?	al respirar profundo?
Do you use nitroglycerin (under the tongue)?	¿Usa usted nitroglicerina (debajo de la lengua)?
How many times a day/week/month?	¿Cuántas veces al día/semana/mes?
Is that more or less than before?	¿Es más o menos que antes?
Have you taken nitroglycerin now?	¿Tomó usted nitroglicerina en este momento?
How long ago (minutes/hours)?	¿Cuánto hace que la tomó (minutos/horas)?
How many?	¿Cuántas tomó?
Did it make the pain better?	¿Le alivio el dolor?

Children

Are your child's immunizations up to date?	¿Las inmunizaciones de sus hijos están al día?
Was your child sick right before the rash started?	¿Su hijo/a estuvo enfermo/a exactamente antes de que la erupción empezara?
	¿Su hijo/a estuvo enfermo/a exactamente antes de que el **salpullido** empezara?
	¿Su hijo/a estuvo enfermo/a exactamente antes de que las **pintas rojas en su piel** empezaran?
Did he/she have a cough, red eyes, or runny nose?	¿Él/ella tiene tos, ojos rojos o flujo nasal?
	¿Él/ella tiene tos, ojos rojos o **catarro**?
	¿Él/ella tiene tos, ojos rojos o **gripe**?
Did he/she have a high fever or sore throat?	¿Él/ella tiene fiebre alta o garganta irritada?

Constipation

How long have you had constipation?	¿Cuánto tiempo hace que usted está constipado/a?
	¿Cuánto tiempo hace que usted está **estreñido**/a?
Weeks, months, years?	¿Semanas, meses, años?
Are you constipated all the time or just sometimes?	¿Está usted constipado/a todo el tiempo o solamente de vez en cuando?
	¿Está usted **estreñido/a** todo el tiempo o solamente **algunas veces**?
	¿Está usted **estreñido/a** todo el tiempo o solamente **a veces**?
Do you pass gas?	¿Pasa usted gases estomacales?
Do you pass mucus with your stools?	¿Tiene usted moco en sus heces?
	¿Tiene usted mucosidad en su **excreta**?
	¿Tiene usted flema en su **excremento**?

Constipation

Do you have abdominal pain or cramping?	¿Tiene dolor abdominal o retorcijones?
	¿Tiene dolor **de barriga** o retorcijones?
When you have a bowel movement, does it get better, or worse?	¿Después que usted defeca se siente usted mejor o peor?
	¿Después que usted **ensucia** se siente usted mejor o peor?
	¿Después que usted **va al baño** se siente usted mejor o peor?
Do you have nausea or vomiting?	¿Tiene usted nausea or vomitos?
Are you able to control your bowels?	¿Puede usted controlar sus intestinos?
	¿Le alcanza el tiempo para llegar al baño?
How many times in a week do you have a bowel movement?	¿Cuántas veces a la semana usted defeca?
	¿Cuántas veces a la semana usted **ensucia**?
	¿Cuántas veces a la semana usted **va al baño**?
How many times a week is normal for you?	¿Cuántas veces a la semana es lo normal para usted?
Are your stools soft?	¿Sus heces son suaves?
	¿Su **excreta** es suave?
	¿Su **excremento** es suave?
Hard?	¿Duras?
Like rocks?	¿Como roca?
Are your stools thin like a pencil?	¿Sus heces son flacas como un lápiz?
	¿Su **excreta** es flaca como un lápiz?
	¿Su **excremento** es delgado como un lápiz?
Do you have constipation some days and diarrhea other days?	¿Tiene usted constipación unos días y en otros tiene diarrea?
	¿Tiene usted **estreñimiento** unos días y en otros tiene diarrea?
Do you have blood in your stools?	¿Tiene usted sangre en sus heces?
	¿Tiene usted sangre en su **excreta**?
	¿Tiene usted sangre en su **excremento**?

Constipation

Are your stools black and sticky, like tar?	¿Son sus **heces** negras y pegajosas, como tar?
	¿Es su **excreta** negra y pegajosa, como **alquitrán**?
	¿Es su **excremento** negro y pegajoso, como **brea**?
Do you use laxatives?	¿Usa usted laxantes?
Which ones?	¿Cuáles?
How often—every day?	¿Qué tan a menudo, todos los días?
For how long (weeks, months, years)?	¿Por cuanto tiempo (semanas, meses, años)?
How many glasses of water do you drink each day?	¿Cuántos vasos de agua usted toma cada día?
	¿Cuántos vasos de agua usted **consume** cada día?
	¿Cuántos vasos de agua usted **bebe** cada día?

Cough

Do you have a cough?	¿Tiene usted tos?
Is this a new cough?	¿Es su tos reciente?
How long have you had it (days, weeks, months, years)?	¿Cuánto tiempo hace que la tiene (días, semanas, meses, años)?
Did it start suddenly or slowly?	¿Le empezó de repente o despacio?
Do you cough up phlegm?	¿Esta usted tosiendo flema?
Is it clear?	¿Es clara?
White?	¿Blanca?
Yellow?	¿Amarilla?
Green?	¿Verde?
Brown?	¿Café?
	¿Marrón?
	¿Carmelito?
	¿Castaño?
Bloody?	¿Sangrienta?

Cough

Do you frequently have a lot of phlegm in your throat?	¿Tiene usted frecuentemente mucha flema en su garganta?
Do you feel like you have to clear your throat frequently?	¿Siente usted la necesidad de despejarse su garganta frecuentemente?
	¿Siente usted la necesidad de **limpiarse** su garganta frecuentemente?
	¿Siente usted la necesidad de **toser** frecuentemente?
	¿Siente usted la necesidad de **aclararse** su garganta frecuentemente?
Do you have associated hoarseness?	¿Tiene usted ronquera asociada con su flema?
Do you have wheezing?	¿Tiene usted resollos al respirar?
	¿Tiene usted **silbidos** al respirar?
For how long (hours, days, weeks)?	¿Por cuanto tiempo (horas, días, semanas)?
Do you have difficulty breathing?	¿Tiene usted dificultad respirarando?
When active or walking?	¿Cuando está activo/a o caminando?
When resting?	¿Cuando está descansando?
Does your cough wake you up at night?	¿Su tos lo despierta por las noches?
Has it been getting worse recently?	¿Recientemente se le está empeorando su tos?
How long has it been getting worse (days, weeks, months)?	¿Cuánto tiempo hace que se le ha empeorando (días, semanas, meses)?
Is your cough worse . . .	¿Ha empeorado su tos . . .
when you breathe deeply?	cuando respira profundo?
at night?	por la noche?
when you lie down?	cuando se acuesta?
when you exercise?	cuando hace ejercicios?
in cold air?	en aire frio?
How many pillows do you use under your head when you sleep?	¿Cuántas almohadas usted utiliza debajo de su cabeza al dormir?
	¿Cuántas almohadas usted **usa** debajo de su cabeza?
	¿Cuántas almohadas usted **pone** debajo de su cabeza?

Cough

Can you breathe normally lying flat?	¿Puede usted respirar normalmente cuando está acostado?
Have you ever had asthma?	¿Ha tenido usted alguna vez asma?
Have you ever had congestive heart failure?	¿Ha tenido usted alguna vez fallo cardiaco congestivo?
Do you have fever/chills?	¿Tiene usted fiebre/escalofríos?
Did you take your temperature with a thermometer?	¿Se toma usted su temperatura con un termómetro?
What was your temperature?	¿Cuál fue su temperatura?
Do you have frequent heartburn?	¿Tiene usted ardor de estómago?
Is it worse lately?	¿Se le ha empeorado últimamente?
Do you have sinus pain?	¿Tiene usted dolor en sus senos nasales?
Do you have hay fever/allergies?	¿Tiene usted fiebre de heno/alergias?
	¿Tiene usted **catarro anual en la nariz y los ojos**/alergias?
Do you take allergy medicine?	¿Está usted tomando medicamentos para la alergia?
Which ones?	¿Cuáles son?
Did you have a cold or flu recently?	¿Ha tenido recientemente catarro o influenza?
	¿Ha tenido recientemente **resfriado** o influenza?
	¿Ha tenido recientemente **gripe** o influenza?

Depressed Mood

Have you ever been treated for depression?	¿Ha sido usted tratado alguna vez por depresión?
How long ago (months, years)?	¿Cuánto tiempo atrás (meses, años)?
	¿Cuánto tiempo **hace** (meses, años)?
What medicine were you on?	¿Qué medicamentos estaba usted tomando?
	¿Qué **medicinas** estaba usted tomando?
Did it work well?	¿Estos medicamentos, le trabajaron?
	¿Estas **medicinas**, le trabajaron?

Depressed Mood

How many days a week do you feel depressed?	¿Cuántos días a la semana se sentía usted deprimido(a)?
For how long (days, weeks, months, years)?	¿Por cuanto tiempo (días, semanas, meses, años)?
Have you lost interest or pleasure in doing things?	¿Ha usted perdido interés o placer en hacer actividades?
	¿Ha usted perdido interés o placer en hacer **cosas**?
Have you lost or gained a lot of weight recently?	¿Ha usted perdido o ganado mucho peso recientemente?
How many pounds?	¿Cuántas libras?
Do you sleep well?	¿Duerme usted bien?
Too much or too little?	¿Duerme usted mucho o poco?
How many hours a night do you sleep, in total?	¿Cuántas horas por noche duerme usted?
Is your energy level normal?	¿Su estado de energía está normal?
Increased?	¿Alto?
Decreased?	¿Reducio?
	¿Bajo?
	¿Disminuido?
	¿Pobre?
Do you often feel worthless or guilty?	¿Se siente usted a menudo que no vale nada o culpable?
Do you have difficulty concentrating or making decisions?	¿Tiene usted dificultad concentrándose o tomando decisiones?
Are you able to remember most things well?	¿Puede usted acordarse bien de las cosas?
Are you nervous most days of the week?	¿Se siente usted nervioso(a) la mayoría de los días de la semana?
Do you feel anxious most of the time?	¿Se siente usted ansioso(a) la mayoría del tiempo?
Have you ever been treated for anxiety?	¿Ha sido usted alguna vez tratado por ansiedad?
Do you feel irritable frequently?	¿Se siente usted irritable la mayoría del tiempo?

Depressed Mood

Do you have thoughts of wanting to hurt or kill yourself or others?	¿Ha usted tenido pensamientos de querer herir o matar a otros al igual que a usted?
Do you have a plan?	¿Tiene usted un plan en específico?
Do you have a way to carry out your plan?	¿Tiene usted la forma de llevar a cabo su plan?
Have you ever tried to hurt yourself or someone else?	¿Ha usted tratado de herir o matar a otra persona al igual que a usted?
Are you afraid that you might try this time?	¿Tiene usted miedo de que pueda tratar de hacerlo esta vez?

Diarrhea

Do you have diarrhea?	¿Tiene usted diarrhea?
Did it start suddenly?	¿Le empezaron de momento?
Did it start gradually?	¿Le empezaron gradualmente?
	¿Le empezaron **despacio**?
How long have you had it (hours, days, weeks, months)?	¿Cuánto tiempo hace que usted tiene diarrea (horas, días, semanas, meses)?
Do you have diarrhea all the time or just sometimes?	¿Usted tiene diarrea todo el tiempo o solamente de vez en cuando?
	¿Usted tiene diarrea todo el tiempo o solamente **algunas veces**?
	¿Usted tiene diarrea todo el tiempo o solamente **a veces**?
Do you have constipation some days and diarrhea other days?	¿Está usted constipado/a algunos días y otros tiene diarrea?
	¿Está usted **estreñido/a** algunos días y otros tiene diarrea?
How many bowel movements do you have each day?	¿Cuántas veces usted defeca al día?
	¿Cuántas veces usted **ensucia** al día?
	¿Cuántas veces usted **va al baño** al día?
Are your stools well formed?	¿Sus heces están bien formadas?
	¿Su **excreta** está bien formada?
Are they loose?	¿están sueltas?
Are they like water?	¿están acuosas?
	¿Como si fuera agua?

Diarrhea

Do you have blood in your stools?	¿Tiene usted sangre en sus heces? ¿Tiene usted sangre en su **excreta**? ¿Tiene usted sangre en su **excremento**?
Do you have mucus in your stools?	¿Tiene usted moco en sus heces? ¿Tiene usted mucosidad en su **excreta**? ¿Tiene usted flema en su **excremento**?
Are your stools greasy or oily?	¿Son sus heces grasosas o grasientas? ¿Está su **excreta** grasosa o grasienta? ¿Está su **excremento** grasosa o grasienta?
Do you have abdominal pain?	¿Tiene usted dolor abdominal? ¿Tiene usted dolor **de barriga**?
Point to where the pain is.	Apúnteme con su dedo donde le duele.
Is the pain better after you have a bowel movement?	¿Su dolor se mejora después de que usted defeca? ¿Su dolor se mejora después de que usted **ensucia**? ¿Su dolor se mejora después de que usted **va al baño**?
Do you have rectal pain when you have a bowel movement?	¿Tiene usted dolor en el recto al defecar? ¿Tiene usted dolor en el recto al **ensuciar**? ¿Tiene usted dolor en el recto al **ir al baño**?
Is the diarrhea worse when you eat foods containing milk or wheat?	¿Se empeora su diarrea cuando usted come comidas que contienen leche o trigo?
Have you traveled outside the country recently? Where?	¿Ha usted viajado fuera del país recientemente? ¿Adónde fue?
Have you taken antibiotics recently?	¿Ha usted tomado antibióticos recientemente?
Did you eat out recently?	¿Ha comido usted fuera de su casa recientemente?
Do you take laxatives?	¿Toma usted laxantes?

Dizziness

Do you have dizziness?	¿Tiene usted mareos?
Are you dizzy now?	¿Está usted mareado(a) en estos momentos?
Do you feel lightheaded, or does it feel like things are spinning around you?	¿Se siente usted que se quiere desmayar o siente que las cosas le dan vueltas a su alrededor?
Do you faint during these spells?	¿Se desmaya usted durante esos momentos?
Do you feel like you might faint but do not?	¿Se siente que se quiere desmayar pero no se desmaya?
How long have you had dizzy spells (hours, days, weeks, months)?	¿Cuánto tiempo hace que usted tiene estas sensaciones de mareo (horas, días, semanas, meses)?
How long does it last each time (minutes, hours)?	¿Cada vez que ocurren cuanto tiempo duran (minutes, horas)?
Does it come on suddenly?	¿Aparecen de repente sin aviso?
Does it come on without warning or slowly over a few hours?	¿Aparecen de repente o despacio por unas cuantas horas?
Does it get worse when you . . .	¿Se empeoran cuando usted . . .
roll over in bed?	se da vuelta en su cama?
stand up suddenly?	se para repentinamente?
turn your head to look up?	vira la cabeza y mira hacia arriba?
change positions?	al cambiarse de posiciones?
Are you able to do some things during the dizziness?	¿Puede usted hacer algo durante estos periodos de mareos?
Or do you have to lie down?	¿O usted tiene que acostarse?
How many episodes have you had in the past week(s), month(s)?	¿Cuántos episodios ha tenido usted durante la pasada(s) semana(s), mes(es)?
When you are dizzy, do you have associated . . .	¿Cuándo usted está mareada, también tiene . . .
nausea/vomiting?	nâusea/vómitos?
diarrhea?	diarrea?
intense sweating?	sudores intensivos?
	sudores **masivos**?
Do you have fullness in one ear before the dizziness starts?	¿Siente usted que tiene uno de sus oídos lleno antes de empezarle los mareos?

Dizziness

Do you have ringing in the ear?	¿Siente usted un zumbido en sus oídos?
	¿Siente usted un **campanilleo** en sus oídos?
	¿Siente usted un **repique** en sus oídos?
Do you have loss of hearing in one ear?	¿Tiene pérdida de audición en un oído?
During the dizziness, do you have . . .	¿Durante su mareo, tiene usted . . .
	¿Durante su **vertigo**, tiene usted . . .
a headache?	dolor de cabeza?
numbness or tingling on one side?	entumecimiento u hormigueo en un lado?
double vision?	visión doble?
difficulty forming words?	dificultad formando palabras?
Do you have discharge from your ear?	¿Tiene usted descargas por su oído?
	¿Le está **saliéndo líquido** por su oído?
Do you have bleeding from your ear?	¿Le están sangrando su oído?

Dyspepsia

Have you ever had stomach ulcers?	¿Ha usted alguna vez tenido úlceras estomacales?
Have you ever vomited blood?	¿Ha usted alguna vez vomitado sangre?
When was the last time (days/weeks/months/years)?	¿Cuándo fue la ultima vez (días/semana/meses/años)?
Do you smoke?	¿Usted fuma?
Do you drink alcohol?	¿Usted toma alcohol?
	¿Usted **consume** alcohol?
	¿Usted **bebe** alcohol?
What kind?	¿Qué tipo?
How much in a day, week?	¿Cuánto toma por día, semana?
Do you take ibuprofen, Motrin™, or similar medicines?	¿Toma usted ibuprofen, Motrin™ o medicamentos similares?
Every day?	¿Todos los días?
For how long (days/weeks/months/years)?	¿Por cuanto tiempo (días/semana/meses/años)?
Did the pain start suddenly?	¿El dolor le empezó de repente?

Dyspepsia

Did the pain start gradually?	¿El dolor le empezó gradualmente? ¿El dolor le empezó **despacio**?
How long does it last?	¿Cuánto tiempo le duro?
Point to where the pain is.	Apúnteme con su dedo donde le duele.
How long have you had this problem?	¿Cuánto tiempo hace que usted tiene este problema?
Is it constant?	¿Es constante?
Does it come and go?	¿Viene y se va?
Is the pain burning, stabbing, or crampy?	¿El dolor se siente candente, punzante o como si fueran retorcijones?
Is it worse . . . before you eat? while you eat? after you eat? when lying down? with stress? after eating milk products?	¿Se empeora . . . ? antes de comer? cuando come? después de comer? cuando se acuesta? cuando tiene tensión? cuando come productos lácteos? cuando come productos **que contienen leche**?
Does the pain feel better when you eat? When you don't eat? When you pass stool?	¿Se le mejora el dolor cuando come? ¿Cuando no come? ¿Cuando defeca? ¿Cuando **ensucia**? ¿Cuando **va al baño**?
Have you tried any medicines to help this problem? What are they?	¿Ha usted tratado medicamentos para ayudarle con el problema? ¿Ha usted tratado **medicinas** para ayudarle con el problema? ¿Cuáles son?
Does the pain wake you from sleep?	¿El dolor lo despierta?
Do you have nausea, vomiting?	¿Tiene usted nausea, vomitos?
Do you have a cough, hoarseness?	¿Tiene tos, ronquera?

Dyspepsia

Do you have black, sticky stools, like tar?	¿Son sus heces negras y pegajosas, como tar? ¿Está su **excreta** negra y pegajosa, como **alquitrán**? ¿Está su **excremento** negro y pegajoso, como **brea**?
Do you have difficulty with swallowing?	¿Tiene dificultad al tragar?
Do you have constipation?	¿Está usted constipada? ¿Está usted **estreñida**?

Dyspnea

Do you have difficulty breathing?	¿Tiene dificultad respirando?
Is it difficult to breathe through your nose or through your mouth? For how long (days/weeks)? Do you have a stuffy nose? Do you have a runny nose? Do you have a sore throat? Do you have an earache? Do you have fever or chills? Do you have sinus pain or pressure?	¿Tiene usted dificultad respirando por su nariz o por su boca? ¿Por cuánto tiempo (días/semanas)? ¿Tiene la nariz tapada? ¿Tiene flujo nasal? ¿Tiene **catarro**? ¿Tiene **gripe**? ¿Le duele la garganta? ¿Tiene dolor en sus oídos? ¿Tiene fiebre o escalofríos? ¿Tiene dolor o presión en sus senos nasales?
How long have you been having difficulty breathing?	¿Cuánto tiempo hace que tiene dificultad respirando?
Is it constant?	¿Es constante?
Does it come and go?	¿Le viene y se va?
Is it difficult to breathe when you are resting? Do you have pain when you breathe deeply? Where? Do you have pain in your leg? Have you been traveling recently?	¿Le es difícil respirar cuando descansa? ¿Tiene usted dolor cuando respira profundo? ¿Dónde? ¿Tiene dolor en su pierna? ¿Ha viajado últimamente?

Dyspnea

How many hours were you sitting?	¿Por cuantas horas estuvo sentado/a?
Have you had surgery recently?	¿Ha tenido alguna operación recientemente?
Do you have difficulty breathing when walking?	¿Usted tiene dificultad respirando cuando camina?
How far can you walk before you have difficulty breathing?	¿Qué tan lejos usted puede caminar antes de sentir dificultad al respirar?
Less than one block?	¿Más de dos bloques?
One block?	¿Más de dos cuadras?
More than two blocks?	¿Más de dos manzanas?
How many pillows do you use under your head when you sleep?	¿Cuántas almohadas usted utiliza debajo de su cabeza al dormir?
	¿Cuántas almohadas usted **usa** debajo de su cabeza?
	¿Cuántas almohadas usted se **pone** debajo de su cabeza?
Can you breathe normally lying flat?	¿Usted puede respirar normalmente cuando está acostado?
Do you have difficulty breathing at night?	¿Usted tiene dificultad respirando por la noche?
Do you wake up feeling like you have stopped breathing?	¿Se despierta sintiéndose como que no puede respirar?
Has anyone told you that you had stopped breathing while sleeping?	¿Le ha dicho alguien que usted deja de respirar mientras duerme?
Do you snore?	¿Usted ronca?
Do you feel rested when you wake up in the morning?	¿Se siente descansado/a cuando despierta?
Do you fall asleep unintentionally in the daytime?	¿Se queda dormida sin querer durante el día?
Do you have swelling in your legs?	¿Usted tiene hinchazón en las piernas?
	¿Usted tiene **inflamación** en las piernas?
For how long?	¿Qué tiempo hace que están hinchadas?
Is it more or less than usual?	¿Es más o menos de lo usual?
	¿Es más o menos de lo **corriente**?
	¿Es más o menos de lo **normal**?

Dyspnea

Do you smoke?	¿Usted fuma?
Did you used to smoke?	¿Usted fumaba?
Do you have a cough?	¿Tiene tos?
How long have you had it?	¿Por cuánto tiempo la ha tenido?
Do you cough up sputum?	¿Toce esputo?
	¿Toce **flema**?
A lot or a little each time?	¿Mucha o poca?
Is it clear?	¿Es clara?
White?	¿Blanca?
Yellow?	¿Amarilla?
Green?	¿Verde?
Do you cough up blood?	¿Tose sangre?
Do you have night sweats?	¿Suda por la noche?
Does your cough wake you up at night?	¿Lo/la despierta la tos por la noche?
Do you have any wheezing?	¿Tiene usted resollo?
	¿Tiene usted **silbidos**?
Do you have a history of asthma?	¿Tiene usted un historial de asma?
	¿ **Ha tenido** asma?
	¿ **Ha sufrido** de asma?
Do you have emphysema?	¿Tiene enfisema?
Do you use medications for your lungs?	¿Toma medicamentos para los pulmones?
	¿Toma **medicinas para poder respirar mejor**?

Dysuria

Do you have burning or pain when urinating?	¿Tiene usted dolor o quemazón al orinar?
How many days?	¿Cuántos días?
Did it start suddenly?	¿El dolor le empezó de repente?
Did it start slowly?	¿El dolor le empezó despacio?
Do you urinate more often than usual?	¿Usted orina más a menudo de lo acostumbrado?

Dysuria

Do you pass more or less urine than usual each time?	¿Cada vez que orina, está usted orinando mas o menos de lo acostumbrado?
Does your bladder feel empty or full after urinating?	¿Su vejiga se siente vacia o llena después de orinar?
Do you feel the need to urinate more urgently than usual?	¿Siente usted la necesidad de orinar con más urgencia de lo acostumbrado?
Does your urine look . . .	¿Su orine luce . . . ¿Su orine **se mira** . . .
dark?	oscuro?
light?	claro?
red?	rojo?
cloudy?	turbio?
brown?	café? **marrón**? **brown**?
Have you had back pain since this started?	¿Tiene usted dolor de espalda desde que esto empezó?
Do you have nausea or vomiting? Fever or chills?	¿Tiene usted nauseas o vómitos? ¿Fiebre o escalofríos?
Have you had sex without a con dom recently?	¿Ha tenido usted sexo recientemente sin utilizar preservativos? ¿Ha tenido usted sexo recientemente sin utilizar **condones**?
Do you have vaginal itching or discharge?	¿Tiene usted picazón o descargas vaginales?
Do you have discharge from your penis?	¿Tiene usted descargas por su pene?
Have you ever had kidney stones?	¿Ha tenido usted piedras en los riñones?

Fever

How many days ago did the fever start?	¿Cuántos días hace que le empezó la fiebre?
How high is the fever?	¿Qué tan alta es la fiebre?
Is it constant?	¿Es constante?
Does it come and go?	¿Viene y se va?
Do you have shaking chills with the fever?	¿Tiene usted escalofríos con temblores y fiebre?
Do you have night sweats?	¿Tiene usted sudores nocturnos?
	¿Usted **suda por la noche**?
Have you lost weight recently?	¿Ha perdido peso recientemente?
How many pounds?	¿Cuántas libras?
	¿Cuántos **kilogramos**?
Over how many weeks, months?	¿En cuantas semanas, meses?
Is your appetite normal?	¿Su apetito está normal?
Increased?	¿Aumentado?
Decreased?	¿Reducido?
	¿Bajo?
	¿Desminuido?
	¿Pobre?
Do you feel very tired since the fever began?	¿Se siente usted muy cansado/a desde que la fiebre le empezó?
Do you have a headache or stiff neck?	¿Tiene dolor de cabeza o siente su cuello rígido?
	¿Tiene dolor de cabeza o siente su cuello **duro**?
Do you have difficulty in speaking since the fever began?	¿Tiene dificultad hablando desde que le empezó la fiebre?
Weakness in your arms or legs?	¿Debilidad en sus brazos o piernas?
Seizures?	¿Convulsiones?
Do you have any confusion?	¿Se siente usted confundido/a?
Do you have a cough?	¿Tiene usted tos?
Stuffy nose?	¿Nariz tapada?
Sore throat?	¿Garganta irritada?
Sinus pain?	¿Dolor en sus sienes nasales?
Do you cough up sputum or blood?	¿Está usted tosiendo esputo o sangre?
	¿Está usted tosiendo **flema** o sangre?

Fever

Do you have chest pain?	¿Tiene usted dolor de pecho?
Do you have difficulty breathing?	¿Tiene usted dificultad al respirar?
Do you have any new rashes?	¿Tiene usted alguna erupción nueva? ¿Tiene usted algún **salpullido** nuevo?
Do you have burning with urination?	¿Siente usted quemazón al orinar?
Do you have blood in your urine?	¿Tiene usted sangre en la orina?
Do you have diarrhea?	¿Tiene usted diarrea?
Do you have abdominal pain?	¿Tiene usted dolor abdominal? ¿Tiene usted dolor **de barriga**?
Have your eyes or skin turned yellow?	¿Están sus ojos o piel amarillo/a?
Have you been around anyone else who is sick?	¿Ha estado usted alrededor de alguien que está enfermo?
Have you been in the hospital recently?	¿Ha estado usted en el hospital recientemente?
Have you traveled outside the country recently?	¿Ha usted viajado recientemente fuera del país?
Have you had any sexual intercourse without a condom recently?	¿Ha usted tenido relaciones sexuales sin preservativos recientemente? ¿Ha usted tenido relaciones sexuales sin **condones** recientemente?
Do you use intravenous drugs?	¿Usa usted drogas intravenosas? **¿Usted se inyecta drogas?**
Do you share needles?	¿Usted comparte agujas?
Have you ever had surgery on your heart valves?	¿Ha usted tenido alguna cirugía en las válvulas cardiacas? ¿Ha usted tenido alguna cirugía en las válvulas **del corazon**?
Do you have HIV?	¿Tiene usted VIH (virus de inmunodeficiencia humana)?
Are you taking steroids?	¿Está usted tomando esteroides?

Genitourinary Discharge

Do you have a vaginal/ penile discharge?	¿Tiene usted descargas vaginales/ por el pene? ¿ **Le está saliendo** descargas vaginales/ por el pene?
Is it white?	¿Son blancas?
Yellow?	¿Amarillas?
Green?	¿Verdes?
Clear?	¿Claras?
Bloody?	¿Sangrientas?
How many days have you had it?	¿Cuántos días hace que usted tiene o ha visto estas descargas?
Did it start suddenly?	¿Le empezaron de repente?
Did it start slowly?	¿Le empezaron lentamente?
Do you have burning with urination?	¿Tiene usted quemazón al orinar?
Do you have blood in your urine?	¿Tiene usted sangre en la orina?
Do you have any vaginal/penile ulcers or lesions?	¿Tiene usted úlceras o lesiones vaginales/en el pene?
Do you have any rashes on your palms or feet?	¿Tiene usted algún tipo de erupción en la palma de sus manos o en sus pies? ¿Tiene usted algún tipo de **salpullido** en la palma de sus manos o en sus pies? ¿Tiene usted algún tipo de **pintas rojas en su piel** en la palma de sus manos o en sus pies?
Are you sexually active?	¿Está usted sexualmente activo?
How many days, weeks, months ago was the last time you had sex?	¿Cuándo fue la última vez que usted tuvo sexo días/semanas/meses?
With your spouse or partner?	¿Con su esposo/a o compañero/a?
With someone new?	¿Con alguien nuevo?
Do you have more than one sexual partner?	¿Tiene usted más de un compañero sexual?
Did you use a condom?	¿Usa usted preservativos? ¿Usa usted **condones**?

Genitourinary Discharge

Does your partner have this same problem?	¿Tiene su compañero el mismo problema ya mencionado?
Do you have fever/chills?	¿Tiene usted fiebre/escalofríos?
Do you have nausea/vomiting?	¿Tiene usted nausea/vómitos?
Do you have abdominal pain?	¿Tiene usted dolor abdominal?
	¿Tiene usted dolor **de barriga**?
Do you have a history of sexually transmitted infections (syphilis, gonorrhea, HIV, herpes)?	¿Tiene usted un historial de infecciones transmitidas sexualmente, como por ejemplo: sífilis, gonorrea, VIH (virus de immunideficiencia humana), herpes u otras?
	¿ **Ha tenido** usted un historial de infecciones transmitidas sexualmente, como por ejemplo: sífilis, gonorrea, VIH (virus de immunideficiencia humana), herpes u otras?
	¿ **Ha sufrido** usted un historial de infecciones transmitidas sexualmente, como por ejemplo: sífilis, gonorrea, VIH (virus de immunideficiencia humana), herpes u otras?
Were you treated?	¿Fue usted tratado/a?

Headache

Do you have a headache?	¿Tiene usted dolor de cabeza?
Is it throbbing?	¿Es pulsante?
Aching?	¿Adolorido?
Stabbing?	¿Punzante?
Sharp?	¿Agudo?
Dull?	¿Sordo?
Squeezing?	¿Apretado?
	¿ **Como si le estuvieran exprimiendo su cabeza**?
Like a band around your head?	¿Como una banda alrededor de la cabeza?

Headache

Does it hurt to brush your hair?	¿Le duele cuando se peina?
How long do your headaches usually last (in minutes, hours, days)?	¿Usualmente, cuánto tiempo duran sus dolores de cabeza (en minutos, horas, días)?
During your headache . . .	¿Durante su dolor de cabeza . . .
does the light hurt your eyes?	le duelen sus ojos al mirar a la luz?
do you have nausea or vomiting?	tiene usted nausea o vomitos?
do you see stars or spots in your vision?	ve usted estrellas o puntos?
	ve usted estrellas o **manchas**?
do you lose your vision?	pierde usted su visión?
	pierde usted su **vista**?
do you have weakness or paralysis in your arms or legs?	tiene usted debilidad o parálisis en sus brazos o piernas?
Which side?	¿Cuál lado?
How long does it last (minutes or hours)?	¿Cuánto tiempo le dura (minutos o horas)?
do you have numbness or tingling?	tiene usted entumecimiento o hormigueo?
Where?	¿Dónde?
do you lose consciousness?	¿pierde usted su conocimiento?
Are you very sleepy after the headache ends?	¿Se siente muy dormido después de que termina su dolor de cabeza?
	¿Se siente muy **soñoliento/a** después de que termina su dolor de cabeza?
	¿Se siente muy **agotado/a** después de que termina su dolor de cabeza?
	¿Se siente **con ganas de dormir** después de que termina su dolor de cabeza?
How long does the sleepiness last?	¿Cuánto dura su estado de soñoliencia?
Do you have any strange sensations right when the headache starts?	¿Siente usted alguna sensación rara al empezarle su dolor de cabeza?
What medicine do you take for your headache?	¿Qué medicamento toma usted para su dolor de cabeza?
	¿Qué **medicina** toma usted para su dolor de cabeza?

Headache

Does it make the headache go away?	¿Este medicamento, le quita su dolor de cabeza? ¿Esta **medicina**, le quita su dolor de cabeza?
How many headaches do you get each month?	¿Cuántos dolores de cabeza usted tiene por mes?
Does anyone in your family have migraines?	¿Alguien padece de migrañas en su familia?
Has a doctor ever told you that you have migraines?	¿Algún doctor le ha dicho a usted que padece de migrañas?
Do you get the headaches after eating certain foods or around the time of your period?	¿Le dan dolores de cabeza después de que usted come algún tipo de comida o durante su menstruación? ¿Le dan dolores de cabeza después de que usted come algun tipo de comida o durante su **período**?

Insomnia

Do you have problems sleeping?	¿Tiene usted problemas durmiendo?
How long have you had this problem (days, weeks, months)?	¿Cuánto tiempo hace que usted tiene éste problema (días, semanas, meses)?
Do you have problems falling asleep? What time do you go to bed each night? Same time each night?	¿Tiene usted problemas durmiéndose? ¿A qué hora usted se va a la cama todas las noches? ¿A la misma hora todas las noches?
How many minutes/hours does it take you to fall asleep?	¿Cuántos minutos/horas usted necesita para dormirse?
Do you have problems with waking up frequently during the night? How many times each night? What times do you wake up?	¿Tiene usted problemas despertándose frecuentemente por la noche? ¿Cuántas veces por noche? ¿A qué hora usted se despierta?
Do you have problems falling back to sleep after you wake up in the night? How many minutes/hours does it take to fall back to sleep?	¿Tiene usted problemas volviéndose a dormir después de que se despierta por la noche? ¿Cuántos minutos/horas le toma para dormirse de nuevo?

Insomnia

Do you have problems with waking up too early in the morning?	¿Tiene usted problemas levantándose muy temprano en la mañana?
What time do you get up each day?	¿A qué hora usted se levanta cada día?
Same time each day?	¿A la misma hora todos los días?
How many hours do you sleep each night?	¿Regularmente cuántas horas usted duerme cada noche?
How many nights each week do you have problems sleeping?	¿Cuántas noches por semana usted tiene problemas durmiendo?
Do you feel rested when you get up in the morning?	¿Se siente usted descansado/a cuando se levanta por la mañana?
Do you sleep alone or with someone else?	¿Usted duerme solo/a o con alguien?
Does your partner keep you awake?	¿Su compañero la mantiene despierto/a?
Do you snore loudly?	¿Ronca usted muy fuerte?
Have you ever been told you stop breathing while sleeping?	¿Alguien le ha dicho que usted para de respirar cuando duerme?
Are you frequently sleepy during the day?	¿Se siente usted dormido durante el día?
	¿Se siente usted **soñoliento/a** durante el día?
	¿Se siente usted **agotado/a** durante el día?
	¿Se siente usted **con ganas de dormir** durante el día?
Do your legs frequently feel restless, like you have to move them?	¿Frecuentemente siente sus piernas inquietas, con la necesidad de moverlas?
More often at night?	¿Más a menudo por la noche?
Does it feel like a crawling sensation?	¿Siente una sensación de algo subiéndole?
Burning sensation?	¿Una sensacion ardiente?
	¿Una sensacion **quemante**?
Tingling sensation?	¿Una sensacion de hormigueo por sus piernas?
	¿Una sensacion de hormigueo **en sus** piernas?

Insomnia

Does the feeling go away or feel better when you move your legs?	¿Estas sensaciones ya mencionadas se mejoran cuando usted mueve sus piernas?
What time do you usually go to bed?	¿A qué hora usted usualmente se acuesta?
What time do you usually get up?	¿A qué hora usted usualmente se levanta?
Do you do any of these things while in bed?	¿Hace usted algunas de las siguientes actividades en la cama?
Read?	¿Lee?
Watch TV?	¿Mira televisión?
Eat?	¿Come?
Do you take naps during the day?	¿Toma usted siestas durante el día?
What time?	¿A qué hora?
How many minutes/hours each nap?	¿Cuántos minutos/horas por siesta?
Do you drink coffee?	¿Toma usted café?
Do you drink tea?	¿Toma usted té?
Do you drink sodas with caffeine?	¿Toma usted sodas que contienen cafeína?
Do you smoke?	¿Usted fuma?
Do you drink alcohol?	¿Usted toma alcohol?
	¿Usted **consume** alcohol?
	¿Usted **bebe** alcohol?
Do you eat right before bedtime?	¿Come usted antes de acostarse?
How many hours before you go to bed?	¿Cuántas horas antes de acostarse?
Is it a heavy meal?	¿Es una comida pesada?
	¿Es una comida **fuerte**?
Do you have heartburn?	¿Padece usted de ardor de estómago?
Is it worse while you are lying down?	¿Se empeora cuando usted está acostado/a?
Is your bedroom dark, quiet, and peaceful while you are sleeping?	¿Está su cuarto oscuro, callado, y tranquilo al usted dormir?
Do you take medicine to help you sleep?	¿Toma usted medicamentos para ayudarle a dormir?
	¿Toma usted **medicinas** para ayudarle **con su sueño**?
Which one?	¿Cúales?
Does it help?	¿Le ayudan?

Insomnia

Instructions on Sleep Hygiene

I want you to follow these instructions for sleeping.	Quiero que usted siga estas instrucciones para dormir.
Do not go to bed until you are tired and ready to go to sleep.	No se acueste a dormir hasta que usted esté cansado/a y listo/a para dormir.
Do not do anything in bed other than sleeping and sex (no reading, eating, or watching TV).	No haga nada en la cama a menos que sea dormir o hacer el sexo (no lea, coma o mire televisión).
If you wake up in the middle of the night and can't go back to sleep, get out of bed and do something (read, watch TV) until you are ready to fall asleep again.	Si se levanta durante la noche ya que no puede dormir, levántese de la cama y haga algo como leer o mirar televisión hasta que usted se sienta listo/a para dormirse.
Get out of bed at the same time each day (whether or not you are still sleepy).	Levántase a la misma hora todos los días aunque todavía se sienta dormido. Levántase a la misma hora todos los días aunque todavía se sienta **soñoliento**. Levántase a la misma hora todos los días aunque todavía se sienta **agotado/a**. Levántase a la misma hora todos los días aunque todavía se sienta **con ganas de dormir**.
Do not take naps.	No tome siestas.
Do not eat a heavy meal within 2 hours or more before bedtime.	No coma muy pesado por lo menos 2 horas o más antes de acostarse/**irse a la cama**. No coma **fuerte** por lo menos 2 horas o más antes de acostarse.
You can eat a light snack before bedtime, like toast, warm milk, or herbal tea.	Usted puede comer algo ligero antes de irse a la cama como una tostada, leche tibia, o té de hierbas.
Do not drink anything with caffeine after 5:00 pm.	No tome nada que contenga cafeína después de las cinco p.m.
Do not drink alcohol.	No tome bebidas alcohólicas. No **consuma** bebidas alcoholicas. No **beba** bebidas alcoholicas.

Insomnia

Regular activity during the day, like walking, will help you sleep better.	Actividades regulares durante el día, como caminar, le ayudaran a dormir mejor.
Playing soft music at bedtime can be relaxing.	Oír música suave antes de acostarse le ayudará a relajarse.
Try to keep your bedroom dark and quiet while sleeping.	Trate de mantener su cuarto lo más oscuro y callado en el proceso de dormir.

Motor Vehicle Collision

Were you in a motor vehicle accident?	¿Estuvo usted en un accidente automovilístico? ¿Estuvo usted en un accidente **de carro**? ¿Estuvo usted en un accidente **de auto**?
How many hours/days ago?	¿Hace cuántas horas/días?
In a car?	¿En un carro? ¿En un **auto**? ¿En un **automóvil**? ¿En un **vehiculo**?
In a bus?	¿En un autobús?
In a train/subway?	¿En un tren/metro?
Were you the driver?	¿Estaba usted manejando?
Were you a passenger? Front/back seat? Driver's side?	¿Era usted el pasajero? ¿En el asiento de atrás o en el de alante? ¿Del lado del conductor? ¿Del lado del **chofer**?
Was the car moving or stopped?	¿Estaba el carro en movimiento o parado? ¿Estaba el **auto** en movimiento o parado? ¿Estaba el **automóvil** en movimiento o parado? ¿Estaba el **vehiculo** en movimiento o parado?

Motor Vehicle Collision

Did you run into another car?	¿Usted choco?
Did another car run into you?	¿Lo chocaron?
Did you get hit from behind?	¿Le pegaron por detrás? ¿Le **dieron** por detrás?
On the driver's side?	¿Por el lado del conductor? ¿Por el lado del **chofer**?
On the passenger's side?	¿Por el lado de pasajero?
From the front?	¿Por el frente?
Was it a head-on collision?	¿Fue un choque frente a frente?
Was the other driver driving toward you?	¿El otro conductor estaba manjando/**guiando** hacia usted? ¿El otro conductor estaba manjando/**guiando** directamente hacia usted?
Were you wearing a seatbelt?	¿Tenia su cinturón de seguridad puesto?
Was it a shoulder strap?	¿Era cinturón de seguridad de hombro?
Was it a lap belt?	¿Era solo de la cintura?
Do you have abdominal pain?	¿Tiene dolor abdominal? ¿Tiene dolor **de barriga**?
Do you have blood in your urine?	¿Tiene sangre en la orina?
Did you hit your head?	¿Se golpeo la cabeza?
Did you lose consciousness?	¿Perdió el conocimiento?
Do you have a headache?	¿Tiene dolor de cabeza?
Do you have blurred or double vision?	¿Tiene visión borrosa o doble?
Do you feel dizzy?	¿Se siente mareado/a?
Do you have nausea/vomiting?	¿Tiene usted nausea/vómitos?
Did you hit your chest?	¿Se golpeo su pecho?
On the steering wheel?	¿En el volante? ¿En el **timón**?
Do you have chest pain?	¿Tiene usted dolor de pecho?
Does it hurt to take a deep breath?	¿Le duele cuando respira profundo? ¿Le duele cuando respira **hondo**?
Are you having difficulty breathing now?	¿Tiene dificultad respirando?
Do you have neck pain?	¿Tiene dolor en su cuello?

Motor Vehicle Collision

Do not move your head.	No mueva la cabeza.
We need to x-ray your neck before we can remove the brace.	Necesitamos tomarle unos rayos x antes de que le quitemos el collarin. Necesitamos tomarle unas **placas** antes de que le quitemos el **cuello ortopèdico**.
Show me where you hurt.	Enséñeme donde le duele. **Muéstreme** donde le duele.
After the accident, were you able to walk away from the car without help?	¿Pudo alejarse del carro caminando después del accidente sin ayuda? ¿Pudo alejarse del **auto** caminando después del accidente sin ayuda? ¿Pudo alejarse del **automóvil** caminando después del accidente sin ayuda? ¿Pudo alejarse del **vehículo** caminando después del accidente sin ayuda?
Were you taken to the ER?	¿Lo/la llevaron a la sala de emergencia?
Which hospital?	¿A cuál hospital?
Did they take x-rays?	¿Le tomaron rayos x? ¿Le tomaron **placas**?
Did they take a head CT?	¿Le tomaron una tomografía computarizada (CT)?
Were the results normal or abnormal?	¿Los resultados fueron normales o atípicos? ¿Los resultados fueron normales o **irregulares**? ¿Los resultados fueron normales o **anormales**? ¿Los resultados fueron normales o **le encontraron algo malo**?
Do you have the medical records from that visit?	¿Tiene los documentos médicos de esa visita?

Motor Vehicle Collision

You need to bring me your medical records, including results of tests done.	Necesita traer sus archivos médicos, incluya los resultados de los examenes que le han hecho.

Nausea/Vomiting

Do you have nausea?	¿Tiene usted nausea?
Are you vomiting?	¿Ha estado usted vomitando?
How many days ago did it start?	¿Cuántos días hace que empezó?
Did it start suddenly?	¿Le empezó de repente?
Did it start gradually?	¿Le empezó gradualmente?
	¿Le empezó **despacio**?
Did you start with just nausea and then vomiting?	¿Le empezó primero con nausea seguido por vómitos?
	¿Le empezó primero con nausea **y después con** vómitos?
Did you start with vomiting?	¿Le empezó con vómitos?
Is the vomiting projectile?	¿Sus vómitos salen como un proyectil?
	¿Sus vómitos salen **como una bala**?
Does anyone else at home have the same symptoms?	¿Alguien más en su casa tiene los mismos síntomas?
Do you have diarrhea?	¿Tiene usted diarrea?
Do you have abdominal pain?	¿Tiene usted dolor abdominal?
	¿Tiene usted dolor **de barriga**?
Is it crampy?	¿Con retorcijones?
Sharp?	¿Agudo?
Burning?	¿Candente?
Aching?	¿Dolorido?
Show me where the pain is.	Enséñeme donde le duele.
	Muéstreme donde le duele.
Does it feel better when you lie down?	¿Lo siente mejor cuando se acuesta?
	¿ **Se le mejora** cuando se acuesta?
Does it feel better when you sit up?	¿Lo siente mejor cuando se sienta?
	¿ **Se le mejora** cuando se sienta?

Nausea/Vomiting

Does the pain go to your back?	¿Se le va el dolor a la espalda? ¿**El dolor se le pasa** a la espalda?
How many times have you vomited today? How many times since it began?	¿Cuántas veces ha vomitado hoy? ¿Cuántas veces desde que este problema le empezó?
Are you vomiting up blood?	¿Está usted vomitando sangre?
Does it have green bile?	¿Contine su vómitos bilis verde?
Have you eaten out or eaten unusual foods lately?	¿Ha comido usted últimamente en un restaurante o ha comido comidas un poco atípicas? ¿Ha comido usted últimamente en un restaurante o ha comido comidas un poco **irregulares**? ¿Ha comido usted últimamente en un restaurante o ha comido comidas un poco **raras**? ¿Ha comido usted últimamente en un restaurante o ha comido comidas un poco **fuera de lo normal**?
Did you become ill a few hours after eating something?	¿Se enfermó horas después de comer estas?
Did you eat food that was canned or preserved at home?	¿Ha comido usted comidas enlatadas o preservadas hechas en su casa?
Do you have ear pain? (For children): Does the child pull on his/her ear? (For children): Have you/the child recently had a cold or flu?	¿Tiene usted dolor de oídos? ¿El niño se hala sus oídos? ¿El niño se hala sus **orejas**? ¿Usted o su niño han tenido recientemente catarro o influenza? ¿Usted o su niño han tenido recientemente **resfriado** o influenza? ¿Usted o su niño han tenido recientemente **gripe** o influenza?

Nausea/Vomiting

Are you pregnant?	¿Está usted embarazada? ¿Está usted en **estado**? ¿Está usted **encinta**?
Is there a chance that you are pregnant?	¿Hay alguna posibilidad de que usted pudiese estar embarazada? ¿Hay alguna posibilidad de que usted pudiese estar en **estado**? ¿Hay alguna posibilidad de que usted pudiese estar **encinta**?
Have you had a hysterectomy?	¿Tuvo usted una histerectomía?
Does it feel like the room is spinning around you?	¿Siente usted que el cuarto le está dando vueltas?
Do you feel full sooner than normal when eating?	¿Se siente usted llena más rápido de lo normal cuando come?
Do you have a headache?	¿Tiene usted dolor de cabeza?
Do you have a fever?	¿Tiene usted fiebre?
Do you have a stiff neck?	¿Tiene usted el cuello tenso?
Does the light hurt your eyes?	¿Le hace daño la luz en sus ojos?
Has your skin or eyes turned yellow?	¿Se ha vuelto su piel o sus ojos amarillos?

Pain

Calf Pain

Do you have pain in your calf?	¿Le duele su pantorrilla?
How many days/weeks/months ago did it start?	¿Hace cuántos días/semanas/meses le comenzó?
Did it start suddenly?	¿Le comenzó de repente?
Did it start gradually?	¿Le comenzó gradualmente? ¿Le comenzó **despacio**?
Both or just one?	¿En las dos o solo en una?
Which one?	¿En cúal?
Is it swollen?	¿Está hinchada? ¿Está **inflamada**?
Is it red?	¿Está roja? ¿Está **enrojecida**?

Pain

Is it painful to touch?	¿Le duele cuando se la toca?
Have you traveled recently in a car or plane?	¿Ha viajado en carro o avión recientemente?
	¿Ha viajado en **auto** o avión recientemente?
	¿Ha viajado en **automóvil** o avión recientemente?
	¿Ha viajado en **vehículo** o avión recientemente?
How many hours were you sitting?	¿Por cuántas horas estuvo sentado/a?
Have you had surgery recently?	¿Ha tenido una operación recientemente?
How many days/weeks ago?	¿Hace cuántos días/semanas?
Do you have chest pain?	¿Tiene dolor en el pecho?
Do you have difficulty breathing?	¿Tiene dificultad al respirar?
Are you coughing up blood?	¿Ha tosido sangre?
Have you ever had blood clots in your arms or legs before?	¿Ha tenido alguna vez coágulos de sangre en sus brazos o piernas?
Do you get cramps in your legs at night?	¿Le dan calambres en las piernas por la noche?
Do you get pain in your calves with walking?	¿Tiene dolor en sus pantorrillas cuando camina?
Is it an ache?	¿Es adolorido?
Is it a cramp?	¿Es de tipo calambre?
Show me where you get it.	Enséñeme donde lo tiene.
	Muéstreme donde lo tiene.
Does it go away when you rest?	¿Se le pasa cuando descansa?
	¿Se **le va** cuando descansa?
	¿Se **le desaparece** cuando descansa?
How many minutes does it take to go away?	¿Cuántos minutos pasan antes de que el dolor o el calambre se le hayan pasado?
How far can you walk before you get the pain?	¿Qué tan lejos puede caminar sin que le duela?
	¿Cuánta distancia puede caminar antes de que le duela?

Pain

In feet?	¿En pies?
In blocks?	¿En manzanas? ¿En **cuadras**?
In miles?	¿En millas?
Do you get the same pain at rest?	¿Le duele igual cuando descansa?
Are your feet cold all the time?	¿Tiene los pies fríos en todo momento?
Do your feet or toes ever turn blue?	¿Se le han puesto alguna vez sus pies o dedos de los pies azul?
Is the skin on your legs more shiny than usual?	¿Le brilla la piel de sus piernas más de lo usual? ¿Le brilla la piel de sus piernas más de lo **corriente**? ¿Le brilla la piel de sus piernas más de lo **normal**? ¿Le brilla la piel de sus piernas más de lo **común**?
Have you lost some of the hair on your legs?	¿Ha perdido pelo en sus piernas?
Do you have numbness or tingling in your feet or legs?	¿Se le adormecen o siente homigueo en las piernas o pies? ¿Se le adormecen o le dan **cosquilleo** en las piernas o pies?
Have you had a test for circulation in your legs?	¿Ha tenido un examen para la circulación de sus piernas? ¿Ha tenido una **prueba** para la circulación de sus piernas?
Was it normal/abnormal?	¿Fue normal/atípico? ¿Fue normal/**irregular**? ¿Fue normal/**anormal**?
How long ago (months/years) was the test?	¿Hace cuánto tiempo (meses/años) que fue su examen? ¿Hace cuánto tiempo (meses/años) que fue su **prueba**?

Pain

Do you smoke?	¿Usted fuma?
How many cigarettes/packs a day?	¿Cuántos cigarros/cajetillas al día?
	¿Cuántos cigarros/**paquetes** al día?
Did you used to smoke more?	¿Fumaba usted más?
For how many years?	¿Por cuántos años?
Do you have high blood pressure?	¿Tiene hipertensión?
	¿Tiene **alta presión sanguinea**?
Do you have heart disease?	¿Tiene enfermedad cardiaca?
	¿Tiene enfermedad **del corazón**?
Have you had bypass surgery or angioplasty on your heart?	¿Ha tenido alguna operación de desviación cardiaca o angioplastia coronaria?
	¿Ha tenido alguna operación de desviación en **el corazón** o angioplastia **cardiaca**?
Have you recently started to exercise or increased the intensity of your exercise?	¿Ha comenzado a hacer ejercicio o ha hecho ejercicio más intenso últimamente?
Are you taking any cholesterol medicine?	¿Está tomando algún medicamento para el colesterol?
Which one?	¿Cuál?
	¿Qué medicamento?
	¿Qué medicina?

Ear Pain

Do you have ear pain?	¿Tiene usted dolor de oído?
Which one?	¿Cuál oído?
Inside or outside?	¿Adentro o afuera?
How long have you had it (hours, days, weeks)?	¿Cuánto tiempo hace que tiene el dolor de oídos (horas, días, semanas)?
Did it come on suddenly or slowly?	¿El dolor le vino de repente o lentamente?
Does it feel...?	¿Lo siente...?
Like pressure?	¿Presión?
Like burning?	¿Quemante?
Like aching?	¿Adolorido?
Sharp?	¿Agudo?

Pain

Clogged?	¿Atascado? ¿ **Obstruido**?
Does it itch?	¿Prurito? ¿So siente con?
Do you have a fever?	¿Tiene usted fiebre?
Do you have discharge from your ear? Did the pain get better when the discharge started?	¿Tiene usted descargas por su oído? ¿Le está **saliéndo líquido** por su oído? ¿Se le mejoró el dolor después que la descarga empezó?
Is your hearing worse since the pain started?	¿Le ha empeorado su audición después que el dolor empezó?
Is the pain worse . . . at night? in the morning? when you swallow? when you pull or push on the ear? when you eat hot foods/cold foods?	¿El dolor es peor . . . por la noche? en la mañana? cuando traga? cuando tira o empuja su oído? cuando come comida caliente o fria?
Do you have a toothache? Show me where it hurts.	¿Tiene usted dolor en sus dientes? Enséñeme donde le duele. **Muéstreme** donde le duele.
Were you sick with a cold or flu before the earache started?	¿Ha estado usted enferma/o con catarro o influenza antes de que el dolor de oidos empezara? ¿Ha estado usted enferma con **resfriado** o influenza antes de que el dolor de oidos le empezara? ¿Ha estado usted enferma con **gripe** o influenza antes de que el dolor de oidos le empezara?
Have you been swimming?	¿Ha estado usted nadando?
Do you put anything inside your ears to clean them (Q-tips)?	¿Se introduce/mete algo dentro de sus oídos para limpiárselos (Q-tips)?
Did you fly in an airplane right before your earache started?	¿Estuvo usted viajando en avión antes de que su dolor de oídos le empezara?

Pain

Do you grind your teeth?	¿Rechina sus dientes mientras duerme?
Does your jaw click or lock when you open it?	¿Su quijada chasquea o se cierra cuando usted la abre?

Hip Pain

Do you have hip pain?	¿Tiene usted dolor de cadera? ¿Tiene usted dolor de **cintura**?
Point to where it hurts.	Enséñeme donde le duele. **Apúnteme** donde le duele.
How long has it been hurting (days, weeks, months)?	¿Cuánto tiempo hace que le están doliendo (días, semanas, meses)?
Is the pain constant, or does it come and go? How long does the pain last each time (minutes, hours, days)?	¿El dolor es constante o viene y se va? ¿Cada vez que tiene el dolor, cuánto tiempo le dura (minutos, horas, dias)?
Does it feel...? Sharp? Dull? Is it burning? Is it aching?	¿Lo siente...? ¿agudo? ¿Mate? **¿Sordo?** ¿Está ardiente? ¿Está adolorido?
Does the pain go anywhere? Point to where the pain goes.	¿Se le riega el dolor a otras partes? Enséñeme adonde va el dolor se le va. **Apúnteme** adonde se le va el dolor.
Do you have pain while at rest? Does the pain wake you up at night?	¿Tiene usted dolor al descansar? ¿La despierta el dolor por la noche?
Do you have pain with walking?	¿Tiene usted dolor cuando camina?
Is the pain worse with . . . walking? standing? sitting? lying down?	¿El dolor es peor cuando está. . . caminando? parado/a? sentado/a? acostado/a?

Pain

Does it click or pop with movement?	¿Chasquea (como un refresco) al abrirse con movimiento? ¿Chasquea (como una **gaseosa**) al abrirse con movimiento?
Have you had an accident or injury to that hip?	¿Ha usted tenido un accidente o lesión en su cadera? ¿Ha usted tenido un accidente o **trauma** en su cadera? ¿Ha usted tenido un accidente o **problema** en su cadera? ¿Ha usted tenido una lesión o **herida** en su cadera? ¿Ha usted tenido una lesión o **daño** en su cadera?
How long ago (days, weeks, months, years)?	¿Cuánto tiempo hace (días, semanas, meses, años)?
Did you fall recently? How long ago (days, weeks)?	¿Se ha usted recientemente caído/a? ¿Cuánto tiempo hace (días, semanas)?
Have you had surgery on this hip before?	¿Ha usted tenido cirugía en su cadera? ¿Ha usted tenido cirugía en su **cintura**?
Did you have a hip replacement?	¿Tuvo usted un reemplazo de caderas? ¿Tuvo usted un reemplazo de **cintura**?
Have you tried any over-the-counter medicines for the pain? Acetaminophen ibuprofen, Motrin™? Do they relieve the pain? Totally? Partially?	¿Ha usted tratado algún medicamento sin receta médica para el dolor? ¿Acetaminofén, ibuprofen, Motrin™? ¿Le ayudan con el dolor? ¿Completamente? ¿Parcialmente?
Are you taking any other medicine for pain? Show me.	¿Está usted tomando otros medicamentos o medicinas para el dolor? Enséñemelos. **Muéstremelos**.

Pain

Have you taken steroids before?	¿Ha anteriormente usado usted esteroides?
Many times?	¿Muchas veces?
For how many weeks/months/years?	¿Por cuántas semanas/meses/años?
Do you smoke?	¿Usted fuma?
Do you drink alcohol?	¿Usted toma alcohol? ¿Usted **consume** alcohol? ¿Usted **bebe** alcohol?
How many drinks per week?	¿Cuántos tragos por semana?
For how many years?	¿Por cuántos años?
Did you drink more heavily in the past?	¿Tomaba usted más fuertemente en el pasado? ¿Tomaba usted más **pesadamente** en el pasado? ¿Tomaba usted **mucho más** en el pasado?
Have you tried ice packs/heating pad?	¿Ha usted tratado una bolsa de hielo/una almohadilla de calentamiento? ¿Ha usted tratado una bolsa de hielo/una **placa** de calentamiento?
Did it help?	¿Le ayudó?
Did you use an electric heating pad?	¿Ha usted utilizado una almohadilla de calentamiento? ¿Ha usted utilizado una **placa** de calentamiento?

Knee Pain — Dolor de Rodillas

Do you have knee pain?	¿Tiene usted dolor de rodilla?
Show me where it hurts.	Enséñeme donde le duele. **Muéstreme** donde le duele.
How long have you had it (in days, weeks, months, years)?	¿Cuánto tiempo hace que le duele (en días, semanas, años)?
Did it start suddenly?	¿Le empezó de repente?
Did it start slowly?	¿Le empezó despacio?

Pain

Have you ever injured your knee?	¿Se ha usted lastimado alguna vez su rodilla?
How long ago (days, weeks, months, years)?	¿Qué tiempo hace que se lastimo su rodilla (días, semanas, meses, años)?
Were you in a car accident?	¿Fue en un accidente de carro?
	¿Fue en un accidente de **auto**?
	¿Fue en un accidente de **automobil**?
	¿Fue en un accidente de **vehículo**?
Did you injure it during exercise or playing sports?	¿Usted se lastimo su rodilla haciendo ejercicios o jugando algún deporte?
Did you twist your knee?	¿Se torcio su rodilla?
Did your knee hit something?	¿Se dio usted en su rodilla?
In the front?	¿Al frente?
On the side?	¿Al lado?
In the back?	¿En la parte de atrás?
Did you fall on your knee?	¿Se calló usted en su rodilla?
Is the pain aching?	¿Es su dolor adolorido?
Sharp?	¿Agudo?
Burning?	¿Como si le estuvieran quemando?
Throbbing?	¿Con palpitaciones?
Does your knee...	Su rodilla . . .
Lock up?	¿Se le cierra?
Pop?	
Click?	
Does your knee suddenly give out?	¿Su rodilla, le falla repentinamente?
Do you have swelling in your knee?	¿Tiene hichazon en su rodilla?
	¿Tiene **inflamación** en su rodilla?
How long has it been swollen (hours/days/weeks)?	¿Qué tiempo hace que está hinchada (horas/días/semanas)?
Did it swell immediately or slowly?	¿Se le hincharón de repente o despacio?
Does it feel hot or normal?	¿Su rodilla se siente caliente o normal?
Is it red?	¿Está roja?
Do you have a fever?	¿Tiene usted fiebre?

Pain

Do you have stiffness in your knee?	¿Tiene usted rigidez en su rodilla?
Mostly in the mornings?	¿Mayormente en la mañana?
After you have been sitting for a while?	¿Después de haber estado sentado durante un rato?
How many minutes or hours does the stiffness last?	¿Cuántos minutos u horas dura su rigidez en su rodilla?
Does sitting make it better or worse?	¿Al estar sentado/a se siente mejor o peor?
Standing?	¿Al estar parado/a?
Walking?	¿Caminando?
Do you take any medicine for the pain?	¿Está tomando usted algún medicamento o medicinas para su dolor?
Which medicine?	¿Qué medicamentos?
	¿Qué **medicinas**?
Does it make it better?	¿Lo/a hacen sentir mejor?
Have you ever been told you have arthritis in your knees?	¿Le han dicho alguna vez que usted tiene arthritis en sus rodillas?
Have you ever had an x-ray of your knee?	¿Le han tomado alguna vez rayos x/ **placas** de su rodilla?
How long ago (days/weeks/months/years)?	¿Cuándo fue (días/semanas/meses/años)?
Have you ever had your knee injected with steroids?	¿Le han inyectado alguna vez esteroides en su rodilla?
How long ago (days/weeks/months/years)?	¿Cuándo fue (días/semanas/meses/años)?

Low Back Pain

Do you have back pain?	¿Tiene usted dolor de espalda?
Did it start suddenly?	¿Le empezó de repente?
Did it start slowly and gradually get worse over time?	¿Le empezó despacio y gradualmente se le ha empeorado?
Is it constant, or does it come and go?	¿Es constante o viene y se va?
Show me where the pain is.	Enséñeme donde le duele.
	Muéstreme donde le duele.
Is the pain mostly in your back?	¿Es su dolor mayormente en su espalda?

Pain

Does the pain radiate . . .	¿Se riega su dolor . . .
down your leg?	hacia su pierna?
Which leg?	¿Cuál pierna?
down the inside or outside of your leg?	hacia adentro o afuera de su pierna?
down the front or back of your leg?	al frente o detrás de su pierna?
past your knee?	más abajo de su rodilla?
to your foot?	hacia su pie?
to the top or bottom of the foot?	arriba o abajo de su pie?
How long have you had it (in days, weeks, months, years)?	¿Cuánto tiempo lleva con éste dolor (en días, semanas, meses, años)?
Have you had similar episodes of back pain before?	¿Anteriormente ha tenido usted episodios similares de dolor de espalda?
	¿Anteriormente ha tenido usted **momentos** similares de dolor de espalda?
Did you have an x-ray at that time?	¿Le han hecho rayos x durante éstos episodios?
	¿Le han hecho **placas** durante éstos episodios?
MRI?	¿Resonancia magnética?
Other test?	¿Otros tipos de exámenes?
Do you know the results?	¿Sabe los resultados de estas pruebas?
Did it show any abnormality?	¿Muestran anormalidad los resultados de estas pruebas?
Have you been treated for back pain with medications before?	¿Ha sido usted tratado(a) antes con medicamentos por su dolor de espalda?
	¿Ha sido usted tratado(a) antes con **medicinas** por su dolor de espalda?
Which medication?	¿Qué medicamentos?
	¿Qué **medicinas**?
Is the pain aching?	¿Su dolor se siente adolorido?
Ripping?	¿Desgarrado?
Like electric shocks?	¿Como un choque eléctrico?

Pain

Have you had any recent accident or injury to your back?	¿Recientemente ha tenido usted algún accidente o lesión en su espalda? ¿Recientemente ha tenido usted algún accidente o **trauma** en su espalda? ¿Recientemente ha tenido usted algún accidente o **problema** en su espalda? ¿Recientemente ha tenido usted algún accidente o **herida** en su espalda? ¿Recientemente ha tenido usted algún accidente o **daño** en su espalda?
Have you ever had surgery on your back? How many years ago?	¿Ha tenido usted en su vida cirugía en su espalda? ¿Cuántos años hace?
Does it get better or worse with . . . standing? sitting? lying down? walking? bending forward?	¿Se mejora o empeora cuando está . . . ? parado/a? sentado/a? acostado/a? caminando? inclinándose hacia el frente? **flexionándose** hacia el frente? **doblándose** hacia el frente?
Is the pain worse when you cough? Sneeze? Lift?	¿El dolor se empeora cuando tose? ¿Estornuda? ¿Levanta algo?
Are you able to control your bowels?	¿Puede usted controlar sus intestinos?
Are you able to control your bladder?	¿Puede usted controlar su vejiga?
Do you have numbness in your leg or foot? Tingling? Burning?	¿Tiene usted entumecimiento en sus piernas o pies? ¿Hormigueo? ¿Quemazón?
Do you have weakness in your legs?	¿Tiene usted debilidad en sus piernas?
Do you have paralysis in your legs?	¿Tiene usted parálisis en sus piernas?
Do you have a fever or chills?	¿Tiene usted fiebre o escalofríos?
Do you have nausea or vomiting?	¿Tiene usted nausea o vómitos?

Pain

Do you have pain or burning when urinating?	¿Tiene usted dolor o quemazón al orinar?
Are you taking any medicines for the pain?	¿Está tomando usted algún medicamento para su dolor?
	¿Está tomando usted alguna **medicina** para su dolor?
Show me.	Enséñeme lo que está tomando.
	Muéstreme lo que está tomando.
Are your activities limited by your back pain?	¿Están sus actividades limitadas por su dolor de espalda?
How long have they been limited?	¿Qué tiempo hace que están limitadas?
More than a week/month?	¿Más de una semana/mes?
How many minutes/hours can you . . .	¿Cuántos minutos/horas usted puede . . .
stand?	estar parado?
sit?	estar sentado?
walk?	caminar?
How many pounds can you lift?	¿Cuántas libras usted puede levanter?

Peripheral Edema

How long have you had swelling in your legs (days, weeks, months)?	¿Cuánto tiempo hace que usted tiene hinchazón en sus piernas (días/semanas/meses)?
	¿Cuánto tiempo hace que usted tiene **inflamación** en sus piernas (días/semanas/meses)?
Did it start suddenly or slowly?	¿Le empezó de repente o lentamente?
Do you have swelling in just one leg?	¿Tiene usted hinchazón en una pierna solamente?
	¿Tiene usted **inflamación** en una pierna solamente?
Is the leg painful?	¿Le duele la pierna?

Peripheral Edema

Have you traveled recently in a car or plane?	¿Ha viajado en carro o avión recientemente?
	¿Ha viajado en **auto** o avión recientemente?
	¿Ha viajado en **automóvil** o avión recientemente?
	¿Ha viajado en **vehículo** o avión recientemente?
How many hours were you sitting?	¿Por cuántas horas estuvo sentado?
Did you have surgery recently?	¿Tuvo usted cirugía recientemente?
How many days/weeks ago?	¿Hace cuántos días/semanas?
Do you smoke?	¿Usted fuma?
Have you ever had a blood clot in your leg?	¿Ha usted tenido alguna vez un coágulo en su pierna?
Do you have . . .	¿Tiene usted . . .
congestive heart failure?	fallo cardíaco congestivo?
heart disease?	enfermedades del corazón?
liver disease?	enfermedades del hígado?
kidney disease?	enfermedades del riñón?
thyroid disease?	enfermedades de la tiroide?
Is the swelling constant, or does it come and go?	¿La hinchazón es constante o viene y se va?
	¿La **inflamación** es constante o viene y se va?
Does the swelling go down when you are sleeping?	¿Se le baja la hinchazón cuando usted está durmiendo?
	¿Se le baja la **inflamación** cuando usted está durmiendo?
Do you have difficulty breathing?	¿Tiene usted dificultad respirando?
At rest?	¿Al descansar?
With walking?	¿Cuando camina?
Did your breathing become worse with the swelling?	¿Se le empeora su respiración con la hinchazón?
	¿Se le empeora su respiración con la **inflamación**?

Peripheral Edema

Do you have a cough that is new?	¿Su tos es nueva?
	¿Su tos es **reciente**?
Do you cough up pink phlegm?	¿Tose usted flema de color rosada?
Do you have any wheezing?	¿Está usted resollando?
	¿Está usted **respirando con un silbido**?
Is it worse at night?	¿Se empeora en la noche?
How many pillows do you use under your head when you sleep?	¿Cuántas almohadas usted utilisa debajo de su cabeza cuando duerme?
	¿Cuántas almohadas usted **usa** debajo de su cabeza?
	¿Cuántas almohadas usted **pone** debajo de su cabeza?
How long have you slept on [number] pillows?	¿Cuánto tiempo hace que usted duerme con [numero] almohadas?
Is that more than before?	¿Esta cantidad es más que antes?
Can you breathe normally lying flat?	¿Puede usted dormir normalmente acostado en su espalda sin almohadas?
	¿Puede usted dormir normalmente acostado con su espalda **hacia la cama**?
Are you taking any new medications?	¿Está usted tomando algún medicamento nuevo?
	¿Está usted tomando alguna **medicina** nueva?
Show me.	Enséñemelo/a.
	Muéstremelo/a.
Did the swelling begin after you started the medication?	¿La hinchazón le empezó antes de que usted empezara a tomar este o estos medicamento(s)?
	¿La **inflamación** le empezó antes de que usted empezara a tomar esta o estas **medicina(s)** ?

Peripheral Edema

Have you run out of any medication since before the swelling started?	¿Se le ha/han acabado algún/algunos medicamento(s) antes de que la hinchazón le empezara? ¿Se le ha/han **terminado** algunas **medicina(s)** antes de que la hinchazón le empezara? ¿Se le ha/han **agotado** algúna/algunas **medicina(s)** antes de que la **inflamación** le empezara?
Do you take a diuretic (water pill)?	¿Toma usted algún diurético (píldora para aumentar su orina o orinar más)?
Have you run out?	¿Se le acabaron? ¿Se le **terminaron**? ¿Se le **agotaron**?
How long ago (days, weeks)?	¿Cuándo fue (días/semanas)?
Do you drink alcohol?	¿Usted toma alcohol? ¿Usted **consume** alcohol? ¿Usted **bebe** alcohol?
How many drinks each day/week?	¿Cuántos tragos por día/semana?
Do you have a history of drinking a lot?	¿Hace mucho que usted toma bebidas alcohólicas?
Have you had yellow skin or eyes?	¿Ha tenido usted ojos o piel amarilla?
Do you have any abdominal pain or swelling?	¿Tiene usted dolor abdominal o hinchazón en su abdomen? ¿Tiene usted dolor **de barriga** o **inflamación** en su **barriga**?
Have you ever had swelling like this before?	¿Ha usted tenido alguna vez este tipo de hinchazón? ¿Ha usted tenido alguna vez este tipo de **inflamación**?
How long ago (months/years)?	¿Cuánto tiempo hace (meses/años)?

Rash

How long have you had the rash (in days, weeks)?	¿Cuánto tiempo hace que usted tiene erupción (en días, semanas)?
	¿Cuánto tiempo hace que usted tiene **salpullido** (en días, semanas)?
	¿Cuánto tiempo hace que usted tiene **pintas rojas en su piel** (en días, semanas)?
Did it start suddenly?	¿Le empezó de repente?
Did it start gradually over days?	¿Le empezó gradualmente hace unos cuantos días?
Have you ever had a rash like this before?	¿Ha usted tenido alguna vez erupción?
	¿Ha usted tenido alguna vez **salpullido**?
	¿Ha usted tenido alguna vez **pintas rojas en su piel**?
Show me where it started.	Enséñeme donde le empezaron.
	Muéstreme donde le empezaron.
Did it spread?	¿Se le rego para otras partes?
Fast?	¿Rápido?
Slowly?	¿Despacio?
Is the rash getting any better?	¿Se le está mejorando la erupción?
	¿Se le está mejorando el **salpullido**?
	¿Se le está mejorando las **pintas rojas en su piel**?
Worse?	¿Se le están empeorando?
Does it itch?	¿Le pica?
A lot?	¿Mucho?
A little?	¿Poco?
Is it very painful?	¿Le es muy dolorosa la erupción?
	¿Le es muy doloroso el **salpullido**?
	¿Le es muy doloroso las **pintas rojas en su piel**?

Rash

Is it red?	¿Son rojas?
Was it red when it started?	¿Eran color rojo cuando le empezaron?
Did it turn red later?	¿Se volvieron rojo más tarde? ¿Se **cambiaron** a rojo mas tarde?
Did you feel itching or burning before the rash started?	¿Sintió usted picazón o quemazón antes de que le empezara la erupción? ¿Sintió usted picazón o quemazón antes de que le empezara **el salpullido**?
Is there any drainage from the rash?	¿La erupción está drenando? ¿**El salpullido** está **supurando**?
Is it clear, yellow, or red?	¿Es claro, amarillo o rojo? ¿Es **incoloro**, amarillo o rojo?
Do you have a fever?	¿Tiene usted fiebre? ¿Tiene usted **calentura**?
Were you sick before the rash started?	¿Estuvo usted enfermo/a antes de que le empezara?
Did you have a sore throat or high fever?	¿Tuvo usted la garganta irritada o fiebre alta?
Have you started any new medicines in the past few weeks?	¿Empezó usted a tomar algún medicamento nuevo en las pasadas semanas?
Do you have any difficulty breathing?	¿Tiene usted alguna dificultad respirando?
Do you have swelling in your tongue?	¿Tiene su lengua inchada?
Lips?	¿Labios?
Face?	¿Cara?
Do you have a cat or dog that goes outside?	¿Tiene usted un gato o perro que entra y sale de su casa?
Did you do any yard or garden work a few days before the rash started?	¿Estuvo usted trabajando en su patio o jardín días antes de que la erupción le empezara? ¿Estuvo usted trabajando en su patio o jardín días antes de que el **salpullido** le empezara? ¿Estuvo usted trabajando en su patio o jardín días antes de que **las pintas rojas en su piel** le empezaran?

Rash

Have you been sexually active in the past year?	¿Ha estado usted sexualmente activo/a en los pasados años?
Do you use or inject any illegal/illicit drugs (like cocaine, heroin, or methamphetamine)?	Usted usa o se invecta drogas ilegales/ilícitas (como cocaína, heroína, o metanfetaminas)?
Does anyone else in your house have the same rash?	¿Alguien más en su casa tiene el mismo tipo de erupción? ¿Alguien más en su casa tiene el mismo tipo de **salpullido**? ¿Alguien más en su casa tiene el mismo tipo de **pintas rojas en su piel**?
Have you used any new soap, detergent, deodorant, or lotions recently?	¿Ha usted recientemente utilizado un nuevo jabón, detergente, desodorante o lociones? ¿Ha usted recientemente **usado** un nuevo jabón, detergente, desodorante o lociones?
Show me.	Enséñemela(s). Muéstremela(s).
Have you used any creams or ointments to make it better?	¿Usted a utizado alguna crema o ungüento para mejoralse? ¿Usted a **usado** alguna crema o **unción** para mejoralse? ¿Usted a **usado** alguna crema o **untadura** para mejoralse?
Do you have them with you?	¿La(s) tiene con usted?
Show me please.	Enséñemelo(s). **Muéstremelo(s)**.
Did it make the rash better or worse?	¿Le mejoro o empeoro la erupción? ¿Le mejoro o empeoro el **salpullido**? ¿Le mejoro o empeoro **las pintas rojas en su piel**?
Does the sun make it worse or better?	¿El sol le empeora o le mejora?

Sore Throat

Do you have a sore throat?	¿Tiene usted su garganta irritada? ¿Tiene usted su garganta **adolorida**?
How long have you had it (hours, days, weeks)?	¿Cuánto tiempo hace que la tiene irritada (horas, días, semanas)? ¿Cuánto tiempo hace que la tiene **adolorida** (horas, días, semanas)?
Does it hurt to swallow?	¿Le duele al tragar?
Are you able to swallow? Solids, liquids?	¿Puede usted tragar? ¿Cosas solidas, cosas líquidas? ¿Cosas **duras**, cosas líquidas?
Does it feel like something is stuck in your throat?	¿Siente como si tuviera algo atorado en su garganta?
Have you started drooling? How long ago (minutes, hours)?	¿Ya empezó a babearse? ¿Ya empezó a **salirle saliva por la boca**? ¿Cuánto tiempo hace (minutos, horas)?
Do you have sinus pressure or pain? Where?	¿Tiene usted presión o dolor en los senos nasales? ¿Dónde?
Do you have a lot of phlegm in your throat?	¿Tiene usted mucha flema en su garganta?
Do you have to clear your throat frequently?	¿Tiene usted frecuentemente que despejarse su garganta? ¿Tiene usted frecuentemente que **aclararse** su garganta? ¿Tiene usted frecuentemente que **toser**?
Do you have a cough?	¿Tiene usted tos?
Do you have swollen glands? Where? For how long (days, weeks, months)?	¿Tiene alguna glándula inflamada? ¿Dónde? ¿Por cuánto tiempo (días, semanas, meses)?
Do you have heartburn?	¿Tiene ardor estomacal?
Do you get an acid taste in your mouth?	¿Tiene usted sabor a ácido en su boca?

Sore Throat

Have you had any hoarseness since this started?	Ha tenido usted **carraspera** desde que esto le empezo/**comenzo**
Do you have a fever/chills?	¿Tiene usted fiebre/escalofríos?
Do you smoke/chew tobacco?	¿Usted fuma o masca tabaco?
Have you lost weight recently? Intentionally? How many pounds?	¿Recientemente, usted a perdido peso? ¿Intencionadamente? **¿Deliberadamente?** ¿Cuántas libras?
Does anyone at home have these same symptoms?	¿Alguien más en su casa tiene los mismos síntomas?
Are you sexually active?	¿Está usted sexualmente activo(a)?
Have you had oral sex recently? With or without a condom?	¿Recientemente, usted a tenido sexo oral? ¿Con o sin preservativos? ¿Con o sin **condones**?
Is your appetite normal recently?	¿Su apetito está normal recientemente?
Is your appetite decreased recently?	¿Su apetito se le a reducio recientemente? ¿Su apetito se le ha **bajado** recientemente? ¿Su apetito se le ha **disminuido** recientemente? ¿Su apetito está **pobre** recientemente?

Upper Respiratory Infection

Did you start to feel sick suddenly or more gradually over days?	¿Empezó a sentirse enfermo/a inmediatamente o gradualmente en unos cuantos días? ¿Empezó a sentirse enfermo/a inmediatamente o gradualmente **sobre** unos cuantos días?
Show me where you feel sick.	Enséñeme donde usted se siente mal. **Muéstreme** donde usted se siente mal.
Do you feel congested? Mostly in your head and nose? Mostly in your chest?	Usted se siente congestionado/a. ¿Mayormente en su cabeza y nariz? ¿Mayormente en su pecho?

Upper Respiratory Infection

How long have you been sick (in days, weeks)?	¿Qué tiempo hace que usted se siente enfermo/a (en días o semanas)?
Do you have a headache?	¿Tiene dolor de cabeza?
Show me where.	Enséñeme adonde. **Muéstreme** adonde.
Is it a dull, sharp, throbbing, or squeezing pain?	¿El dolor es obtuso, agudo, palpitante o apretado? ¿El dolor es obtuso, agudo, **pulsante** o **retorcijado**?
Does the light hurt your eyes?	¿Le molesta la luz en su sojos?
Do you have an earache?	¿Tiene dolor de oído?
Show me which ear.	¿Enséñeme cual oído? ¿**Muéstreme** cual oído?
Do you have any drainage from your ear?	¿Le está drenando su oído?
Is the drainage clear, yellow, or bloody?	¿El drenaje es claro, amarillo or ensangrentado? ¿El drenaje es claro, amarillo or **sangriento**? ¿El drenaje es claro, amarillo or **sanguinolento**?
Do you have itchy eyes?	¿Tiene picazón en sus ojos?
Do you have watery eyes?	¿Tiene sus ojos aguados?
Do you have a runny nose?	¿Su nariz le está chorreando? **¿Tiene mucha moquera en su nariz?**
Is the mucus clear, white, yellow, green, or bloody?	¿El moco es claro, blanco, amarillo, verde o ensangrentado? ¿El **moco** es claro, blanco, amarillo, verde o **sangriento**? ¿La **flema** es clara, blanca, amarilla, verde o **sanguinolenta**?
Do you have facial pain?	¿Tiene dolor facial? ¿Tiene dolor **en la cara**?
Show me where.	¿Enséñeme adonde? ¿**Muéstreme** adonde?
Do you have tooth pain?	¿Tiene dolor de diente? ¿Tiene dolor de **muela**?

Upper Respiratory Infection

Is your head or facial pain worse when you bend over?	¿Su dolor facial o en su cara es peor cuando usted se inclina?
	¿Su dolor facial o en su cara es peor cuando usted se **dobla**?
Do you have a sore throat?	¿Le duele su garganta?
	¿Le **molesta** su garganta?
Does it hurt to swallow?	¿Le duele al tragar?
	¿Le molesta cuando traga?
Do you have a hoarse voice?	¿Está ronco?
	¿Está **afónico**?
	¿Está **enronquecido**?
	¿Está **carrasposo**?
Have you lost your voice?	¿Perdió usted su voz?
Do you have a cough?	¿Tiene tos?
Do you cough up mucus?	¿Usted tose moco?
	¿Usted tose **flema**?
A lot of mucus or only a little?	¿Mucho moco o solo un poco?
	¿Mucho **mucus** o solo un poco?
	¿Mucha **flema** o solo un poco?
Is the color of the mucus clear, white, yellow, green, brown, or bloody?	¿El color de su moco es claro, blanco, amarillo, verde, o marón?
	¿El color de su **moco** es claro, blanco, amarillo, verde, o **brown**?
	¿El color de su **flema** es claro, blanco, amarillo, verde, o **carmelita**?
Is it a dry cough?	¿Es una tos seca?
Do you have wheezing (a whistling sound when you breathe in or out)?	¿Tiene usted resollo (un sonido en forma de silbido cuando usted respira hacia adentro o hacia afuera)?
	¿Tiene usted resoplo (un sonido en forma de silbido cuando usted respira hacia adentro o hacia afuera)?

Upper Respiratory Infection

Do you have difficulty breathing?	¿Tiene usted dificultad respirando?
Through your nose?	¿Atravez de su su nariz?
Through your mouth?	¿Atravez de su su boca?
At rest?	¿Al descansar?
With activity?	¿Con actividad?
Do you have a fever or chills?	¿Tiene usted fiebre o escalofríos?
Do you have nausea or vomiting?	¿Tiene usted nausea o vomitos?
Every day?	¿Todos los días?
How many times?	¿Cuántas veces?
Are you able to eat?	¿Puede comer?
Are you able to drink fluids?	¿Puede tomar líquidos?
	¿Puede **beber** líquidos?
Do you have muscle aches?	¿Tiene usted dolor muscular?
Show me where.	¿Enséñeme donde?
	¿**Muéstreme** donde?
Have you taken any medicines to make you feel better?	¿Ha usted tomado algún medicamento para mejorarse?
	¿Ha usted tomado **alguna medicina** para **sentirse** mejor?
Aspirin?	¿Aspirina?
Tylenol™ (acetaminophen)?	¿Tylenol™ (acetaminofén)?
Ibuprofen (Motrin™, Aleve™ or similar)?	¿Ibuprofeno (Motrin™, Aleve™ o algo similar)?
Do you have it with you?	¿Lo tiene con usted?
Please show me.	Por favor enséñemelo/a(s).
	Por favor **muéstremelo/a(s)**.
Does it make you feel better?	¿Lo hacen sentir mejor?

Weight Loss

Have you been trying to lose weight?	¿Ha estado usted tratando de perder peso?
Are you on a special diet to lose weight?	¿Está usted en alguna dieta especial para perder peso?
How many pounds have you lost? In how much time (weeks/months)?	¿Cuántas libras ha usted perdido? ¿En cuánto tiempo (semanas/meses)?
Have you gained or lost weight before as an adult?	¿Ha perdido o ganado usted anteriormente, como adulto, peso?
Have you ever had cancer?	¿Ha tenido cancer?
Do you have thyroid disease?	¿Tiene usted problemas con su tiroides?
Do you have HIV?	¿Tiene usted VIH (virus de inmunodeficiencia humana)?
Do you have a family history of diabetes?	¿Tiene usted un historial familiar de diabetes?
Has your appetite increased?	¿Le ha aumentado su apetito? **¿Tiene usted más apetito?**
Do you have excessive thirst?	¿Tiene usted sed excesiva?
Do you have excessive urination?	¿Ha estado usted orinando excesivamente?
Do you have diarrhea? Are the stools greasy?	¿Tiene usted diarrea? ¿Están sus heces grasienta? ¿Está su **excreta** grasosa?
Do your stools float?	¿Sus heces flotan? ¿Su **excreta** flota? ¿Su **excremento** flota?
Do you have blood in your stools?	¿Tiene usted sangre en sus heces? ¿Tiene usted sangre en su **excreta**? ¿Tiene usted sangre en su **excremento**?
Do you have excessive sweating?	¿Está usted sudando excesivamente? ¿Está usted sudando **mucho**?
Do you have palpitations?	¿Tiene usted palpitaciones (en su corazón)?
Are you hot more than usual?	¿Se siente usted con más calor de lo usual? ¿Se siente usted con más calor de lo **normal**? ¿Se siente usted con más calor de lo **corriente**?

Weight Loss

Do you feel tired all the time?	¿Se siente usted más cansado de lo usual? ¿Se siente usted más cansado de lo **normal**? ¿Se siente usted más cansado de lo **corriente**?
Do you feel nervous or irritable or have tremors?	¿Se siente usted nervioso/a, irritable o tiene temblores?
Are you sleeping well?	¿Está usted durmiento bien, sin problemas?
Are you sleeping poorly?	¿Está usted durmiendo poco o mal?
Have you been exercising more than usual?	¿Ha estado usted haciendo ejercicio más de lo usual? ¿Ha estado usted haciendo ejercicio más de lo **corriente**? ¿Ha estado usted haciendo ejercicio más de lo **normal**?
Has your appetite decreased?	¿Se le ha reducido su apetito? ¿Se le ha **bajado** su apetito? ¿Se le ha **disminuido** su apetito? ¿Su apetito está pobre?
Do you have difficulty swallowing?	¿Tiene usted dificultad tragando?
Do you feel full with less food lately?	¿Últimamente, se siente usted lleno/a con menos comida? ¿Últimamente, se siente usted lleno/a **comiendo menos**?
Do you have nausea/vomiting?	¿Tiene usted nauseas/vómitos?
Do you have constipation?	¿Está usted constipado/a? ¿Está usted **estreñido/a**?
Do you have blood in your stools?	¿Tiene usted sangre en sus heces? ¿Tiene usted sangre en su **excreta**? ¿Tiene usted sangre en su **excremento**?
Do you have black, sticky stools (like tar)?	¿Están sus heces negras o pegajosas (como tar)? ¿Está su **excremento** negro o pegajoso (como **alquitran**)? ¿Está su **excreta** negra o pegajosa (como **brea**)?

Weight Loss

Do you have abdominal pain?	¿Tiene usted dolor abdominal?
	¿Tiene usted dolor **de barrig**a?
Do you have a fever/chills?	¿Tiene usted fiebre/escalofríos?
Do you have a cough?	¿Tiene usted tos?
Do you cough up blood?	¿Está usted tosiendo sangre?
For how many days/weeks/months?	¿Cuántos días/semanas/meses hace?
Do you smoke?	¿Usted fuma?
Do you have any enlarged lymph nodes or masses?	¿Tiene usted algún nódulo inflamado o alguna masa?
Are you sexually active?	¿Está usted sexualmente activo(a)?
When was the last time you had sex without a condom?	¿Cuándo fue la última vez que usted tuvo sexo sin usar un preservativo?
	¿Cuándo fue la última vez que usted tuvo sexo sin usar un **condón**?
Have you ever been tested for HIV?	¿Le han hecho a usted alguna vez la prueba del VIH (virus de inmunodeficiencia humana)?
How long ago (months/years)?	¿Cuándo fue (meses/años)?
Was it positive or negative?	¿Fue positiva o negativa?
Do you use intravenous drugs?	¿Usted se inyecta drogas?
Do you feel depressed?	¿Se siente usted deprimido/a?
[If yes, see Depressed Mood in this chapter].	
Have you ever been treated for depression?	¿Ha sido usted tratado por depresión?

Chapter 6

Active Medical Conditions

This chapter includes many of the chronic medical conditions most commonly encountered in clinical practice. Frequently, patients will present with no specific "chief complaint," but rather as a routine follow-up for a chronic medical condition, say hypertension or diabetes. In this case the "OLD CARTS" method of history taking (see Chapter 5, "History of Present Illness for Common Symptoms") no longer applies. Instead, the clinician needs a "snapshot" idea of where a patient is in their disease process.

You will likely encounter these scenarios in a variety of settings. Certainly in outpatient office visits, but also in emergency room or inpatient encounters where you need to assess the status of existing comorbidities and determine how they may impact the patient's current medical problem.

In this chapter, you will find a sequence of questions for each disorder. It may not be necessary to ask all the questions for each condition. Ask the relevant questions that you feel are necessary to gauge the status of each disorder. If a patient has an essentially negative response for many of the questions, you may want to move on to the next problem. However, when a patient gives several positive responses, you may need to delve further with more questions. How detailed you get will depend on the patient's responses.

This chapter is especially handy as a quick reference for the office-based clinician seeing patients for "routine" follow-up visits.

Asthma/COPD

Do you smoke?	¿Usted fuma?
How many cigarettes a day?	¿Cuántos cigarrillos al día?
Did you have asthma as a child?	¿Usted tuvo asma en su niñez?
Have you ever been intubated for your asthma/emphysema?	¿Ha sido usted alguna vez entubado/a por su asma o enfisema?
How many times?	¿Cuántas veces?
How long ago was the last time (months, years)?	¿Cuándo fue la última vez (meses, años)?
Have you taken steroids for your asthma/emphysema?	¿Ha usted tomado esteroides debido a su asma o enfisema?
Have you been to the ER for your asthma/emphysema recently?	¿Ha usted estado en la sala de emergencia debido a su asma o enfisema recientemente?
How long ago (days, weeks, months)?	¿Cuánto tiempo hace (días, semanas, meses)?
How many times have you gone in the past year?	¿Cuántas veces usted estuvo en la sala de emergencia el pasado año?
Have you been hospitalized for your asthma/emphysema recently?	¿Ha sido usted hospitalizado(a) por su asma o enfisema recientemente?
How long ago (days, weeks, months)?	¿Cuánto tiempo hace (días, semanas, meses)?
What medicines do you take for your asthma/emphysema?	¿Qué medicinas usted toma para su asma o enfisema?
Show me your inhalers.	Enséñeme sus inhaladores.
	Muéstreme sus inhaladores.
How many times a day do you use this inhaler?	¿Cuántas veces al día usted utiliza este inhalador?
	¿Cuántas veces al día usted **usa** este inhalador?

Asthma/COPD

Show me how you use it.	Enséñeme como usted lo utiliza.
	Muéstreme como usted lo **usa.**
Do you have a peak flow meter at home?	¿Tiene usted un medidor de flujo máximo en su casa?
Do you test your breathing each day?	¿Se examina usted su respiración cada día?
Do you use oxygen?	¿Usa usted oxígeno?
How many hours a day?	¿Cuántas horas por día?
How many liters?	¿Cuántos litros?
Do you have a dog or cat at home?	¿Tiene usted perros o gatos en su casa?
Is your asthma worse...?	¿Su asma está peor ...
	Su asma ha empeorado . . .
During exercise?	Durante ejercicios
	Cuando hace ejercicios
In cold air?	¿Cuándo hace frio?
Around pets?	¿Alrededor de sus animales domésticos?
Perfumes/strong odors?	¿Con perfumes/olores fuertes?
Cigarette smoke?	¿Con humo del cigarrillo?
Do you have difficulty breathing when walking?	¿Tiene usted dificultad respirando al caminar?
How far can you walk before you have difficulty breathing?	¿Qué tanto usted camina antes de sentir dificultad al respirar?
Do you wake up at night coughing?	¿Se levanta usted por la noche tosiendo?
How many times a day/week/month?	¿Cuántas veces por día/semanas/meses?
Do you have problems with coughing now?	¿Tiene usted en este momento problemas de toser?
How long have you been coughing (days, weeks)?	¿Cuánto hace que usted esta tosiendo (días, semanas)?
Are you wheezing now?	¿Está usted en este momento resollando al respirar?
	¿Está usted en este momento **silbando** al respirar?
How long have you been wheezing (days, weeks)?	¿Cuánto tiempo hace que usted está resollando al respirar (días, semanas)?
	¿Cuánto tiempo hace que usted está **silbando** al respirar (días, semanas)?

Asthma/COPD

How many times a day/week/month do you use your rescue inhaler?	¿Cuántas veces al día/semana/mes usted utiliza el inhalador de auxilio? ¿Cuántas veces al día/semana/mes usted **usa** el inhalador de auxilio?
Are you using your rescue inhaler more than you used to?	Está usted utilizando su inhalador de auxilio más de lo que usted lo **usaba** **Está usted utilizando su inhalador de auxilio mas de lo comun comparadolo como lo utilizaba antes?**
Do you have problems breathing now?	¿Tiene usted en este momento problemas respirando?
Is your breathing...	Su respiración . . .
Better than usual?	¿Está mejor de lo usual?
Worse than usual?	¿Peor de lo usual?
The same as usual?	¿Igual de lo usual? ¿Igual de lo **normal**?
Have you missed school/work because of your asthma/emphysema?	¿Ha usted faltado a la escuela/trabajo debido a su asma o enfisema?
How many times in the past 3 months?	¿Cuántas veces en los pasados tres meses?

Chronic Hepatitis

Do you have hepatitis B or C?	¿Tiene usted hepatitis B o C?
Have you ever been treated with interferon?	¿Ha sido usted tratado/a con interferones?
How long ago (month/years) was your last treatment?	¿Cuándo fue su último tratamiento (mes/años)?
Are you still undergoing treatment?	¿Está usted todavía recibiendo tratamiento?
For how many months were you treated?	¿Por cuántos meses fue usted tratado/a?
Was it successful?	¿Resultó el tratamiento?
Did the virus clear from your blood?	¿Ya está usted sano/a de su virus? ¿Ya está usted **curado/a** de su virus?

Chronic Hepatitis

Do you have abdominal pain or swelling?	¿Tiene usted dolor abdominal o hinchazón?
	¿Tiene usted dolor **en la barriga** o hinchazón?
Point to where the pain is.	Marque donde siente el dolor.
	Apúnteme donde siente el dolor.
Are your stools brown?	¿Sus heces son de color café?
	¿Su **excreta** es de color **marrón**?
	¿Su **excremento** es de color **brown**?
Clay colored?	¿Color barro?
Yellow?	¿Amarilla?
Black?	¿Negra?
Green?	¿Verde?
Is your appetite normal?	¿Su apetito está normal?
Decreased?	¿Reducido?
	¿**Bajo**?
	¿**Disminuido**?
	¿**Pobre**?
Increased?	¿Aumentado?
Do you have nausea/vomiting?	¿Tiene usted nausea/vómitos?
Do you have a fever?	¿Tiene usted fiebre?
Do you have yellow skin or eyes?	¿Su piel u ojos están amarillos?
Do you have generalized itching?	¿Tiene usted picazón por todas partes?
What color is your urine?	¿De qué color es su orina?
Yellow?	¿Amarilla?
Coca-cola™ colored?	¿Color Coca-cola™?
Do you have problems with bleeding or easy bruising?	¿Tiene usted problemas sangrando a menudo o se amagulla la piel fácilmente?
	¿Tiene usted problemas sangrando a menudo o **de moretones en** su piel fácilmente?

Chronic Hepatitis

Do you drink alcohol?	¿Usted toma alcohol? ¿Usted **consume** alcohol? ¿Usted **bebe** alcohol?
How many days/ weeks/months/ years ago was the last time?	¿Cuántos días/semanas/meses/años) fue la ultima vez?
Do you understand that alcohol may damage your liver?	¿Entiende usted que el alcohol puede dañarle el higado?
Do you need help in quitting?	¿Necesita usted ayuda para abandonar este hábito?
Do you use any recreational or illegal drugs?	¿Utiliza usted fármacos recreativos o drogas ilegales? ¿ **Usa** usted fármacos recreativos o drogas **ilícitas**?
How many days/ weeks/months/ years ago was the last time?	Cuántos días/semanas/meses/años) fue la ultima vez?
You cannot be treated for hepatitis if you continue to use drugs or drink alcohol.	¿Usted no puede seguir siendo tratado por hepatitis si continua utilizando fármacos, drogas ilegales o tomando alcohol? ¿Usted no puede seguir siendo tratado por hepatitis si continúa **usando** fármacos, drogas ilegales o **consumiendo** alcohol? ¿Usted no puede seguir siendo tratado por hepatitis si continua utilizando fármacos, drogas ilegales, o **bebiendo** alcohol?
Do you take Tylenol/acetaminophen often?	¿Toma usted Tylenol/acetaminofén regularmente?

Chronic Pain

How bad is your pain (one is almost no pain, and ten is you need to be in the ER)?	¿Qué tan mal es su dolor (uno es casi sin dolor, y diez es necesario que usted vaya para la sala de emergencia?
Is your pain constant?	¿Es su dolor constante?
Does it come and go?	¿Va y viene?
Is it worse...	¿Es peor ...
In the morning?	¿en la mañana?
In the afternoon?	¿en la tarde?
In the evening	¿al atardecer?
At night?	¿en la noche?
Does it feel. . .	¿Se siente . . .
achy?	dolorido?
throbbing?	que le vibra?
sharp?	agudo?
cramping?	con calambre?
Like burning?	candente?
Like stabbing?	punzante?
Like numbness?	entumecido?
Like tingling?	con hormigueo?
Does it radiate?	¿Se le riega?
Show me where.	Enséñeme a donde se le riega. Muéstreme a donde se le riega.
How many times a day does your pain bother you?	¿Cuántas veces al día su dolor le molesta? ¿Cuántas veces al día su dolor le **mortifica**?
One?	¿Una?
Two?	¿Dos?
Three?	¿Tres?
More than three?	¿Más de tres veces?
All day?	¿Todo el día?
Show me your pain medicines.	¿Enséñeme los medicamentos que usted toma para el dolor? ¿**Muéstreme** los medicamentos que usted toma para el dolor?

Chronic Pain

Is your pain level better since you started these medicines?	¿El nivel de su dolor está mejor que antes desde que empezó con estas medicinas?
Worse?	¿Peor?
No different?	¿Igual?
Is your ability to function better since you started these medicines?	¿Su habilidad de funcionar está mejor desde que empezó estos medicamentos?
	¿Su forma de funcionar está mejor desde que empezó estas **medicinas**?
Worse?	¿Peor?
No different?	¿Igual?
	¿No hay diferencia?
Is your pain/quality of life/mood/sleep better than before?	¿Es su dolor/calidad de vida/humor/dormir mejor que antes?
	¿Es su dolor/calidad de vida/**disposición**/dormir mejor que antes?
Worse?	¿Peor?
No different?	¿Igual?
Do you think the medicine is helping?	¿Usted cree que el medicamento le está ayudando?
	¿Usted cree que **la medicina** le está ayudando?
What other things are you doing to relieve your pain?	¿Qué otras cosas usted está haciendo para aliviar su dolor?
Ice?	¿Poniéndole hielo?
Heat (wet or dry)?	¿Poniéndole calor (mojado o seco)?
Meditation?	¿Meditando?
Hypnosis?	¿Usando hipnosis?
Acupuncture?	¿Acupuntura?
Exercise?	¿Ejercicios?
Do you take any over-the-counter medicines for your pain?	¿Está usted tomando medicamentos sin recetas para su dolor?
Show me.	Enséñeme.
	Muéstreme.
Bring everything you take for your pain to each visit.	Traiga a cada visita todo lo que usted toma para su dolor.

Chronic Pain

Are you exercising?	¿Está usted haciendo ejercicios?
What type?	¿Qué tipo?
Walking?	¿Caminando?
Swimming?	¿Nadando?
Cycling?	¿Montando bicicleta?
Weights?	¿Alzando pesas?
Stretching?	¿Haciendo ejercicios de estiramiento?
Chair or floor exercises?	¿Haciendo ejercicios de silla o de piso?
How many minutes/hours each time?	¿Cuántos minutos/horas cada vez que hace ejercicios?
How many days a week?	¿Cuántos días a la semana?
Is it helping your pain?	¿Le están ayudando con su dolor?
Have you seen a physical therapist?	¿Se ha usted tratado con un terapista físico?
Are you still seeing the physical therapist?	¿Todavía sigue usted hiendo a el/la terapista físico?
Do you have constipation?	¿Está usted constipado/a? ¿Está usted **estreñido/a**?
Are you able to do your daily activities?	¿Puede usted hacer sus tareas diarias? ¿**Es capaz de** hacer sus tareas diarias?
Cooking?	¿Cocinar?
Cleaning?	¿Limpiar?
Bathing?	¿Bañarse?
Dressing?	¿Vestirse?
Have you seen a psychiatrist?	¿Ha usted visto al psiquiatra?
On a regular basis?	¿Regularmente?
Have you gained or lost weight?	¿Ha usted ganado o perdido peso?
Are you trying to lose weight?	¿Está usted tratando de perder peso?
Do you smoke?	¿Usted fuma?
Have you been told to stop smoking?	¿Le han dicho alguna vez que pare de fumar?
Do you want to quit smoking?	¿Quiere usted dejar de fumar?
It may be more difficult to control your pain when you smoke.	Le va a ser mas difícil controlar su dolor cuando usted esté fumando.

Chronic Pain

Do you feel your pain is at a level you can tolerate?	¿Usted cree/piensa que su dolor está en un nivel en lo cual puede tolerar?

Chronic Back Pain Instructions

Sleep on a firm mattress.	Duerma en una cama más firme.
If you sleep on your back, put a pillow under your knees.	Si usted duerme en su espalda, póngase una almohada debajo de sus rodillas.
If you sleep on your side, bend your knees and hips, and put a pillow between your knees.	Si usted duerme de lado, doble sus rodillas y caderas, y ponga una almohada entre sus rodillas.
You can use an ice pack, hot water bottle, or heated moist towel for your back pain.	Usted puede utilizar una bolsa de hielo, agua caliente en botella o una toalla húmeda caliente para su dolor de espalda. Usted puede **usar** una bolsa de hielo, agua caliente en botella o una toalla húmeda caliente para su dolor de espalda.
Do not put it directly on your skin.	No la ponga directamente en su piel.
Do not use it for more than 20 minutes at a time.	No lo utilice por más de veinte minutos a la vez. No los **use** por más de veinte minutos a la vez.
Do not sleep on heat or ice.	No duerma aplicándose el calor o el frió.

Congestive Heart Failure

Have you been to the ER recently for your heart failure?	¿Ha estado usted recientemente en la sala de emergencia debido a su insuficiencia cardíaca congestiva?
How long ago (days, weeks, months)?	¿Cuánto tiempo hace (días, semanas, meses)?
Do you have chest pain?	¿Tiene usted dolor del pecho?
Do you have chest pain now?	¿Tiene usted dolor del pecho en este momento?
How many times a day/week/month?	¿Cuántas veces al día/semana/mes?
Is it your usual (typical) chest pain?	¿Es su típico dolor del pecho?

Congestive Heart Failure

Do you use nitroglycerin (under the tongue)?	¿Utiliza usted nitroglicerina (la pastilla que se pone abajo de la lengua)? ¿**Usa** usted nitroglicerina (la pastilla que se pone abajo de la lengua)?
How many times a day/week/month do you use nitroglycerin?	¿Cuántas veces al día/semana/mes usted utiliza nitroglicerina? ¿Cuántas veces al día/semana/mes usted **usa** nitroglicerina?
Is that more or less than before?	¿La usa más o menos que antes?
How many pillows do you use under your head when you sleep?	¿Cuántas almohadas usted utiliza debajo de su cabeza al dormir? ¿Cuántas almohadas usted **usa** debajo de su cabeza? ¿Cuántas almohadas usted **pone** debajo de su cabeza?
How many months/years have you slept on [number] pillows?	¿Cuántos meses o años hace que usted está dormiendo con [number] de almohadas?
Can you breathe normally lying flat?	¿Usted peude respirar normalmente acostado?
Do you have difficulty breathing at night?	¿Usted tiene dificultad respira por la noche?
Do you have swelling in your legs?	¿Usted tiene hinchazón en las piernas? ¿Usted tiene **inflamación** en las piernas?
For how long (days, weeks, months)?	¿Cuánto tiempo hace que están así (días, semanas, meses)? ¿**Qué tiempo** hace que están así (días, semanas, meses)?
Is it more or less than usual?	¿Es más o menos de lo usual? ¿Es más o menos de lo **corriente**? ¿Es más o menos de lo **normal**?

Congestive Heart Failure

Do you have difficulty breathing when walking?	¿Tiene usted dificultad respirando al caminar?
How many blocks/miles can you walk before you have difficulty breathing?	¿Cuántos bloques/millas puede usted caminar antes de empezar a tener dificultad respirando?
	¿Cuántos **cuadras/kilómetros** puede usted caminar antes de empezar a tener dificultad respirando?
	¿Cuántos **manzanas/kilómetros** puede usted caminar antes de empezar a tener dificultad respirando?
Do you have a cough?	¿Tiene usted tos?
Do you cough up blood?	¿Está usted tosiendo sangre?
Do you have problems with fainting or dizziness?	¿Tiene usted problemas con desmayos o mareos?
Do you have palpitations (a feeling of your heart racing or skipping beats)?	¿Tiene usted palpitaciones (se siente que el corazón le corre o le brinca latidos)?
How many seconds/minutes do they last?	¿Cuántos segundos/minutos le dura?
How many times a day or week do you get them?	¿Cuántas veces al día o a la semana le aparece o tiene este problema?
Do you have a scale at home?	¿Tiene usted una balanza en su casa?
	¿Tiene usted **una pesa** en su casa?
Do you weigh yourself?	¿Se pesa usted?
You need to buy a scale and weigh yourself every day.	Usted necesita comprarse una balanza y pesarse todos los días.
	Usted necesita comprarse **una pesa** y pesarse cada día.
If you gain more than 2 pounds in one day, you need to call or come in to be seen.	Si usted aumenta más de dos libras en un día, usted necesita llamar o venir aqui para ser visto.
Do you eat out frequently?	¿Come usted a menudo fuera de su casa?
Do you eat salty foods?	¿Come usted comida alta en sal?
Do you eat canned foods?	¿Come usted comidas enlatadas?
Do you eat packaged foods?	¿Come usted comidas empacadas?
Do you eat fast foods?	¿Come usted comida rápida?

Congestive Heart Failure

Do you eat bacon?	¿Come usted tosino?
Do you eat sausage?	¿Come usted salchicha?
	¿Come usted **embutidos**?
Do you eat ham?	¿Come usted jamón?
Do you eat lunch meats?	¿Come usted carne para bocadillos o sándwiches?
Do you eat cheese?	¿Come usted quesos?
Do you eat chips?	¿Come usted frituras?
How many times a week?	¿Cuántas veces por semana?
Try to eat these foods . . .	Trate de comer este tipo de comidas . . .
less than once/twice a week.	menos de una o dos veces por semana.
less than once/twice a month.	menos de una o dos veces por mes.
only rarely.	raramente.

Coronary Artery Disease

Have you been to the ER recently for chest pain?	¿Ha estado usted recientemente en la sala de emergencia debido a dolor de pecho?
Do you have chest pain?	¿Tiene usted dolor de pecho?
Do you have chest pain now?	¿Tiene usted en este momento dolor de pecho?
How many minutes/hours ago did it start?	¿Cuántos minutos/horas fue que le empezó?
How often do you get chest pain?	¿Qué tan a menudo tiene usted dolor de pecho?
Every day?	¿Todos los días?
	¿Cada día?
How many times a day?	¿Cuántas veces al día?
Every week?	¿Cada semana?
How many times a week?	¿Cuántas veces por semana?
Is it more than before?	¿Es más que antes?
Is it less than before?	¿Es menos que antes?

Coronary Artery Disease

Is it like your usual (typical) chest pain?	¿Es el usual (típico) dolor de pecho?
Do you get it with activity/rest?	¿Le dan cuando usted está activo/descansando?
How much activity?	¿Qué tanto de actividad?
One block?	¿Al caminar un bloque?
One mile?	¿Al caminar una milla?
A flight of stairs?	¿Al subir las escaleras?
Do you use nitroglycerin?	¿Utiliza usted nitroglicerina?
	¿**Usa** usted nitroglicerina?
Under the tongue?	¿Debajo de su lengua?
As a patch?	¿De parche?
How many times a day/week/month do you use nitroglycerin?	¿Cuántas veces al día/a la semana/al mes utiliza usted nitroglicerina?
	¿Cuántas veces al día/a la semana/al mes **usa** usted nitroglicerina?
Is that more or less than before?	¿Es más o menos que antes?
How many blocks/miles/flights of stairs can you walk?	¿Cuántos bloques/millas/escalones puede usted caminar?
	¿Cuántas **cuadras**/millas/escalones puede usted caminar?
	¿Cuántas **manzanas**/kilómetros/escalones puede caminar?
How many times a week do you exercise (walking/cycling/swimming)?	¿Cuántas veces a la semana hace usted ejercicios (caminar/montar bicicleta/nadar)?
How many minutes each time?	¿Cuántos minutos cada vez?
How many pillows do you use under your head when you sleep?	¿Cuántas almohadas usted utiliza debajo de su cabeza al dormir?
	¿Cuántas almohadas usted **usa** debajo de su cabeza?
	¿Cuántas almohadas usted **pone** debajo de su cabeza?
How long have you slept with (number) pillows?	¿Cuánto hace que usted duerme con [number] de almohadas?
Can you breathe normally lying flat?	¿Puede usted respirar normalmente al estar acostado sin alomadas?

Coronary Artery Disease

Do you have difficulty breathing at night?	¿Tiene usted dificultad respirando en la noche?
Do you have swelling in your legs?	¿Tiene usted hinchazón en las piernas?
	¿Tiene usted **inflamación** en las piernas?
For how long (days, weeks, months)?	¿Por cuánto tiempo (días, semanas, meses)?
Is it more than usual?	¿Es más o menos de lo usual?
	¿Es más o menos de lo **corriente**?
	¿Es más o menos de lo **normal**?
Is it less than usual?	¿Es menos de lo usual?
	¿Es menos de lo **corriente**?
	¿Es menos o de lo **normal**?
Do you have difficulty breathing when walking?	¿Tiene usted dificultad respirando al caminar?
How far can you walk before you have difficulty breathing?	¿Qué tan lejos puede usted caminar antes de tener dificultad al respirar?
Can you walk up stairs?	¿Puede usted subir las escaleras?
How many flights of stair can you walk up?	¿Cuántos escalones puede usted subir?
Do you have pain in your calves when walking?	¿Tiene usted dolor en las pantorrillas al caminar?
Show me where.	Enséñeme a donde.
	Muéstreme a donde.
Is it an aching or cramping pain?	¿Es de tipo dolorido o de tipo calambre?
How far can you walk before you feel pain?	¿Qué tan lejos puede usted caminar antes de que le duela?
Do you have problems with fainting or dizziness?	¿Tiene usted problemas de desmayo o de mareos?
Do you have any palpitations (a feeling of your heart racing or skipping beats)?	¿Tiene usted palpitaciones (siente que su corazón está en una carrera o que brinca latidos)?
How many seconds or minutes do they last?	¿Cuántos segundos o minutos le duran?
Do you smoke?	¿Usted fuma?
How many cigarettes a day?	¿Cuántos cigarrillos al día?

Coronary Artery Disease

Do you eat foods low in cholesterol?	¿Come usted comidas bajas en colesterol?
Fat?	¿Grasas?
Salt?	¿Sal?
Do you eat out frequently?	¿Come usted frecuentemente fuera de su casa?
Sit down restaurants?	¿En restaurantes?
Fast food?	¿Comidas rápidas?

Depression

Is your mood better than before?	¿Está su humor mejor que antes?
	¿Está **su disposición** mejor que antes?
Worse than before?	¿Peor que antes?
About the same?	¿Más o menos igual?
Are you taking your medicines every day?	¿Está usted tomando sus medicamentos todos los días?
Do you think the medicines are helping your mood?	¿Usted cree que los medicamentos le están ayudando con su humor?
	¿Usted cree que los medicamentos le están ayudando con su disposición?
Do you think your mood could be better?	¿Usted cree que su humor podría mejorar?
	¿Usted cree que **su disposición** podría mejorar?
Are you taking more pleasure in your normal activities?	¿Le da a usted más placer llevar a cabo sus actividades normales?
Are you taking less pleasure in your normal activities?	¿Le da a usted menos placer llevar a cabo sus actividades normales?
Are you able to concentrate on a task better than before?	¿Puede usted concentrase en una tarea mejor que antes?
Is your memory better than before?	¿Está su memoria mejor que antes?
Worse?	¿Peor?
The same?	¿Más o menos igual?

Depression

Is your appetite normal?	¿Está su apetito normal?
Decreased?	¿Reducido?
	¿Bajo?
	¿Disminuido?
	¿Pobre?
Increased?	¿Aumentado?
Do you sleep well?	¿Duerme usted bien?
Too much?	¿Duerme mucho?
Too little?	¿Duerme poco?
How many hours a night do you sleep in total?	¿Cuántas horas en total usted duerme en la noche?
Do you have thoughts of wanting to hurt or kill yourself or others?	¿Tiene usted pensamientos de querer lastimarse o matarse o hacer lo mismo con otras personas?
Do you have a plan?	¿Tiene usted algún plan de como hacerlo?
	¿Tiene usted algun plan de como **lograrlo**?
Do you have a way to carry out your plan?	¿Tiene usted o sabe la forma en la cual va a llevar a cabo su plan?
Have you ever tried to kill yourself or hurt someone else?	¿Ha tratado de matarse o de lastimar usted a otra persona?

Diabetes

Do you take pills for your diabetes?	¿Toma usted pastillas para su diabetes?
Do you take insulin?	¿Usted se inyecta insulina?
What type of insulin (70/30, NPH, Lantus)?	¿Qué tipo de insulina (setenta/treinta, NPH, Lantus)?
How much insulin do you use in the morning?	¿Cuánta insulina utiliza usted en la mañana?
	¿Cuánta insulina **usa** usted en la mañana?
Afternoon?	¿Tarde?
Evening?	¿Al anochecer?
At bedtime?	¿Antes de acostarse?
Do you have excessive thirst?	¿Tiene usted sed excesiva?
	¿Tiene usted mucha sed?

Diabetes

Do you have excessive hunger?	¿Tiene usted hambre excesiva? **¿Tiene usted mucha hambre?**
Do you have excessive urination?	¿Orina usted excesivamente? **¿Orina usted mucho?**
Do you have any rashes/ulcers?	¿Tiene usted erupción/úlceras? ¿Tiene usted **salpullido**/úlceras? ¿Tiene usted **pintas rojas en su piel**/úlceras?
For how many days/weeks/months?	¿Por cuánto tiempo días/semanas/meses?
Are you checking your glucose level?	¿Se está usted revisando sus niveles de azúcar?
Before breakfast?	¿Antes del desayuno?
Before lunch?	¿Antes de almuerzo?
Before dinner?	¿Antes de la cena?
Before bedtime?	¿Antes de acostarse?
You need to check your glucose level every time before you use insulin.	Usted necesita revisarse su nivel de azúcar cada vez que se inyecte con insulina. Usted necesita revisarse su nivel de **glucosa** cada vez que se inyecte con insulina.
Do you have your glucometer?	¿Tiene usted su glucómetro o medidor de azúcar? ¿Tiene usted su glucómetro o medidor de **glucosa**?
Let me see it.	Déjeme verlo.
Do you have your logbook?	¿Tiene usted su diario de sus niveles de azúcar?
Let me see it.	Déjeme verlo.
Please bring your glucometer and logbook to each visit.	Por favor traiga se glucómetro y diario en toda sus visitas.
How many times a week/month is your glucose level less than 80?	¿Cuántas veces a la semana/mes son sus niveles de azúcar menos de 80? ¿Cuántas veces a la semana/mes son sus niveles de **glucosa** menos de 80?
Does it happen mostly before breakfast?	¿Estos niveles usualmente ocurren antes del desayuno?
In the afternoon?	¿En la tarde?

Diabetes

Before dinner?	¿Antes de la comida?
	¿Antes de la **cena**?
Late at night?	¿Tarde en la noche?
What time?	¿A qué hora?
Does it happen when you forget to eat or when you eat late?	¿Ocurre cuando usted se olvida de comer o cuando come tarde?
Are your sugars mostly above 150?	¿Está su azúcar mayormente por arriba de ciento cincuenta?
200?	¿Doscientos?
Higher?	¿Más alta?
Do you follow a diabetic diet?	¿Sigue usted una dieta diabética?
Are you taking your medicines regularly?	¿Se está usted tomando sus medicamentos regularmente?
Do you have symptoms like sweating, shaking, or confusion?	¿Tiene usted síntomas como de sudor frío, temblor o confusión?
Do you check your sugar when this happens?	¿Se revisa usted su azúcar cuando esto pasa?
What is the level?	¿Cuál es su nivel?
What time of day does this usually happen?	¿A qué hora del día usualmente esto pasa?
	¿A qué hora del día usualmente esto **sucede**?
Do you eat your meals at about the same time each day?	¿Come usted sus comidas alrededor de la misma hora todos los días?
Do you eat snacks between meals?	¿Come usted meriendas entre comidas?
Do you eat a snack before bedtime?	¿Come usted algún bocadillo antes de acostarse?
Do you exercise (walk/cycle/swim)?	¿Hace usted ejercicios como (caminar/montar bicicleta/nadar)?
How many times a week?	¿Cuántas veces a la semana?
How many minutes each time?	¿Cuántos minutos cada vez que usted hace ejercicio?
Do you eat a snack before or after exercise?	¿Come usted algún bocadillo antes o después de hacer ejercicios?
You need to eat a snack [number] minutes before exercise/after exercise.	Usted necesita comerse un bocadillo, [number] minutos antes o después de hacer ejercicios.

Diabetes

Are you checking your feet every day?	¿Se está usted revisando sus pies regularmente?
Do you have numbness or tingling in your feet?	¿Tiene usted entumecimiento o comezón en sus pies?
Do you wear shoes or slippers at all times?	¿Usted tiene usa zapatos o sandalias en todo momento?
	¿Usted tiene puestos zapatos o **zapatillas** en todo momento?
	¿Usted tiene puestos zapatos o **pantuflas** en todo momento?
	¿Usted tiene puestos zapatos o **chancletas** en todo momento?
Do you have blurry vision?	¿Tiene usted visión borrosa?
Does it come and go?	¿Viene y se va?
When was your last eye exam (months/years)?	¿Cuándo fue su último examen de ojos (meses/años)?
Do you have impotence problems?	¿Tiene usted problemas con su erección o de impotencia?
For how long?	¿Por cuánto tiempo?

For exercise and nutrition questions, see Chapter 11, "Health Behaviors History and Education."

Gastroesophageal Reflux Disease

Do you have problems with heartburn?	¿Tiene usted problemas de acidez gástrica o ardor de estómago?
Is it better with medicine?	¿Se mejora con el medicamento?
Are you taking the medicine regularly?	¿Está usted tomando el medicamento regularmente?
Does your food come back up into your throat?	¿Se le regresa la comida a la garganta?
Do you get an acid taste in your mouth?	¿Tiene sabor ácido en su boca?
Do you have abdominal pain?	¿Tiene usted dolor abdominal?
	¿Tiene usted dolor **en la barriga**?
Is it associated with eating?	¿El dolor está relacionado al comer?
	¿Al comer le duele?
Does it happen before meals?	¿Le duele antes de comer?

Gastroesophageal Reflux Disease

During meals?	¿Cuándo come?
After meals?	¿Después de comer?
Have you ever had stomach ulcers?	¿Ha usted tenido alguna vez úlceras estomacales?
Is your appetite normal?	¿Su apetito está normal?
Decreased?	¿Reducido?
	¿**Bajo**?
	¿**Disminuido**?
	¿**Pobre**?
Increased?	¿Aumentado?
Do you have nausea?	¿Usted tiene nauseas?
Do you have vomiting?	¿Está usted vomitando?
	¿Está usted arrojando?
Is it green?	¿Su vomito es verde?
Yellow?	¿Amarillo?
Bloody?	¿Con sangre?
Like coffee grounds?	¿Cómo granos de café?
Clear?	¿Claro?
Containing solids?	¿Sólidos?
Are you vomiting blood?	¿Ha vomitado sangre?
	¿Ha **usted arrojado** sangre?
Is it bright red?	¿Es su vomito color rojo vivo?
	¿Es su vomito color rojo **intenso**?
Dark like coffee grounds?	¿Como granos de café?
Do you have blood in your stools?	¿Tiene usted sangre en las heces?
	¿Tiene usted sangre en la **excreta**?
	¿Tiene usted sangre en el **excremento**?
Do you have any black, sticky stools like tar?	¿Están sus heces negras o pegajosas como tar?
	¿Está su **excremento** negro o pegajoso como **alquitrán**?
	¿Está su **excreta** negra o pegajosa como **brea**?
Are you losing/gaining weight?	¿Está usted perdiendo o ganando peso?
Do you have a cough?	¿Tiene usted tos?
Is it worse at night?	¿Se le empeora por la noche?

Gastroesophageal Reflux Disease

Do you drink beverages with caffeine (coffee, tea, soda)?	¿Toma usted bebidas que contienen cafeína (como café, té, o sodas)? ¿**Consume** usted bebidas que contienen cafeína (como café, té, o sodas)? ¿**Bebe** usted bebidas que contienen cafeína (como café, té, o sodas)?
Do you smoke?	¿Usted fuma?
Do you eat chocolate/peppermints?	¿Come usted chocolate/mentas?
Do you drink alcohol? These may make your reflux worse.	¿Toma usted alcohol? ¿**Consume** usted alcohol? ¿**Bebe** usted alcohol? Estas ya mencionadas, le pueden agravar su reflujo.
It may help to sleep with your head raised.	Le podría ayudar si durmiera con la cabeza levantada o levantar la cabezera de la cama.
Try not to eat [number] hours before going to bed. You may have a light snack before bedtime to keep your sugar level up.	Trate de no comer [number] horas antes de acostarse. Usted puede comer un bocadillo ligero antes de irse a la cama para mantener su nivel de azúcar elevado. Usted puede comer **un aperitivo** ligero antes de irse a la cama para mantener su nivel de azúcar elevado.

Hypertension

How many years have you had high blood pressure?	¿Cuántos años hace que usted tiene alta presión?
Do you have a blood pressure monitor at home?	¿Tiene usted un aparato para vigilar su presión sanguínea en su casa?
Do you check your blood pressure at home/a pharmacy/a fire station?	¿Usted se revisa su presión sanguínea en su casa/farmacia/estación de bomberos?
	¿Usted se revisa su presión sanguínea en su casa/farmacia/**parque** de bomberos?
Do you write it down?	¿Usted la escribe y sigue su progreso?
I want you to keep a log of your blood pressure and bring it with you each visit.	¿Yo quiero que usted lleve un registro/diario de su presión sanguínea y que lo traiga con usted a cada visita?
Do you have chest pain?	¿Tiene usted dolor del pecho?
How many times a day/week/month?	¿Cuántas veces al día/semana/mes?
Do you get it with activity/rest?	¿Le da cuando está activo/a o descansando?
How much activity?	¿Cuánta actividad?
Walking one block?	¿Al caminar un bloque?
Walking one mile?	¿Al caminar una milla?
Walking one flight of stairs?	¿Subiendo las escaleras?
How many times a week do you exercise (walking/cycling/swimming)?	¿Cuántas veces a la semana usted hace ejercicio (caminando/montando bicicleta/nadando)?
How many minutes each time?	¿Cuántos minutos cada vez que hace ejercicios?
How many pillows do you use under your head when you sleep?	¿Cuántas almohadas usted utiliza debajo de su cabeza al dormir ?
	¿Cuántas almohadas usted **usa** debajo de su cabeza al dormir?
	¿Cuántas almohadas usted **pone** debajo de su cabeza al dormir?
How long have you slept with [number] pillows?	¿Cuánto hace que usted duerme con [number] de almohadas?
Can you breathe normally lying flat?	¿Puede usted respirar normalmente al estar acostado sin almohadas?

Hypertension

Do you have difficulty breathing at night?	¿Tiene usted dificultad respirando en la noche?
Do you have swelling in your legs?	¿Tiene usted hinchazón en las piernas?
For how long (days, weeks, months)?	¿Por cuánto tiempo (días, semanas, meses)?
Do you have difficulty breathing when walking?	¿Tiene usted dificultad respirando al caminar?
How far can you walk before you have difficulty breathing?	¿Qué tan lejos puede usted caminar antes de tener dificultad respirando?
Do you feel dizzy or faint when you sit up, stand up, or change positions?	¿Se siente mareado o que se va a desmayar cuando se sienta, se para o cambia de posiciones?
In order to give your body a chance to adjust, you need to stand up or change positions more slowly.	Para darle a su cuerpo una oportunidad de adaptarse, necesita usted pararse o cambiar posiciones más despacio.
Do you have any palpitations (a feeling of your heart racing or skipping beats)?	¿Tiene usted palpitaciones (siente que su corazón está en una carrera o que le brinca latidos)?
How many seconds/minutes do they last?	¿Cuántos segundos/minutos le duran?
Do you have severe headaches?	¿Tiene usted dolores de cabeza severos?
Do you have blind spots in your vision?	¿Tiene usted puntos ciegos en su visión?
Do you have difficulty speaking or walking now?	¿Tiene usted en este momento dificultad hablando o caminando?
Do you have paralysis or weakness on one side of your body that is new?	¿Tiene usted o a notado recientemente parálisis o debilidad en una mitad de su cuerpo?
Do you smoke?	¿Usted fuma?
How many cigarettes a day?	¿Cuántos cigarrillos al día?
Do you eat salty foods?	¿Come usted comidas altas en sal?
Canned foods?	¿Comidas enlatadas?
Packaged foods?	¿Comidas empacadas?
Fast foods?	¿Comidas rápidas?
Bacon?	¿Tocino?
Sausage?	¿Embutidos?
	¿**Salchichas**?
Ham?	¿Jamón?

Hypertension

Lunch meats?	¿Carne para sándwiches?
Cheese?	¿Queso?
Chips?	¿Frituras?
How many times a week?	¿Cuántas veces a la semana?
Try to eat these foods . . .	Trate de comer estas comidas . . .
less than once/twice a week.	Menos de una o dos veces por semana.
less than once/twice a month.	Menos de una o dos veces por mes.
only rarely.	Raramente.
Do you eat out frequently?	¿Come usted frecuentemente fuera de su casa?
Fast food?	¿Comidas rápidas?

For exercise and nutrition questions, see Chapter 11, "Health Behaviors History and Education."

Obesity

How long have you been overweight?	¿Cuántos años hace que usted tiene exceso de peso?
	¿Cuántos años hace que usted **ha estado en** exceso de **sobrepeso**?
Since childhood?	¿Desde su niñez?
	¿Desde su **infancia**?
Are other members of your family overweight or obese?	¿Hay otros miembros de su familia que tienen exceso de peso?
	¿Hay otros miembros de su familia que estan **sobrepesados**?
Do you feel that you need to lose weight?	¿Piensa o se siente usted que tiene que perder peso?
Do you believe that losing weight would be better for your health?	¿Cree usted que perdiendo peso podría mejorar o beneficiar su salud?
Have you tried to lose weight previously?	¿Ha usted tratado de perder peso anteriormente?
Did you follow any special diet to lose weight?	¿Sigue usted alguna dieta en especial para perder peso?
Weight Watchers?	¿Método nutricional o dieta Weight Watchers (club de adelgazamiento)?
Atkins?	¿Método nutricional o dieta Atkins?
Jenny Craig?	¿Método nutricional o Dieta Jenny Craig?

Obesity

Low carb?	¿Método nutricional o dieta baja en carbohidratos?
Low calorie?	¿Método nutricional o dieta baja en calorías?
Did you follow an exercise program to lose weight?	¿Sigue usted algún plan de ejercicio para bajar de peso?
Walking?	¿Caminar?
Swimming?	¿Nadar?
Cycling?	¿Ciclismo?
	¿**Montar bicicleta**?
Aerobics?	¿Ejercicio aeróbico?
Exercise classes?	¿Clases para hacer ejercicios?
Were you successful in losing weight?	¿Turo usted exitoso perdiendo peso?
	¿Fue usted exitoso perdiendo peso?
	¿Lo logró?
How many times in the past did you seriously try to lose weight?	¿Cuántas veces seriamente en el pasado usted trato de perder peso?
Do you think that you eat too much?	¿Cree usted que come demasiado?
Do you eat out frequently? Fast food?	¿Come usted afuera frecuentemente? ¿Come comida rápida o platos preparados?
	¿Come usted **en restaurantes** frecuentemente? ¿Come comida rápida o platos preparados?
How many times a week?	¿Cuántas veces por semana?
Do you exercise now?	¿Está usted hoy en día haciendo ejercicio?
	¿Ha está usted **actualmente** haciendo ejercicio?
What type of exercise?	¿Qué tipo de ejercicio?
Walking?	¿Caminar?
Swimming?	¿Nadar?
Cycling?	¿Ciclismo?
	¿**Montar bicicleta**?
Aerobics?	¿Ejercicio aeróbico?
Exercise classes?	¿Clases para hacer ejercicios?
How many minutes a day?	¿Cuántos minutos por día?

Obesity

How many times a week?	¿Cuántas veces por semana?
Do you eat snacks?	¿Come usted meriendas? ¿Come usted **bocadillos**? ¿Come usted **entremeses**?
How many times a day?	¿Cuántas veces por día?
Do you eat junk food?	¿Come usted comida chatarra o de valor alimenticio bajo?
How many times a day/week?	¿Cuántas veces por día o por semana?
Do you eat when you are not hungry?	¿Come usted aun cuando usted no tiene apetito? ¿Come usted **hasta** cuando usted no tiene ganas de comer?
When you are sad?	¿Come cuando está triste? ¿Come cuando está **afligido**?
Stressed?	¿Estresado? ¿ **Nervioso/a**?
Depressed?	¿Deprimido/a? ¿ **Abatido/a**?
Happy?	¿Contento/a?
Lonely?	¿Cuando se siente solo/a?
Have you ever seen a dietician?	¿Ha usted visto e ido a una dietista?
How many months/years ago was the last time?	¿Cuántos meses o años fue la última vez?
Do you ever eat food and then intentionally vomit to get rid of the food?	¿Ha usted comido e intencionalmente arrojado o vomitado para así librarse o deshacerse de la comida?
Do you ever binge by eating large quantities of food, and then feel guilty afterwards?	¿Ha usted alguna vez comido con desenfreno/una gran cantidad de comida, y después se ha sentido culpable por la cantidad que comió?
Have you ever been diagnosed with or treated for an eating disorder?	¿Ha sido usted alguna vez diagnosticado o tratado debido a un trastorno alimenticio?
Bulimia or anorexia nervosa?	¿Como por ejemplo bulimia o anorexia nervosa?
Have you ever had weight loss surgery?	¿Ha usted tenido o se ha hecho cirugía para perder peso?

Obesity

Is weight loss surgery something you want to consider?	¿Es la cirugía para perder peso algo que usted quiere o ha estado considerando?

For exercise and nutrition questions, see Chapter 11, "Health Behaviors History and Education."

Peripheral Vascular Disease — Enfermedad Vascular Periférica

Peripheral Vascular Disease	Enfermedad Vascular Periférica
Are you walking regularly?	¿Está usted caminando regularmente?
How many minutes/blocks/miles each time?	¿Cuántos minutos/bloques/millas cada vez?
	¿Cuántos minutos/**cuadras**/ millas cada vez?
	¿Cuántos minutos/**manzanas/ kilómetros** cada vez?
Do you get pain in your calves with walking?	¿Le da dolor en sus pantorrillas al caminar?
Is it an ache or cramp?	¿Es una molestia en la pantorrilla o calambre?
Show me where you get it.	¿Enséñeme donde le da u ocurre?
	¿**Muéstreme** donde le da u ocurre?
Does it go away when you stop?	¿Este dolor se le va cuando usted para?
How many minutes does it take to go away?	¿Cuántos minutos tarda antes de irse el dolor?
How far can you walk before you feel pain?	¿Qué tan lejos puede caminar antes de darle dolor?
More than a block?	¿Más de un bloque?
	¿Más de una **cuadra**?
	¿Más de **una manzana**?
Less than a block?	¿Menos de un bloque?
	¿Menos de **una cuadra**?
	¿Menos de **una manzana**?
Do you get the same pain in your legs or feet at rest?	Le da este mismo dolor aun cuando está descansando sus piernas o pies?
Are your feet cold all the time?	¿Están sus pies fríos cuando esto ocurre?
	¿Se encuentran sus pies fríos cuando esto ocurre?

Peripheral Vascular Disease

Do your feet or toes ever turn blue?	¿Se le han vuelto morados alguna vez los dedos de sus pies?
Do you have any ulcers on your legs or feet?	¿Tiene usted alguna úlcera en sus piernas o pies?
Do you get chest pain? [If yes, see "Chest Pain" in Chapter 5.	¿Le dan dolores de pecho?
Do you have problems with impotence?	¿Tiene usted problemas de impotencia?
For how many months/years?	¿Por cuántos meses o años?
Do you take aspirin?	¿Toma usted aspirina?
Every day?	¿Todos los días?
Do you take other medicines for your circulation?	¿Toma usted algún otro medicamento para su circulación?
Show me.	¿Enséñemelo? ¿Muéstremelo?
Have you had any surgery to restore circulation in your legs?	¿Ha usted tenido algún tipo de cirugía para restorar la circulación de sus piernas?
How many months/years ago?	¿Cuántos meses o años hace?
Do you smoke?	¿Usted fuma?
How many cigarettes/packs a day?	¿Cuántos cigarrillos/cajetillas por día? ¿Cuántos cigarrillos/**paquetes** por día?
For how many years?	¿Por cuántos años?
Do you want to quit?	¿Quiere usted dejar el vicio de fumar? ¿Quiere usted **abandonar** el vicio de fumar?
Are you willing to use medication to help you quit? (If yes, see "Smoking Cessation," page 182.)	¿Quiere utilizar algún tipo de medicamento para así dejar de fumar? ¿ **Desea** utilizar algún tipo de **medicina** para así dejar de fumar? ¿ **Está de acuerdo usted en usar** algún tipo de **medicina** para así dejar de fumar?

Seizure Disorder

How long have you had a seizure disorder?	¿Cuántos años hace que usted a tenido ataques epilépticos?
	¿Cuántos años hace que usted a tenido **convulsiones**?
Did you have seizures as a child?	¿Tuvo usted en su niñez ataques epilépticos?
	¿Tuvo usted en su niñez **convulsiones**?
Are your seizures a result of head trauma?	¿Sus ataques epilépticos fueron/son a causa de trauma cerebral?
	¿Sus **convulsiones** fueron a causa de trauma cerebral?
Brain injury?	¿Trauma cerebral?
Infection?	¿Infección?
What kind of seizures are they?	¿Qué tipo de ataques epilépticos a padecido usted?
	¿Qué tipo de ataques epilépticos a **sufrido** usted?
	¿Qué tipo de **convulsiones** a **sufrido** usted?
Tonic-clonic or petit mal?	¿Convulsiones tónico-clónica o crísis de ausencia?
Are you aware of the seizure coming on?	¿Se da usted cuenta cuando le va a empezar el ataque epiléptico?
	¿Se da usted cuenta cuando le va a empezar **la convulsión**?
Do you lose control of your bladder or bowels during the seizure?	¿Pierde usted control de su vejiga e intestinos durante el ataque epiléptico?
	¿Pierde usted control de su vejiga e intestinos durante **la convulsión**?
Are you especially sleepy after the seizure?	¿Se siente usted con ganas de dormir después del ataque epiléptico?
	¿Se siente usted con ganas de dormir después de **la convulsión**?

Seizure Disorder

Are you aware of what is happening during the seizure?	¿Sabe usted que está pasando durante el ataque epiléptico? ¿Sabe usted que está pasando durante **la convulsión**?
Do you fall or bite your tongue during the seizure?	¿Se cae o se muerde su lengua durante el ataque epiléptico? ¿Se cae o se muerde su lengua durante **la convulsión**?
How many weeks/months/years ago was your last seizure?	¿Cuántas semanas/meses/años hace que usted tuvo su último ataque epiléptico? ¿Cuántas semanas/meses/años hace que usted tuvo su última **convulsión**?
Were you taking your medicines at the time?	¿Estaba usted tomando su medicamento cuando sucedió?
Are you under the care of a neurologist?	¿Está usted viéndose con algún neurólogo? ¿Está usted **siguiéndose** con algún neurólogo?
How many weeks/months/years ago was the last time you saw the neurologist?	¿Cuántas semanas/meses/años hace que usted vio su neurólogo por última vez?
Are you taking medicines for your seizures?	¿Está usted tomando medicinas para sus ataques epilépticos? Está usted tomando medicamentos para sus **convulsiones**?
Show me.	Enséñemelo. **Muéstremelo.**
Have you taken medicines for your seizures in the past?	¿Ha usted tomado en el pasado medicamentos para sus ataques epilépticos? ¿Ha usted tomado en el pasado medicinas para sus **convulsiones**?
Did the neurologist tell you to stop them or, did you run out?	¿Le dijo a usted el neurólogo que dejase de tomar sus medicamentos o se le acabaron? ¿Le dijo a usted el neurólogo que dejase de tomar sus medicinas o se le **terminaron**?

	¿Le dijo a usted el neurólogo que dejase de tomar sus **medicinas** o se les **agotaron**?
Are you getting seizures more frequently than before?	¿Le están dando ataques convulsivos más frecuentes que antes?
Less frequently than before?	¿Menos frecuentes que antes?
No change in frequency?	¿No han ávido cambios en frecuencia?
Do you drink alcohol?	¿Toma usted alcohol?
	¿**Consume** usted alcohol?
	¿**Bebe** usted alcohol?
Alcohol can make you have seizures more easily.	El alcohol le induce más frecuentes ataques epilépticos.
	El alcohol le **frecuenta** más convulsiones.

Smoking Cessation

Do you smoke/chew tobacco?	¿Usted fuma o masca tabaco?
How many cigarettes each day?	¿Cuántos cigarillos al día?
How many years?	¿Por cuantos años?
Have you ever quit?	¿Ha usted alguna vez dejado de fumar?
For how long (days, weeks, months, years)?	¿Por cuánto tiempo (días, semanas, meses, años)?
Did you use a nicotine patch/gum/inhaler/nasal spray/medication to help you quit?	¿Ha usted utilizado el parche/goma de mascar/aerosol nasal de nicotina/medicamentos para ayudarle a dejar de fumar?
	¿Ha usted **usado** el parche/goma de mascar/aerosol nasal de nicotina/medicamentos para ayudarle a dejar de fumar?
Did you use a pill to help you quit?	¿Toma usted alguna pastilla para ayudarle a dejar de fumar?
Did it help?	¿Le ayudó?
Do you want to quit now?	¿Quiere usted en este momento dejar de fumar?
Do you want to quit now because . . .	¿Quiere usted en este momento dejar de fumar por . . .

Smoking Cessation

of your health?	su salud?
of your family?	familia?
of money?	dinero?
you are tired of smoking?	cansado de fumar?
Do you believe you are ready to quit?	¿Usted cree que está listo para dejar de fumar?
Are you willing to try a nicotine patch/gum/inhaler/nasal spray/medication to help you quit?	¿Está usted dispuesto/a tratar el parche/goma de mascar/inhalador o aerosol nasal de nicotina?
I want you to try the patch/gum/inhaler/nasal spray/medication.	¿Yo quiero que usted trate el parche/goma de mascar/inhalador o aerosol nasal de nicotina?
Do not smoke while wearing the patch.	No fume mientras esté utilizando el parche.
If you must smoke, remove the patch, wait 2 hours, and put the patch back on.	Si necesita fumar, quítese el parche, espere 2 horas y póngase el parche de nuevo.
	Si **debiese** fumar, quítese el parche, espere 2 horas y póngase el parche de nuevo.
You need to use only half a piece of gum at a time.	Cada vez que utilize su goma de mascar solo necesita usar la mitad de esta.
	Cada vez que **use** su goma de mascar solo necesita usar la mitad de esta.
Chew the gum between your teeth until you taste the nicotine, and then hold the gum between your cheek and gums for no more than 30 minutes.	Mastique la goma de mascar entre sus dientes hasta que sepa la nicotina, después mantenga la goma de mascar entre su cachete y su encía por no más treinta minutos.
Use a half piece/whole piece of gum every [number] hours each day.	Use la mitad o la pieza completa de su goma de mascar cada [number] horas todos los días.
Are you using the patch/gum/inhaler/nasal spray/medication now?	¿Está usted utilizando en este momento el parche/goma de mascar/inhalador o aerosol nasal de nicotina?

Smoking Cessation

How many days/weeks/months have you been on the nicotine patch/gum/inhaler/nasal spray/medication?	¿Cuántos días/semanas/meses hace que usted está en el parche/goma de mascar/inhalador o aerosol nasal de nicotina?
What dose of patch are you on (21, 14, 7 milligrams)?	¿Qué dosis de parche está usted utilizando (veintiuno, catorce, o siete miligramos)?
Do you have any rashes from the patch?	¿Tiene usted erupción debido al parche?
	¿Tiene usted **salpullidos** debido al parche?
	¿Tiene usted **pintas rojas en su piel** debido al parche?
Are you bothered by vivid or bad dreams from using the patch?	¿Está usted siendo molestado/a por sueños vividos o malos debido a la utilización del parche?
It may help to take off the patch before you go to bed.	Le podría ayudar removiéndose el parche antes de acostarse.
	Le podría ayudar **quitándose** el parche antes de acostarse.
Are you still smoking?	¿Todavía usted fuma?
How many cigarettes have you smoked this week/month?	¿Cuántos cigarrillos se ha usted fumado esta semana o mes?
How long ago was your last cigarette (days, weeks, months)?	¿Cuánto hace que usted fumó su último cigarrillo (días, semanas o meses)?
Do you have strong cravings?	¿Tiene usted antojos de fumar?
	¿Tiene usted **ganas fuertes** de fumar?
Do you think the patch is working?	¿Usted cree que el parche le está trabajando?
Are you ready to decrease the dose?	¿Está usted listo para bajar la dosis?

Thyroid Disease

Are you hot or cold all the time?	¿Se siente usted en todo momento con mucho calor o frió?
Do you sweat more than usual?	¿Suda usted más de lo usual?
	¿Suda usted más de lo **corriente**?
	¿Suda usted más de lo **normal**?

Thyroid Disease

Is your hair more coarse or dry than usual?	¿Está su pelo más áspero o seco de lo usual? ¿Se siente que su pelo está más **grueso** o seco de lo corriente? ¿Está su pelo más áspero o seco de lo **normal**?
Is your hair thinner than usual?	¿Está su pelo más delgado de lo usual? ¿Está su pelo está más delgado de lo **corriente**? ¿**Siente que** su pelo está más **fino** de lo **normal**?
Have you been losing your hair?	¿Ha estado usted perdiendo cabello? ¿Ha estado usted perdiendo **pelo**?
Do you have dry skin? Itchy skin?	¿Tiene usted su piel seca? ¿Le pica?
Do you have rashes?	¿Tiene erupciones? ¿Tiene **salpullido**? ¿Tiene **pintas rojas en su piel**?
Do you feel tired all the time?	¿Se siente usted cansado/a todo el tiempo?
Are your periods heavier than usual?	¿Su menstruación es más fuerte de lo usual? ¿Su menstruación es más fuerte de lo **corriente**? ¿**Su período** es más fuerte de lo **normal**?
Do you feel nervous?	¿Se siente usted nerviosa/o?
Do you feel irritable?	¿Se siente usted irritable?
Do you have tremors?	¿Tiene temblores?
Do you have insomnia?	¿Tiene insomnio? **¿No puede dormir?**
Do you have constipation or diarrhea?	¿Está usted constipado/a o tiene diarrea? ¿Está usted **estreñido/a** o tiene diarrea?
Do you have palpitations (a feeling of your heart racing or skipping beats)?	¿Tiene usted palpitaciones (siente que su corazón le corre o le brinca latidos)?
Do you have swelling in your legs?	¿Tiene usted hinchazón en sus piernas?

Chapter 7

Comprehensive Adult History

The adult comprehensive history is essentially "the rest of the story." Once you have asked questions concerning the history of the present illness or condition for which the patient is being seen, use this section to fill in the blanks. The adult comprehensive history is an important piece of the clinical picture taken during the workup of a new patient, and often will help in determining whether the current "chief complaint" is new or if the patient has had similar medical conditions or risks for such in the past.

For billing purposes, the comprehensive adult history is termed the PFSH (Past Family Social History) and contains the following elements:

- **Past** medical history includes illnesses, immunizations, operations, injuries, medications, compliance, and treatments.
- **Family** history is important to determine genetic disorders, as well as those diseases which may place the patient at risk. For example, the age at which a patient needs colon cancer screening depends on family history.

Also, knowing that a patient has a family history of early heart disease is essential in determining cholesterol goals.

- **Social** history includes employment and work exposures, education, marital status, substance use, travel and sexual history. Included in this chapter are screening tools for alcohol abuse, domestic violence, and depression. For pediatric social history, see Chapter 10, "Questions for Special Populations."

The comprehensive adult history included here follows the standard format and order taught in most medical history textbooks.

Childhood Illnesses

Have you ever had . . .	¿Ha usted tenido alguna vez . . .
measles?	sarampión?
mumps?	paperas?
whooping cough?	tos ferina?
chicken pox?	varicela?
smallpox?	viruela?
scarlet fever?	escarlatina?
rheumatic fever?	fiebre reumática?
diphtheria?	difteria?
polio?	polio?

Past Medical History

Do you have . . . ?	¿Usted tiene . . . ?
Have you ever had . . . ?	¿Ha usted tenido . . . ?
Have you been told by a doctor you have . . .	¿Le ha dicho algún doctor que usted tiene . . .
arthritis?	artritis?
asthma?	asma?
bladder infections?	infecciones de la vejiga?
blood disease (hemophilia, leukemia, anemia)?	enfermedades de la sangre (hemofilia, leucemia, o anemia)?
bronchitis?	bronquitis?
cancer?	cáncer?
diabetes?	diabetes?

Past Medical History

emphysema?	enfisema?
epilepsy?	epilepsia?
flu?	gripe?
gout?	gota?
hepatitis?	hepatitis?
heart disease (heart attack)?	enfermedades del corazón (ataque al corazón)?
	enfermedades del corazón (**ataque cardiaco**)?
high blood pressure?	alta presión?
kidney disease?	enfermedades renales?
	enfermedades **de los riñones**?
infections?	infecciones?
stones?	piedras?
dialysis?	dialisis?
liver disease?	enfermedades del hígado?
pneumonia?	pulmonía?
rheumatic fever?	fiebre reumática?
seizures?	convulsiones?
thyroid disease?	enfermedades de las tiroides?
TB?	tuberculosis?
stomach ulcers?	úlceras estomacales?
stroke?	accidente cerebrovascular (ACV)?
	derrame cerebral?
	apoplejía?
infarct?	infarto?

What year? ¿En que año?

Immunizations

Have you been vaccinated for...	¿Ha sido vacunado/a contra...
measles?	sarampión?
mumps?	paperas?
rubella?	rubéola
whooping cough?	tosferina?
chicken pox?	varicela?
diphtheria?	difteria?
polio?	polio?
meningitis?	meningitis?
tetanus?	tétano?
shingles (zoster)?	herpes zóster?
pneumonia?	neumonía?
flu?	influenza?
	gripe?
human papillomavirus (for cervical cancer)?	virus de papiloma humano (VHP) (relacionado con cáncer cervical)
hepatitis A?	hepatitis A
hepatitis B?	hepatitis B
What month/year?	¿En qué mes/año?

Accidents/Injuries

Have you ever had major trauma or injury?	Ha tenido usted alguna vez algún trauma or herida?
	Ha tenido usted alguna vez algún trauma or **daño**?
What year was the next to last and last time?	¿En que año fue la penúltima y última vez?
What part of the body? (See "Anatomy" in Chapter 3, "Vocabulary.")	¿En que parte del cuerpo?
Was it broken?	¿Estaba rota?
Did they replace it?	¿Se la reemplazaron?
Did they repair it?	¿Se la repararon?
Do you have any loss of function resulting from the injury?	¿Ha perdido usted alguna función por culpa de esta lesión?
	¿Ha perdido usted alguna función por culpa de este **trauma**?
	¿Ha perdido usted alguna función por culpa de esta **herida**?
	¿Ha perdido usted alguna función por culpa de este **daño**?

Surgical History

Have you ever had surgery?	¿Ha tenido usted alguna vez cirugía?
How many surgeries total?	¿Cuántas cirugías en total?
Starting with the most recent, what year and month was it?	¿Empezando con las más recientes, que año y mes fueron?
What city/state/hospital was it in?	¿En qué ciudad/estado/hospital fueron?
Show me where you had surgery.	Enséñeme donde fue la cirugía.
	Muéstreme donde fue la cirugía.
	Apúnteme donde fue la cirugía.
What kind of surgery?	¿Qué tipo de cirugía?
What part of the body? (See "Anatomy" in Chapter 3, "Vocabulary.")	¿En qué parte del cuerpo?
Did they take it out?	¿Se lo/la sacaron?
Did you have a tumor?	¿Tuvo usted un tumor?

Surgical History

Was it cancer?	¿Era canceroso?
Was it infected?	¿Era infeccioso?
Was it broken?	¿Se lo rompieron?
Did they replace it?	¿Fue reemplazado?
Did they repair it?	¿Se lo repararon?
Did you have anesthesia for it?	¿Al repararlo le pusieron anestesia?
Did you have problems with anesthesia?	¿Tuvo usted problemas con la anestesia?
Have you been told you have a heart murmur?	¿Le han dicho que usted tiene un soplo cardiaco?
	¿Le han dicho que usted tiene un soplo **en el corazón**?
Have you ever had a heart valve replaced or repaired?	¿Le han reemplazado o arreglado alguna vez una válvula cardiaca?
	¿Le han reemplazado o arreglado alguna vez una válvula **del corazón**?
Aorta?	¿La válvula aortica?
Mitral?	¿La mitral?
Pulmonic?	¿La pulmonar?
Tricuspid?	¿La tricúspide?

Hospitalizations

Have you been hospitalized for any medical problems (separate from surgery or injury)?	¿Ha sido usted hospitalizada/o por algún problema médico (que no tenga que ver con cirugía o lesiones)?
	¿Ha sido usted hospitalizada/o por alguna **razón** médica (que no tenga que ver con cirugía o **trauma**)?
	¿Ha sido usted hospitalizada/o por alguna **razón** médica (que no tenga que ver con cirugía o **problema**)?
	¿Ha sido usted hospitalizada/o por alguna **razón** médica (que no tenga que ver con cirugía o **herida**)?
	¿Ha sido usted hospitalizada/o por alguna **razón** médica (que no tenga que ver con cirugía o **daño**)?

Hospitalizations

How many times?	¿Cuántas veces?
What month/year were the last two times?	¿Qué mes/año fue la última y penúltima vez?
What part of the body? (See "Anatomy" in Chapter 3, "Vocabulary.")	¿En qué parte del cuerpo fue?

Medications

See "Medications" in Chapter 4, "Meeting the Patient."

Allergies

Are you allergic to any medicines?	¿Es usted alérgico/a a algún medicamento?
	¿Es usted alérgico/a a alguna **medicina**?
	¿Tiene usted alergia a algún medicamento?
Which medicines?	¿Cuáles medicamentos?
	¿Cuáles **medicinas**?
Do you get a rash from the medication?	¿Ha padecido de erupción con algunos de estos medicamentos ya mencionados?
	¿Ha padecido de **salpullidos** con algunos de estos medicamentos ya mencionados?
	¿Ha padecido de **pintas rojas en su piel** con algunos de estas **medicinas** ya mencionados?
Difficulty breathing or swallowing?	¿Dificultad respirando o tragando?
Swelling?	¿Hinchazón?
	¿Inflamación?
Do you have food allergies?	¿Tiene usted alergia a algún tipo de comida?
Are you allergic to . . .	¿Usted es alérgico/a a . . .
shellfish?	¿Mariscos?
nuts?	¿Nueces?
wheat?	¿Trigo?

Allergies

soy?	¿Soya?
eggs or poultry?	¿Huevos o pollo?
other foods?	¿Otros tipos de comida?
contrast dye?	¿Tintes de contraste?
Are you allergic to any animals?	¿Es usted alérgico/a a algún animal como?
Dogs?	¿Perros?
Cats?	¿Gatos?
Birds?	¿Pájaros?
Horses?	¿Caballos?
Sheep?	¿Ovejas?
Cows?	¿Reses (vacas y toros)?
Other animals?	¿Otros tipos de animales?
Which ones?	¿Cuáles?
Do you have hay fever?	¿Tiene usted fiebre del heno?
	¿Tiene usted **catarro anual de la nariz y de ojos**?
Have you had any skin tests done for the allergies?	¿Usted ha tenido exámenes de la piel para la alergia?
	¿Usted ha tenido **pruebas** de la piel para la alergia?

Family History

Has anyone in your family had . . .	¿Alguien en su familia ha tenido . . .
diabetes?	diabetes?
a heart attack?	ataque al corazón?
	ataque **cardíaco**?
heart disease?	enfermedad del corazón?
a stroke?	accidente cerebro vascular
	derrame cerebral?
	apoplejía?
high blood pressure?	alta presión?
cancer?	¿cáncer?
What kind?	¿Qué tipo?
Breast?	¿De senos?

Family History

Ovarian?	¿De ovario?
Colon?	¿De colon?
Prostate?	¿De próstata?
Skin?	¿De la piel?
mental illness?	enfermedad mental?
Depression?	¿Depresión?
Schizophrenia?	¿Esquizofrenia?
Bipolar disorder?	¿Desorden bipolar?
Psychosis?	¿Psicosis?
Anxiety?	¿Ansiedad
arthritis?	¿artritis?
asthma?	¿asma?
hemophilia?	¿hemofilia?
epilepsy?	¿epilepsia?
emphysema?	¿enfisema?
anemia?	¿anemia?
kidney disease?	¿enfermedad renal?
	¿enfermedad **de los riñones**?
tuberculosis?	¿tuberculosis?
alcoholism?	¿alcoholismo?
drug addiction?	¿adicción a drogas?
Who?	¿Quién?
Mother?	¿Madre?
Father?	¿Padre?
Sister?	¿Hermana?
Brother?	¿Hermano?
Grandmother?	¿Abuela?
Grandfather?	¿Abuelo?
Aunt?	¿Tía?
Uncle?	¿Tío?
What age were they when they . . .	¿Qué edad tenían cuando ellos . . .
were diagnosed?	fueron diagnosticados?
had their first event?	cuándo ellos tuvieron su primer acontecimiento?
died?	murieron?

Social History	Historial Social
Do you work?	¿Usted trabaja?
What kind of job?	¿Qué tipo de trabajo?
Desk job?	¿De escritorio?
Manual labor?	¿Labor manual?
Farm work?	¿Trabajo de granja?
	¿Trabajo de **finca**?
Migrant work?	¿Trabajo de migratorio?
	¿Trabajo de **paso**?
	¿Trabajo de **emigrante**?
Construction?	¿Trabajo de construcción?
Landscape work (yard work)?	¿Trabajo de jardinería (trabajo de patio)?
Janitorial services (cleaning)?	¿Trabajo de limpieza?
	¿Trabajo de **conserje**?
	¿Trabajo de **aseador**?
Factory work?	¿De factoría?
Food server?	¿De camarero/a?
	¿De **mesero/a**?
Taxi driver?	¿De taxista?
Bus driver?	¿De chofer de autobús?
Truck driver?	¿De camionero?
How many hours a day?	¿Cuántas horas al día?
How many days a week?	¿Cuántos días a la semana?
Have you ever worked around...	¿Usted a trabajado alguna vez con los siguientes...
pesticides?	pesticidas?
asbestos?	asbestos?
fumes or toxic chemicals?	vapores o químicos tóxicos?
coal?	carbón crudo?
loud noises?	ruidos fuertes?
	ruidos **estrepitosos**?
	ruidos **altos**?
Did you graduate high school?	¿Usted se graduó de escuela superior?
	¿Usted se graduó de un **instituto de enseñanza secundaria**?

Social History

What is the highest grade level you finished?	¿Cuál fue el nivel de escuela más alto que usted alcanzó? ¿Cuál fue el nivel de escuela más alto que usted **terminó**? ¿Cuál fue el nivel de escuela más alto que usted **acabó**? **¿Hasta qué grado de escuela usted llegó?**
Did you go to college?	¿Usted fue a la universidad?
Can you read and write Spanish?	¿Usted puede leer y escribir en español?
Are you married?	¿Está usted casado/a?
Divorced?	¿Divorciado/a?
Single?	¿Soltero/a?
Separated?	¿Separado/a?
Widowed?	¿Viudo/a?
Do you live in a house?	¿Vive usted en una casa?
Apartment?	¿Apartamento?
Boarding house?	¿Pensión?
Shelter?	¿Refugio para necesitados?
Do you live alone? Whom do you live with?	¿Vive usted solo? ¿Con quién usted vive?
Do you feel safe at home? Do you have problems with domestic violence?	¿Se siente usted seguro en su casa? ¿Tiene usted problemas de violencia doméstica?
Do you smoke?	¿Usted fuma?
Chew tobacco? How many cigarettes per day? For how many years? Have you ever quit? For how long (in days, weeks, months or years) Did you use a nicotine patch/gum/inhaler/nasal spray/medication to help you quit?	¿Masca tabaco? ¿Cuántos cigarrillos por/**al** día? ¿Por cuantos años? ¿Ha usted dejado de fumar alguna vez? ¿Por cuánto tiempo (en días, semanas, meses)? ¿Ha usted utilizado nicotina en parche/goma de mascar/inhalador/aerosol nasal/medicamentos para ayudarle a dejar de fumar?

Social History

	¿Ha usted **usado** nicotina en parche/ goma de mascar/inhalador/ aerosol nasal/**medicinas** para ayudarle a dejar de fumar?
Did it help?	¿Le ayudaron?
Do you want to quit now?	¿Usted quiere dejar de fumar hoy día?
Did you used to smoke?	¿Usted fumaba?
How many months/years ago did you quit?	¿Cuántos meses/años hace que usted dejó de fumar?
	¿Cuántos meses/años hace que usted **paro** de fumar?
Do you drink alcohol?	¿Usted toma alcohol?
	¿Usted **consume** alcohol?
	¿Usted **bebe** alcohol?
What kind (beer, wine, or hard liquor like whiskey, gin, or tequila)?	¿Qué tipo (cerveza, vino, licor fuerte como whisky, gin, tequila?
	¿Qué tipo (cerveza, vino, licor fuerte como: whisky, **ginebra**, tequila?
How much in a day/week/ month (bottles, cans, glasses, ounces, jiggers)?	¿Cuánto toma en un día, semana, mes (botellas, latas, onzas, un poquito)?
	¿Cuánto **consume** en un día, semana, mes (botellas, latas, onzas, un poquito)?
	¿Cuánto **bebe** en un día, semana, mes (botellas, latas, onzas, un poquito)?
Do you use any illegal/illicit drugs like cocaine, heroine, methamphetamines, or marijuana?	¿Utiliza drogas ilegales/ilícitas como: cocaína, heroína, metanfetaminas o marihuana?
	¿**Usa** drogas ilegales/ilícitas como cocaína, heroína, metanfetaminas o **mariguana**?
	¿**Usa** drogas ilegales/ilícitas como cocaína, heroína, metanfetaminas o **cannabis**?
	¿**Usa** drogas ilegales/ilícitas como: cocaína, heroína, metanfetaminas o **tabacón**?

Social History

	¿**Usa** drogas ilegales/ilícitas como cocaína, heroína, metanfetaminas o **yerba**?
Did you ever use these illegal/illicit drugs?	¿Usted alguna vez utilizó algunas de estas drogas ilegales/ilícitas ya mencionadas?
	¿Usted alguna vez **usó** algunas de estas drogas ilegales/ilícitas ya mencionadas?
Which ones?	¿Cuál de ellas?
For how many months/years?	¿Por cuantos meses/años?
How many days/weeks/months/years ago was the last time?	¿Cuántos días/semanas/meses/años fue la última vez?
Did you ever share needles?	¿Usted ha compartido agujas?
	¿Usted ha **intercambiado** agujas?
Are you in rehabilitation?	¿Está usted en rehabilitación?
Have you ever been in rehabilitation for drugs?	¿Ha estado/**sido parte** de un programa de rehabilitación?
How many times have you been in drug rehabilitation?	¿Cuántas veces ha estado/**sido parte** de un programa de rehabilitación?
Have you ever had tuberculosis?	¿Ha usted tenido tuberculosis?
Were you treated?	¿Fue usted tratado?
How many months was the treatment?	¿Por cuántos meses fue usted tratado?
Have you ever had a TB test?	¿Le han hecho alguna vez un examen de la piel para la tuberculosis?
	¿Le han hecho alguna vez una **prueba** de la piel para la tuberculosis?
Was it positive or negative?	¿La prueba fue positiva o negativa?
Have you ever had hepatitis?	¿Usted ha tenido hepatitis?
What kind (A/B/C)?	¿Qué tipo (A/B/C)?
Have you ever had a blood transfusion?	¿Ha usted alguna vez recibido sangre?
Do you have tattoos?	¿Tiene usted tatuajes?
What year did you get them?	¿En qué año se los puso?

Social History

Have you traveled to any countries outside the United States?	¿Ha viajado usted a otro país fuera de los Estados Unidos?
What year and where?	¿En qué año y donde?
What country?	¿Qué país?
Show me.	Enséñeme.
	Muéstreme.
Do you have pets (dog/cat/bird)?	¿Tiene usted animales domésticos (perro/gato/ave)?
What kind of pets?	¿Qué tipo de animal doméstico?
How many pets?	¿Cuántos animales domésticos?
Are they inside or outside pets?	¿Estos animales domésticos viven dentro o afuera de su casa?
Do you have . . .	¿Tiene usted . . .
Have you ever had . . .	¿Ha tenido alguna vez . . .
depression?	depresión?
bipolar disorder (manic depression)?	desorden bipolar (maniaco depresivo)?
schizophrenia?	esquizofrénico?
schizoaffective disorder?	desorden esquizoafectivo?
generalized anxiety disorder?	desorden de ansiedad generalizado?
panic disorder?	desorden de pánico?
psychosis?	psicosis?
Do you see a psychiatrist?	¿Se ve usted con un psiquiatra?
	¿**Va usted a** un psiquiatra?
Have you been treated in the past for depression?	¿Ha usted sido alguna vez tratado por depresión?
Do you have problems with depression now?	¿Tiene usted en este momento problemas de depresión?

Screening Tools

*Screening Questions for Depression**	*Pruebas para determinar depresión*
During the past month have you often felt depressed or hopeless?	¿Se ha sentido usted a menudo deprimido/a o sin esperanza, en el pasado mes?

*Ebell MH. (2004). Routine screening for depression, alcohol problems and domestic violence. *Am. Fam. Phys.* 69(10), 2421-2424.

Social History

During the past month have you often been bothered by little interest or pleasure in doing things?	¿En el pasado mes se ha sentido usted incomodo/a por no tener ánimo o sentir placer en hacer cosas que usted normalmente hace?

If yes to either, go to section on "Depressed Mood" in Chapter 5, "History of Present Illness for Common Symptoms."

*Screening Questions for Alcohol Abuse**	*Preguntas para determinar Abuso de Alcohol*
When was the last time you had more than four/five drinks in one day (women/men)?	¿Cuándo fue la última vez que usted tuvo cuatro/cinco tragos en un día (mujer/hombre)?
Never?	¿Nunca?
In the past three months?	¿En los pasados tres meses?
More than three months ago?	¿Hace más de tres meses?

If answered "in the past three months," consider more in-depth clinical history or CAGE questions.

*Screening Questions for Domestic Violence**	*Preguntas para determinar Violencia domestica*
Have you been hit, kicked, punched, or otherwise hurt by someone in the past year?	¿Le han pegado, pateado, golpeado o maltratado de otra manera por otra persona en el pasado año?
Do you feel safe in your current relationship?	¿Se siente usted segura en su relación actual?
Is there a partner from a previous relationship who is making you feel unsafe now?	¿Tiene usted algún compañero/a de una relación pasada el/la cual en estos momentos le está haciendo sentir inseguro/a? ¿Tiene usted algún compañero/a de una relación **previa** el/la cual en estos momentos le está haciendo sentir inseguro/a?

Sexual History

Are you sexually active?	¿Está usted sexualmente activo/a?
With one partner or more than one partner?	¿Con uno o más de un compañero?
With men?	¿Con hombres?
With women?	¿Con mujeres?
With both?	¿Con ambos?
How many sexual partners have you had in the past year?	¿Cuántos compañeros sexuales ha usted tenido en el pasado año?
How old were you when you first had sex?	¿Qué edad tenía usted cuando tuvo sexo por primera vez?
Do you have a history of sexually transmitted infections?	¿Tiene usted un historial de infecciones sexualmente transmitidas?
	¿**Ha tenido** infecciones sexualmente transmitidas?
	¿**Ha sufrido** de infecciones sexualmente transmitidas?
Syphilis?	¿Sífilis?
Gonorrhea?	¿Gonorrea?
HIV?	¿VIH (virus de inmunodeficiencia humana)?
Herpes?	¿Herpes?
Chlamydia?	¿Clamidia?
Were you treated?	¿Fue usted tratado?
Do you use condoms?	¿Usted utiliza preservativos?
	¿Usted **usa condones**?
Always?	¿Siempre?
Just sometimes?	¿De vez en cuando?
	¿**Algunas veces**?
	¿**A veces**?
Do you use other contraceptives?	¿Usted utiliza otros tipos de contraceptivos?
	¿Usted **usa** otros tipos de contraceptivos?
Pills?	¿Pastillas?
Patches?	¿Parchos?
Intrauterine device?	¿Dispositivos intrauterinos?
Shots?	¿Inyecciones?

Sexual History

Diaphragm?	¿Diafragmas?
Do you have pain with intercourse?	¿Tiene usted dolor al hacer el sexo?
Do you have vaginal intercourse?	¿Tiene usted sexo vaginal?
Do you have oral intercourse?	¿Tiene usted sexo oral?
Do you have anal intercourse?	¿Tiene usted sexo anal?
Do you have a sexual desire?	¿Tiene usted deseo sexual?
Same as before?	¿Igual que antes?
Decreased?	¿Menos?
Are you able to have an orgasm?	¿Puede usted llegar a tener un orgasmo?
	¿**Es capaz de** tener un orgasmo?
Do you have problems with erections?	¿Tiene usted problemas con sus erecciones?
Are you able to get an erection?	¿Puede usted tener una erección?
	¿**Es capaz de** tener una erección?
Sustain an erection to completion?	¿Puede usted sostener su erección hasta el final?
	¿**Es capaz de** sostener su erección hasta **que termine**?
Do you get erections in the night or early morning?	¿Puede usted tener erecciones en la noche o en la mañana?
	¿**Es capaz de** tener erecciones en la noche o en la mañana?
Are you able to ejaculate?	¿Puede usted eyacular?
	¿**Es capaz de** eyacular?

Chapter 8

Review of Systems

The review of systems (ROS) is considered the secondary history and involves asking specific questions targeted to augment the primary history (HPI). These questions are designed to assist you in formulating a differential diagnosis or judging the severity of an illness or disorder.

The ROS is a focused set of questions, organized generally from head to toe, by the major organ systems. In this chapter you will find a complete ROS in the order most commonly used in medical practice.

Use the complete ROS when taking an initial history or admitting a patient to the hospital, or while working up a new patient in an outpatient setting.

However, most often in clinical practice, you may only need the specific ROS questions related to the patient's chief complaint or active medical condition(s). For instance, in many cases when a patient presents with an acute problem, for example at the emergency room or in an urgent care setting, you may need to cover only one or two body systems. Likewise, with patients who present for management of chronic medical conditions whose status has changed, you may need to use one or more body systems targeting that particular disorder.

Constitutional

Do you have a fever, chills?	¿Tiene usted fiebre, escalofríos?
Have you had any sudden changes in weight?	¿Ha tenido usted cambios abruptos de peso?
	¿Ha tenido usted cambios **rápidos** de peso?
Do you have night sweats?	¿Tiene sudores nocturnos?
Have you had a decrease in appetite?	¿Le ha bajado su apetito?
Have you had an increase in appetite?	¿Le ha subido su apetito?
Do you have excessive fatigue?	¿Tiene usted fatiga excesiva?

Skin, Hair, Nails

Do you have any rashes?	¿Tiene usted erupción?
	¿Tiene usted **salpullido**?
	¿Tiene usted **pintas rojas en su piel**?
How long have you had it (weeks, months, years)?	¿Por cuánto tiempo ha tenido este problema (semanas, meses, años)?
Does it itch?	¿Le pican?
Is it red?	¿Son rojas?
Has it spread?	¿Se le han regado?
Did it spread rapidly?	¿Se le han regado rápido?
Did it spread gradually?	¿Se le han regado gradualmente?
	¿Se le han regado **despacio**?
Have you used any new . . .	¿Usted a utilizado algún . . .
	¿Usted a **usado** algún(a) . . .
soaps?	jabón nuevo?

Skin, Hair, Nails

detergents?	detergente nuevo?
deodorants?	desodorante nuevo?
lotions?	loción nueva?
Have you been working outside or in the yard?	¿Ha estado trabajando en el patio u otro lugar afuera?
Have you ever had poison ivy?	¿Usted ha sido expuesto/a a Hiedra venenosa?
	¿Usted ha sido expuesto a Zumaque venenoso?
Do you have problems with dandruff (flaking, itching in your scalp)?	¿Tiene usted problemas de caspa (con descamaciones o con picazón en su cabellara)?
	¿Tiene usted problemas de caspa (con descamaciones o con picazón en su **pelo**)?
What do you use for it?	¿Qué usted utiliza para este problema?
	¿Qué usted **usa** para este problema?
Does it work?	¿Le ha funciona?
Do you have a history of severe sunburns?	¿Tiene usted un historial de quemaduras de sol severas?
	¿**Ha tenido** quemaduras de sol severas?
	¿**Ha sufrido de** un historial de quemaduras de sol severas?
Do you bruise easily?	¿Usted se magulla fácilmente?
	¿Usted recive fácilmente?
Do you have any unusual moles or lesions that worry you?	¿Tiene lunares o lesiones que le preocupen?
Show me.	Enséñeme.
	Muéstreme.
How long have you had it (weeks, months, years)?	¿Por cuánto tiempo las ha tenido (semanas, meses, años)?
Has it changed shape, size, or color recently?	¿Han cambiado forma, tamaño o color recientemente?
Bigger?	¿Más grandes?
Smaller?	¿Más pequeños?
Has it gotten darker?	¿Se le han oscurecido?
Lighter?	¿Se han aclarado?

Skin, Hair, Nails

Do you have any abnormal nail growth?	¿Tiene usted algún crecimiento atípico en sus uñas? ¿Tiene usted algún crecimiento **irregular** en sus uñas? ¿Tiene usted algún crecimiento **anormal** en sus uñas?
Have you had any unusual changes in the color of your skin?	¿Ha tenido usted algún cambio atípico en el color de su piel? ¿Tiene usted algún cambio **irregular** en el color de su piel? ¿Tiene usted algún cambio **raro** en el color de su piel?
Darker/lighter than before?	¿Se le ha oscurecido o aclarado más que antes?
Show me.	Enséñeme. **Muéstreme.**
Do you have any abnormal hair growth?	¿Tiene usted algún crecimiento atípico en su piel? ¿Tiene usted algún crecimiento **irregular** en su piel? ¿Tiene usted algún crecimiento **anormal** en su piel?
Is it more than before?	¿Es más que antes?
Is it less than before?	¿Es menos que antes?
Have you ever had skin cancer?	¿Ha usted tenido cáncer de la piel anteriormente?
Has anyone in your family had skin cancer?	¿Ha tenido alguien en su familia cáncer de la piel?
Mother?	¿Madre?
Father?	¿Padre?
Sister?	¿Hermano?
Brother?	¿Hermano?

HEENT

Head

Do you have frequent or unusual headaches?	¿Tiene usted frecuentes o no muy comunes dolores de cabeza? ¿Tiene usted frecuentes o **fuera de lo normal** dolores de cabeza?
Show me where.	Enséñeme donde. **Muéstreme** donde.
Have you had a severe head injury?	¿Ha usted tenido algúna lesión en su cabeza? ¿Ha usted **sufrido** algún accidente en su cabeza?
Did you lose consciousness when you were injured?	¿Perdió usted el conocimiento cuando fue lesionado? **¿Perdió usted el conocimiento después del accidente?**
Do you have dizziness?	¿Padece usted de mareos **¿Tiene usted mareos?**
Do you lose consciousness?	¿Pierde usted el conocimiento?
Have you lost consciousness in the past 6 months?	¿Ha usted perdido el conocimiento en los pasados seis meses?
How many times?	¿Cuántas veces?

Eyes

Do you have blurred vision?	¿Tiene usted visión borrosa?
Double vision?	¿Doble visión?
Blind spots?	¿Puntos ciegos? ¿**Manchas** ciegas?
Are you able to read as clearly as before?	¿Puede usted leer tan claro como antes? ¿**Es capaz de** leer tan claro como antes?
Do you wear glasses?	¿Usa usted espejuelos? ¿Usa usted **anteojos**? ¿Usa usted **lentes**? ¿Usa usted **gafas**?

HEENT

Contact lenses?	¿Lentes de contacto?
Does the light hurt your eyes?	¿Le molesta la luz en sus ojos?
Do you have itchy or watery eyes?	¿Tiene usted picazón en sus ojos o ojos llorosos? ¿Tiene usted picazón en sus ojos o ojos **acuosos**?
Do you have eye pain?	¿Tiene usted dolor en sus ojos?
Do you have eye discharge? Is it clear? White? Yellow? Are your eyelids stuck together with discharge in the morning?	¿Tiene usted descargas de sus ojos? ¿Es clara? ¿Es blanca? ¿Es amarilla? ¿Están sus parpados pegados con descargas en la mañana?
Do you have glaucoma?	¿Tiene usted glaucoma?
Do you use eyedrops or medicines for your eyes?	¿Utiliza usted gotas o algún otro medicamento para sus ojos? ¿**Usa** usted gotas o alguna otra **medicina** para sus ojos?
Have you had trauma or injury to your eyes? Which one? Can you see out of that eye?	¿Ha usted tenido algúna lesión en sus ojos o se ha lesionado sus ojos? ¿Ha usted tenido algún **trauma** en sus ojos o se ha lesionado sus ojos? ¿Ha usted tenido algún **problema** en sus ojos o se ha lesionado sus ojos? ¿Ha usted tenido alguna **herida** en sus ojos o se ha lesionado sus ojos? ¿Ha usted tenido algún **daño** en sus ojos o se ha lesionado sus ojos? ¿Cuál ojo? ¿Puede usted ver por ese ojo?
How many months/years ago was your last eye exam?	¿Cuándo fue su último examen de ojos, meses/años? ¿Cuándo fue su última **prueba** de ojos, meses/años? ¿Cuándo fue su último **reconocimiento** de ojos, meses/años?

HEENT

Ears

Do you have ear pain?	¿Tiene usted dolor de oído?
Which ear?	¿Enséñeme cuál es el oído?
Inside?	¿Adentro?
Outside?	¿Afuera?
Do you have drainage from your ear?	¿Con o sin descarga?
	¿Con o sin **flujo?**
Is it bloody?	¿Es sangrienta?
	¿Es **sanguinolenta**?
Do you have problems hearing?	¿Tiene usted problemas oyendo?
	¿Tiene usted problemas **escuchando**?
Do you hear ringing in your ears?	¿Oye usted un zumbido en sus oídos?
	¿Oye usted **un campanilleo** en sus oídos?
	¿Oye usted **un repique** en sus oídos?
Sometimes?	¿De vez en cuando?
	¿Algunas veces?
	¿A veces?
Constant?	¿Constantemente?
Do you have vertigo?	¿Tiene usted vértigo?
Like things are spinning around you?	¿Como si todas las cosas alrededor suyas le dieran vueltas?

Nose

Do you have a stuffy nose?	¿Tiene usted su nariz tapada?
Do you have a runny nose?	¿Le está chorreando su nariz?
	¿Tiene su nariz mucho flujo?
Do you have a bloody nose?	¿Su nariz le está sangrando?
Frequently?	¿Frecuentemente?
	¿Amenudo?
Only occasionally?	¿Solo ocasionalmente?
	¿Solo **de vez en cuando**?
Are you able to smell things normally?	¿Puede usted oler normalmente?
	¿Es capaz de oler normalmente?
Do you sneeze a lot?	¿Usted estornuda mucho?

HEENT

Do you have sinus pain or pressure?	¿Tiene usted dolor con presión en sus senos nasales? ¿Tiene usted dolor con presión en **su frente**?
Do you have excessive phlegm at the back of your throat?	¿Tiene usted flema excesiva en la parte de atrás de su garganta?
Do you have to clear your throat more than usual?	Tiene usted que aclararse su garganta más amenudo?
Do you get frequent colds?	¿Se enferma usted a menudo con catarros? ¿Se enferma usted a menudo con **resfriados**? ¿Se enferma usted a menudo con **gripes**?

Mouth and Throat

Do you have tooth pain?	¿Tiene usted dolor en sus dientes? ¿Tiene usted dolor en sus **muelas**?
Do you have loose teeth?	¿Tiene usted dientes sueltos? ¿Tiene usted dientes **débiles**?
Do you have broken teeth?	¿Tiene usted dientes rotos?
Do you have crowns?	¿Tiene usted coronas dentales? ¿Tiene usted **cápsulas artificiales dentales**?
Do you have . . .	¿Tiene usted . . .
swelling in your gums?	hinchazón en sus encías? **inflamación** en sus encías?
pain in your gums?	dolor en sus encías?
bleeding in your gums?	está sangrando por sus encías?
Do you have problems with bad breath?	¿Tiene usted problemas de mal aliento?
Do you wear dentures?	¿Usted tiene o **se pone** dentaduras?
Do they fit well?	¿Están bien ajustadas o **le quedan** bien?
How many months/years ago was your last dental exam?	¿Cuándo fue su último examen dental meses/años? ¿Cuándo fue su última **prueba** dental, meses/años? ¿Cuándo fue su último **reconocimiento** dental, meses/años?

HEENT

Do you have frequent sore throats?	¿Tiene usted frecuentes dolores de garganta?
Do you have problems with hoarseness?	¿Tiene usted problemas de ronquera/ **carraspera/enronquecimiento**?
Do you have a painful tongue?	¿Tiene usted dolor en la lengua?
Do you have mouth ulcers?	**¿Tiene usted úlceras en la boca?**

Neck

Do you have neck pain or stiffness?	¿Tiene usted dolor o rigidez en su cuello?
Do you have lumps in your neck?	¿Tiene usted nódulos en su cuello? ¿Tiene usted **masas** en su cuello? ¿Tiene usted **chichones** en su cuello?
Do you have large or swollen glands?	¿Tiene usted glándulas grandes o inflamadas?
Have you ever had injury or trauma to your neck?	¿Ha usted tenido algún tipo de lesión o trauma en su cuello? ¿Ha usted tenido algún tipo de **problema** o trauma en su cuello? ¿Ha usted tenido algún tipo de **herida** o trauma en su cuello? ¿Ha usted tenido algún tipo de **daño** o trauma en su cuello?

Breasts

Do you have any breast lumps?	¿Tiene usted nódulos en sus senos? ¿Tiene usted **masas** en su **pecho**? ¿Tiene usted **chichones** en su **pecho**?
Which breast?	¿Cuál seno?
Show me.	Enséñeme. **Muéstreme.**
How many days/weeks/ months have you had it?	¿Cuántos días/semanas/ meses ha tenido estos/as?
Has it grown larger?	¿Le han crecido?
Have you ever had a breast biopsy?	¿Ha usted tenido alguna vez una biopsia en sus senos?

Breasts

Was it normal?	¿Fue normal?
Cancerous?	¿Cancerosa?
Do you have breast pain?	¿Tiene usted dolor de senos?
	¿Tiene usted dolor de **pecho**?
Show me where.	Enséñeme donde le duele.
	Muéstreme donde le duele.
Do you have any nipple discharge?	¿Tiene usted algún tipo de flujo?
Is it milky?	¿Es lechoso?
	¿Es **lacteo**?
Is it clear?	¿Es claro?
Is it white?	¿Es blanco?
Is it green?	¿Es verde?
Is it bloody?	¿Es sanguíneo?
How many days/weeks/months/ years have you had it?	¿Por cuantos días/semanas/meses/ años lo ha usted tenido?
Do you examine your breasts every month?	¿Se examina usted sus senos mensualmente?

(See "Breast Self-Exam" in Chapter 11, "Health Behaviors History and Education.")

Respiratory

Do you have lung problems?	¿Tiene usted problemas respiratorios?
What type?	¿De qué tipo?
Asthma?	¿Asma?
Since childhood?	¿Desde su niñez?
	¿Desde su **infancia**?
Emphysema?	¿Enfisema?
Chronic bronchitis?	¿Bronquitis crónica?
Do you smoke?	¿Usted fuma?
Did you used to smoke?	¿Usted fumaba?
Have you ever had tuberculosis?	¿Tuvo usted alguna vez tuberculosis?
When?	¿Cuándo?
How long were you treated?	¿Por cuánto tiempo le trataron?
Have you had pneumonia?	¿Ha tenido usted pulmonía?
When was the last time?	¿Cuándo fue la última vez?

Breasts

Do you have a cough?	¿Tiene usted tos?
How long have you had it?	¿Cuánto hace que la tiene?
Do you cough up sputum?	¿Tose usted esputo?
	¿Tose usted **flema**?
A lot or a little each time?	¿Mucho o un poco cada vez que tose?
Is it clear?	¿Es claro/a?
Is it white?	¿Es blanco/a?
Is it yellow?	¿Es amarillo/a?
Is it green?	¿Es verde?
Do you cough up blood?	¿Tose usted sangre?
Do you have night sweats?	¿Suda usted mucho en la noche?
	¿Suda usted **fuertemente** en la noche?
	¿Suda usted **pesadamente** en la noche?
Do you have any wheezing?	¿Respira usted con dificultad o tiene resuello asmático?
	¿Respira usted con dificultad o tiene **silbido** asmático?
Do you have difficulty breathing?	¿Tiene dificultad respirando?
Do you have pain when you breathe deeply?	¿Tiene usted dolor cuando respira profundo?
Where?	¿Dónde?
How long?	¿Cuánto tiempo?
How many weeks/months/years ago was your last chest x-ray?	¿Cuántos semanas/meses/años hace que usted se hizo una placa radiográfica o **rayos x**'s?
Was it normal?	¿Fue normal?

Cardiac

Do you have . . .	¿Tiene usted . . .
Have you ever had . . .	¿Ha tenido usted alguna vez . . .
high blood pressure?	hipertensión?
	alta presión?
heart disease?	enfermedades cardíacas?
	enfermedades **del corazón**?
a heart attack?	algún ataque al corazón?
	algún ataque **cardíaco**?
When?	¿Cuándo?
heart surgery?	cirugía cardiaca?
	cirugía **del corazón**?
bypass surgery?	alguna operación de desviación?
	alguna operación de **bypass**?
valve replacement?	re-emplazamiento de válvulas cardiacas?
heart failure?	insuficiencia cardíaca?
	falla cardíaca?
When was your last hospitalization or ER visit for your heart failure?	¿Cuándo fue su última hospitalización o visita a la sala de emergencia debido a su insuficiencia cardíaca?
	¿Cuándo fue su última hospitalización o visita a la sala de emergencia debido a su **falla cardíaca**?
rheumatic fever?	fiebre reumática?
heart murmur?	soplo cardíaco?
	soplo **en el corazón**?
Do you have chest pain?	¿Tiene usted dolor de pecho?
How long have you had chest pain (days/weeks/months/years)?	¿Por cuánto tiempo ha tenido dolor en el pecho (días/semanas/meses/años)?
Do you have chest pain now?	¿Tiene usted en este momento dolor de pecho?

(See "Chest Pain" in Chapter 5, "History of Present Illness for Common Symptoms.")

Cardiac

How many times a day/week/month?	¿Cuántas veces al día/semana/mes?
Do you get it with activity?	¿Le da con actividad?
How much activity?	¿Qué tanta actividad?
Walking one block?	¿Caminando un bloque?
	¿Caminando una **cuadra**?
	¿Caminando una **manzana**?
Walking one mile?	¿Caminando una milla?
Walking one flight of stairs?	¿Caminando una subida de escaleras?
At rest?	¿Mientras descansar?
When you lie down?	¿Cuándo se acostarse?
Show me where the pain starts.	Enséñeme donde le comienza al dolor.
	Muéstreme donde le comienza el dolor.
Does the pain stay there?	¿Le permanece ahí el dolor?
	¿Se le queda el dolor ahí?
Does the pain go to your . . .	¿El dolor se le riega hacia su . . .
	¿El dolor se le va al . . .
arm?	brazo?
back?	espalda?
shoulder?	hombro?
jaw?	quijada?
Show me where it goes.	¿Enséñeme hacia donde se le riega?
	Muéstreme a donde se le va.
How long does it last (seconds/minutes/hours)?	¿Cuánto tiempo le dura (segundos/minutos/horas)?
How would you describe the pain?	¿Como usted describiría su dolor?
Sharp?	Cortante?
	Agudo?
Dull?	Mate?
	Obtuso?
	Sordo?
Squeezing?	Apretado?
Pressure?	Presionado?
Aching?	Adolorido?
Tight?	Apretado?

Ripping?	Rasgante? **Rajante**?
Tearing?	Desgarrante?
Throbbing?	Pulsante?
Burning?	Ardiente?
With the chest pain, do you have . . .	¿Con dolor de pecho, tiene . . .
dizziness?	mareos?
nausea?	nauseas?
sweating?	sudores?
anxiety?	ansiedad?
difficulty breathing?	dificultad respirando?
Does the pain go away with . . .	¿Se le quita el dolor . . .
rest?	cuando descansa?
eating?	cuando come?
sitting up?	cuando se para?
antacids?	después de tomar antiácidos?
Do you use nitroglycerin (under the tongue)?	¿Utiliza usted nitroglicerina (la pastilla que se pone abajo de la lengua)? ¿**Usa** usted nitroglicerina (la pastilla que se pone abajo de la lengua)?
How many times a day/week/month?	¿Cuántas veces al día/semana/mes?
Is that more or less than before?	¿La utiliza más o menos que antes?
How many blocks/miles/flights of stairs do you usually walk?	¿Cuántos bloques/millas/subidas de escaleras camina usualmente? ¿Cuántas **cuadras**/millas/subidas de escaleras camina usualmente? ¿Cuántos bloques/**manzanas**/millas, y subidas de escaleras camina usualmente?
How many pillows do you use under your head when you sleep?	¿Cuántas almohadas usted utiliza debajo de su cabeza al dormir? ¿Cuántas almohadas usted **usa** debajo de su cabeza al dormir? ¿Cuántas almohadas usted se **pone** debajo de su cabeza al dormir?
Can you breathe normally lying flat?	¿Usted puede respirar normalmente cuando está totalmente acostado?

Cardiac

Do you have difficulty breathing at night?	¿Usted tiene dificultad respirando por la noche?
Do you have swelling in your legs?	¿Usted tiene hinchazón en las piernas?
	¿Usted tiene **las piernas hinchadas**?
For how long?	¿Qué tiempo hace que están así?
Is it more or less than usual?	¿Es más o menos de lo usual?
	¿Es más o menos de lo **corriente**?
	¿Es más o menos de lo **normal**?
Do you have difficulty breathing when walking?	¿Usted tiene dificultad respirando cuando camina?
How far can you walk before you have difficulty breathing?	¿Qué tan lejos usted puede caminar antes de sentir dificultad al respirar?
Do you have any fainting or dizziness?	¿Ha sentido usted que se va a desmayar o está mareado(a)?
Do you have any palpitations?	¿Tiene usted palpitaciones?
How many seconds/minutes do they last?	¿Cuántos segundos/minutos le duran?
Have you had an ECG this year?	¿Le han hecho un electrocardiograma este año?
Have you ever had a stress test for your heart?	¿Ha tenido un examen de estrés del corazón?
	¿Ha tenido **una prueba** de estrés del corazón?
On a treadmill?	¿En una maquina de andar o correr estática?
	¿En una maquina de andar o correr?
	¿En una **caminadora**?
Was it normal?	¿Fue normal?
Was it abnormal?	¿Fue atípico?
	¿Fue **irregular**?
	¿Fue **anormal**?

Gastrointestinal

Do you have difficulty or pain with swallowing?	¿Tiene usted dificultad o dolor al tragar?
With solids?	¿Al tragar algo solido?
With liquids?	¿Al tragar algo liquido?
With pills?	¿Al tragar pastillas?
Do you feel that something is stuck in your throat?	¿Siente usted como si tuviera algo atorado en su garganta?
	¿Siente usted como si tuviera algo **hincándole** en su garganta?
Do you have heartburn?	¿Tiene usted acidez estomacal?
Does your food come back up into your throat?	¿Se le devuelve la comida a su garganta?
	¿Se le **regresa** la comida a su garganta?
Do you get an acid taste in your mouth?	¿Tiene sabor a ácido en su boca?
Do you have nausea?	¿Usted tiene nauseas?
Vomiting?	¿Ha vomitado?
Is it green?	¿Es verde?
Is it yellow?	¿Es amarillo?
Is it bloody?	¿Contiene sangre?
	¿Está sangrante?
	¿Está sanguinolento?
Is it like coffee grounds?	¿Es como granos de café?
Is it clear?	¿Es claro?
Does it contain solids?	¿Es solido?
Does it smell like stool?	¿Huele a heces?
	¿Huele a **excremento**?
	¿Huele a **material fecal**?
	¿Huele a **deshecho fecal**?
Are you vomiting blood?	¿A vomitado sangre?
	¿A **arrojado** sangre?
Is it bright red?	¿Es rojo vivo?
Is it dark like coffee grounds?	¿Es oscuro como granos de café?

Gastrointestinal

Do you have diarrhea?	¿Tiene diarrea?
Are your stools well formed?	¿Sus heces están bien formadas? ¿Su **excreta** está bien formada? ¿Su **excremento** está bien formado? ¿Su **material fecal** está bien formado?
Hard?	¿Duro?
Loose like water?	¿Está(n) suelto/a como agua?
Are you constipated?	¿Está constipado? ¿Está **estreñido**?
Do you have to strain to pass stool?	¿Tiene problemas para defecar? ¿Tiene problemas para **ensuciar**? ¿Tiene problemas para **ir al baño**?
How many times have you passed stool in the past day/week?	¿Cuántas veces a defecado en el pasado día/semana? ¿Cuántas veces a **ensuciado** en el pasado día/semana? ¿Cuántas veces a **ido al baño** en el pasado día/semana?
When was your last bowel movement?	¿Cuándo fue la última vez que usted defecó? ¿Cuándo fue la última vez que usted **ensució**? ¿Cuándo fue la última vez que usted **fue al baño**?
How many times a week do you have a bowel movement?	¿Cuántas veces a la semana usted defeca? ¿Cuántas veces a la semana usted **ensucia**? ¿Cuántas veces a la semana usted **va al baño**?
Are your stools brown?	¿Son sus heces café? ¿Es su **excreta marrón**? ¿Es su **excremento brown**?
Clay colored?	¿Es/son de color lodo?
Yellow?	¿Es/son amarillo/a(s)?
Black?	¿Es/son negro/a(s)?
Green?	¿Es/son verde(s)?

Gastrointestinal

Do you have blood in your stools?	¿Tiene usted sangre en sus heces? ¿Tiene usted sangre en su **excreta**? ¿Tiene usted sangre en su **excremento**?
Do you have any black, sticky stools like tar?	¿Están sus heces negras o pegajosas como tar? ¿Está su **excremento** negro o pegajoso como **alquitrán**? ¿Está su **excreta** negra o pegajosa como **brea**?
Do you have problems with leaking stool?	¿Tiene usted algún problema con sus heces saliéndosele sin que usted quiera? ¿Tiene usted algún problema con su **excremento chorreándosele** sin que usted quiera? ¿Tiene usted algún problema con su **excreta** saliéndosele sin que usted quiera?
Do you have pain with defecation?	¿Tiene usted dolor al defecar?
Do you have hemorrhoids?	¿Tiene usted hemorroides?
Do you use laxatives? Every day? More than 3 times a week?	¿Utiliza laxantes? ¿**Usa** laxantes? ¿Todos los días? ¿Más de tres veces a la semana?
Do you have abdominal pain or swelling? Point to where the pain is. Does the pain stay there? Does it go anywhere? Point to where it goes. Is it associated with eating?	¿Tiene usted dolor abdominal o hinchazón? ¿Tiene usted dolor **de barriga** o **inflamación**? Enséñeme donde le duele. **Muéstreme** donde le duele. ¿El dolor se le queda ahí? ¿Se le va a otro lado? Enséñeme a donde se le va. Muéstreme a donde se le **pasa**. ¿El dolor está relacionado con comer? **¿Al comer le duele?**

Gastrointestinal

Does it happen before meals?	¿Le duele antes de comer?
During meals?	¿Cuándo come?
After meals?	¿Después de comer?
Is your appetite normal?	¿Su apetito está normal?
Decreased?	¿Reducido? ¿**Bajo**? ¿**Disminuido**? ¿**Pobre**?
Increased?	¿Aumentado?
Are you eating 3 meals a day?	¿Está usted comiendo tres comidas al día?
Are you passing gas normally?	¿Está usted pasando gases normalmente? ¿Está usted pasando **gas por abajo** normalmente?
Do you have more gas than usual?	¿Tiene más gas de lo usual? ¿Tiene más gas de lo **corriente**? ¿Tiene más gas de lo **normal**?
Do you have gallstones?	¿Tiene piedras en la vesícula?
Have you had your gallbladder removed?	¿Le han quitado su vesícula?
Have you had hepatitis? Which type (A/B/C)?	¿Ha tenido hepatitis? ¿Cuál tipo (A/B/C)?
Do you have yellow skin or eyes?	¿Su piel u ojos están amarillo/a(s)?
Have you ever had stomach ulcers?	¿Ha usted tenido alguna vez úlceras estomacales?
Do you have generalized itching?	¿Tiene usted picazón por todas partes?
What color is your urine?	¿De qué color es su orina?

Genitourinary

Do you urinate more often than usual?	¿Está usted orinando más a menudo de lo usual?
	¿Está usted orinando más a menudo de lo **corriente**?
	¿Está usted orinando más a menudo de lo **normal**?
How much urine each time?	¿Cuánto orina usted orina cada vez que va al baño?
A lot?	¿Mucha?
A little?	¿Poco?
Do you have pain or burning with urination?	¿Tiene usted dolor o quemazón cuando orina?
Does your urine smell bad?	¿Su orina huele mal?
Do you have blood in your urine?	¿Tiene usted sangre en la orina?
Do you have abdominal pain?	¿Tiene dolor abdominal?
	¿Tiene dolor **de barriga**?
Point to where the pain is.	Enséñeme donde le duele.
	Muéstreme donde le duele.
Do you have a sense of urgency to urinate?	¿Siente usted una necesidad de urgencia para orinar?
	¿Ir al baño?
Do you have trouble with leaking urine or controlling urination?	¿Tiene usted problemas con su orina, la cual se le sale o chorrea sin querer o controlando su orine?
When you cough or sneeze?	¿Cuándo tose o estornuda?
Do you have the urge to go before you leak?	¿Siente usted urgencia de orinar antes de que le empiece a salir o chorrear su orina?
Do you feel the urge but are unable to get to the bathroom in time?	¿Tiene usted urgencia de orinar pero no es capaz de llegar a tiempo?
Have you ever had kidney stones?	¿Ha tenido piedras en los riñones?
How many months/years ago was the last time?	¿Hace cuántos meses/años fue la última vez?
Do you have a history of frequent bladder or kidney infections?	¿Tiene un historial de infecciones de vejiga o riñones?
	¿**Ha tenido** infecciones de vejiga o riñones?

Genitourinary

	¿**Ha sufrido de** infecciones de vejiga o riñones?
How many times?	¿Cuántas veces?

Female

What age did you begin having periods?	¿A qué edad comenzó su menstruación?
	¿A qué edad comenzó su **período**?
Do you still have periods?	¿Todavía tiene la menstruación?
	¿Todavía tiene **períodos**?
What age did you stop having periods?	¿A qué edad usted dejo de menstruar?
	¿A qué edad usted dejo de tener **períodos**?
Do you have hot flashes?	¿Tiene usted momentos repentinos de mucho calor?
Frequently?	¿Frecuentemente?
Occasionally?	¿Ocasionalmente?
	¿**De vez en cuando**?
Are you taking hormones?	¿Está tomando hormonas?
How many years have you been taking hormones?	¿Por cuántos años ha estado tomando hormonas?
How many days ago was your last period?	¿Hace cuantos días fue su última menstruación?
	¿Hace cuantos días fue su último **período**?
Are they regular?	¿Son regulares?
How many days does the bleeding last?	¿Cuántos días sangra usted durante su menstruación?
How many days between periods?	¿Cuántos días entre períodos?
At what age was your first period?	¿Cuántos días entre menstruaciónes?
How much bleeding?	¿Qué tanto sangra usted durante su período?
A lot?	¿Mucho?
A little?	¿Poco?

How many tampons or pads do you use in a day?	¿Cuántas toallas sanitarias o tampones usted utiliza en un día?
	¿Cuántas toallas sanitarias o tampones usted **usa** en un día?
	¿Cuántas toallas sanitarias o tampones usted se **pone** en un día?
Are your periods very painful?	¿Su menstruación es muy dolorosa?
	¿**Su período** es muy doloroso?
Do you have any vaginal bleeding?	¿Está usted sangrando por la vagina?
Between periods?	¿Entre menstruaciónes?
	¿Entre **períodos**?
How much bleeding?	¿Cuánto sangra?
A lot?	¿Mucho?
A little?	¿Poco?
Do you have vaginal bleeding after intercourse?	¿Tiene sangrado vaginal después de tener relaciones?
Do you have vaginal discharge?	¿Tiene usted descargas o **flujos** vaginales?
What color is it?	¿De qué color son?
Does it have a bad odor?	¿Tienen mal olor?
Do you have vaginal itching?	¿Tiene usted picazón vaginal?
Do you have vaginal sores or lumps?	¿Tiene usted llagas o **nudos** en su vagina?
	¿Tiene usted **ampollas** o **bultos** en su vagina?
	¿Tiene usted **ampollas** o **chichones** en su vagina?
	¿Tiene usted **ampollas** o **masas** en su vagina?
Does it feel like your uterus is falling out of place?	¿Siente que su útero se le está cayendo fuera de su lugar?
	¿Siente que su útero se le está **saliendo** fuera de su lugar?
Have you ever had a sexually transmitted disease?	¿Ha tenido usted alguna vez una enfermedad sexualmente trasmitida?
Which kind?	¿Qué tipo?
Syphilis?	¿Sífilis?
Gonorrhea?	¿Gonorrea?
Chlamydia?	¿Clamidia?
Herpes?	¿Herpes?

Genitourinary

Genital warts?	¿Verrugas genitales?
HIV?	¿VIH?
Pregnancies	*Embarazos*
Have you ever been pregnant?	¿Ha estado embarazada alguna vez? ¿Ha estado **encinta** alguna vez?
How many times?	¿Cuántas veces?
How many times did you deliver?	¿Cuántas veces a dado a luz?
How many were vaginal deliveries?	¿Cuántos de estos han sido partos naturales?
How many were cesarean?	¿Cuántos de estos han sido por cesárea?
Any twins?	¿Ha tenido gemelos?
Triplets?	¿Trillizos?
More?	¿Más de trillizos?
Any breech?	¿Ha tenido un parto en el cual el bebé salió de nalgas?
How many children are living?	¿Cuántos niños están vivos?
Did you have any stillbirths?	¿Ha tenido partos en los cuales el niño no se logro? ¿Ha tenido partos en los cuales el niño no **sobrevivió**?
Did you have any miscarriages?	¿Tuvo algún aborto espontaneo?
Abortions?	¿Abortos en general?
Tubal pregnancies?	¿Embarazos ectópicos?

Male

How many times do you get up to urinate at night?	¿Cuántas veces por la noche usted se levanta a orinar?
Does it take a long time to start urinating?	¿Se tarda usted mucho para empezar a orinar?
Do you have trouble with dribbling?	¿Tiene usted problemas goteándosele su orina?
Do you have a weak stream of urine?	¿Al orinar, su orina sale con poca fuerza?
Do you have any hernias?	¿Tiene alguna hernia?
Show me where.	Enséñeme dónde. **Muéstreme** dónde.
For how long?	¿Por cuánto tiempo?

Genitourinary

Do you have penile sores or discharge?	¿Tiene algún dolor en el pene o descarga?
For how long (days, weeks, months)?	¿Por cuánto tiempo (días, semanas, meses)?
Have you had unprotected sex recently (without a condom)?	¿Ha tenido sexo sin protección últimamente (sin condón)?
	¿Ha tenido sexo sin protección últimamente (sin **preservativo**)?
	¿Ha tenido sexo sin protección últimamente (sin **profiláctico**)?
Does your partner have the same symptoms?	¿Tiene su compañero/a los mismos síntomas?
	¿Tiene su **pareja** los mismos síntomas?
	¿Tiene su **cónyuge** los mismos síntomas?
Do you have any testicular pain or masses?	¿Tiene dolor testicular o masas?
	¿Tiene dolor testicular o **nudos**?
	¿Tiene dolor testicular o **chichones**?

Peripheral Vascular

Do you get pain in your calves with walking?	¿Tiene usted dolor en sus pantorrillas cuando camina?
Is it an ache or cramp?	¿Las tiene adoloridas o siente calambre?
Show me where you get it.	Enséñeme donde le da.
	Muéstreme donde le da.
Does it go away when you stop?	¿Se le va el dolor o el calambre cuando usted se para?
How many minutes does it take to go away?	¿Cuántos minutos le toma antes de que esto suceda?
How far can you walk before you get the pain?	¿Qué tan lejos puede caminar antes de que le dé el dolor?
One block?	¿Un bloque . . . ?
	¿Una cuadra . . . ?
	¿Una manzana. . . ?
Do you get the same pain at rest?	¿Le da el mismo dolor cuando está descansando?

Genitourinary

Are your feet cold all the time?	¿Siente sus pies fríos todo el tiempo?
Do your feet or toes ever turn blue?	¿Se le han puesto sus pies o dedos de color azúl?
Have you ever had a blood clot in the veins in your legs, arms, or lungs?	¿Ha tenido alguna vez un coágulo sanguíneo en las venas de las piernas, brazos o pulmones?
Do you have varicose veins?	¿Tiene venas varicosas?
Do you smoke?	¿Usted fuma?
How many cigarettes/packs a day?	¿Cuántos cigarrillos o cajetillas al día?
	¿Cuántos cigarros o **paquetes** al día?
For how many years?	¿Por cuántos años?

Musculoskeletal

Do you have pain in your joints?	¿Tiene usted dolor en sus articulaciones?
Show me which joints.	Enséñeme cuales articulaciones.
	Muéstreme cuales articulaciones.
For how long?	¿Por cuánto tiempo?
Do you have swollen or red joints?	¿Tiene usted articulaciones hinchadas o rojas?
Do you have joint stiffness?	¿Tiene usted rigidez en las articulaciones?
Is it worse or better in the mornings?	¿Empeora o mejora en las mañanas?
Evenings?	¿En la tarde?
Does the stiffness get better with movement?	¿Siente que la rigidez mejora con movimiento?
Is it worse after sitting for a long time?	¿Siente que empeora después de haber estado sentado por largo tiempo?
Do you have any restriction of motion in your joints?	¿Tiene usted alguna restricción de movimiento en sus articulaciones?
Show me which one.	Enséñeme en cual.
	Muéstreme en cual.
Show me how far you can move it.	Enséñeme que tanto puede mover su articulación.
	Muéstreme que tanto puede mover su articulación.

Musculoskeletal

Have you ever had gout?	¿Ha tenido alguna vez gota?
How long ago was your last attack (weeks, months)?	¿Hace cuanto tiempo sufrió su último ataque (semanas, meses)?
Do you have muscle pain?	¿Tiene usted dolor muscular?
Is it constant or does it come and go?	¿Es constante o le va y viene?
What medicines do you take for the pain?	¿Qué medicamentes está tomando para el dolor?
	¿Qué **medicinas** está tomando para el dolor?
Have you ever had an injury or an accident in that area?	¿Ha sufrido alguna vez de una lesión o accidente en esa área?
	¿Ha sufrido alguna vez de **trauma** o accidente en esa área?
	¿Ha sufrido alguna vez de un **problema** o accidente en esa área?
	¿Ha sufrido alguna vez de una **herida** o accidente en esa área?
	¿Ha sufrido alguna vez de un **daño** o accidente en esa área?
Has the color of your fingers or toes changed in color to blue?	Le ha cambiado el color de los dedos de sus pies o manos a azul?
Purple?	¿Morado?
Black?	¿Negro?
Do you have cold fingers or toes?	¿Siente usted los dedos de sus manos de sus pies fríos?
	¿Siente usted los dedos sus manos y de sus pies **congelados**?

Neurologic

Do you have problems with fainting?	¿Tiene usted problemas de desmayos?
Do you have seizures?	¿Padece usted de convulsiones?
How many years have you had seizures?	¿Por cuantos años ha tenido convulsiones?
How long ago was your last seizure (months/years)?	¿Hace cuando tiempo fue su última convulsión (meses/años)?
Do you have blackouts?	¿Padece usted de desmayos?
Do you have tremors?	¿Tiene usted temblores?
Where?	¿Dónde?
How long have you had them (months/years)?	¿Por cuanto tiempo los ha tenido (meses/años)?
Do you have a tremor when resting?	¿Tiene usted temblores cuando descansa?
Just when you are active?	¿Solamente cuando está activo/a?
	¿Cuando **no está sedentario**?
All the time?	¿Todo el tiempo?
Do you have weakness or paralysis in your arms or legs?	¿Tiene usted debilidad o parálisis en sus brazos o piernas?
Do you have trouble with coordination?	¿Tiene problemas de coordinación?
Are you able to move your arms and legs normally?	¿Puede usted normalmente mover sus brazos y piernas?
	¿**Es capaz de** normalmente mover sus brazos y piernas?
Do you have numbness or tingling?	¿Tiene usted adormecimiento o cosquilleo?

Hematologic

Do you have anemia (low red blood cells)?	¿Tiene usted anemia (baja en glóbulos rojos)?
Do you have a bleeding disorder (like hemophilia)?	¿Tiene usted problemas de sangrado (como hemofilia)?
Do you bruise easily?	¿Se magulla con facilidad?
	¿Se le hacen **moretones** con facilidad?

Hematologic

Do you bleed easily (more than normal)?	¿Sangra usted con facilidad (más de lo normal)? ¿Sangra usted con facilidad (**más de lo común**)?
Do you have problems with getting cuts to stop bleeding?	¿Tiene usted problemas al cortarse para parar de sangrar?
Do you have problems with bleeding gums?	¿Tiene usted problemas en los cuales le sangran las encías?
Have you ever had a blood transfusion?	¿Ha tenido usted alguna vez una transfusión sanguínea?
How many times?	¿Cuántas veces?
Did you ever have a bad reaction to the transfusion?	¿Tuvo alguna vez una reacción adversa a una transfusión? ¿Tuvo alguna vez una reacción **mala** a una transfusión? ¿Tuvo alguna vez una reacción **dañina** a una transfusión? ¿Tuvo alguna vez una reacción **no favorable** a una transfusión?
Do you have any large or swollen lymph glands?	¿Tiene usted crecimiento o inflamación de glándulas linfáticas?
Show me where.	Enséñeme dónde. **Muéstreme** dónde.
How long have they been large?	¿Cuánto tiempo hace que las tiene agrandadas?
Did it come on suddenly?	¿Aparecieron de repente?
Did it come on gradually?	¿Aparecieron gradualmente? ¿Aparecieron de repente o **despacio**?
Is it painful?	¿Son dolorosas?

Endocrine

Do you have thyroid problems?	¿Tiene usted problemas de tiroides?
Is your thyroid too slow?	¿Está su tiroide lenta?
Is your thyroid too fast?	¿Está su tiroide rápida?
Do you have a goiter (large thyroid gland)?	¿Tiene usted bocio (crecimiento de la glándula tiroidea)?
Are you hot all the time?	¿Se siente usted caliente todo el tiempo?
Are you cold all the time?	¿Se siente usted frió/a todo el tiempo?
Have you had any changes in your skin or hair recently?	¿Ha tenido usted algunos cambios en su piel o pelo recientemente?
Are you losing your hair?	¿Está usted perdiendo su pelo?
All over or in patches?	¿Por todos lados o en forma de parches?
For how long?	¿Por cuánto tiempo?
Suddenly?	¿De repente?
Gradually?	¿Gradualmente?
	¿**Despacio**?
Have you had any changes in the size of your hat or gloves (head or hands)?	¿Ha tenido cambios en el tamaño de sus sombrero o guantes (de su cabeza o manos) respectivamente?
Have they gotten bigger?	¿Le han crecido en tamaño su cabeza o manos?
Have they gotten smaller?	¿Le ha disminuido el tamaño su cabeza o manos?
	¿Le ha **bajado** el tamaño su cabeza o manos?
Do you have excessive thirst?	¿Tiene usted sed excesiva?
	¿Tiene usted **mucha sed**?
Do you have excessive hunger?	¿Tiene apetito excesivo?
	¿Tiene usted mucho apetito?
Do you have excessive urination?	¿Está orinando mucho?
	¿Está orinando **en exceso**?
Do you have excessive sweating?	¿Está usted sudando excesivamente?
	¿Está usted sudando **mucho**?
Have you had any sudden weight loss or gain that was unintentional?	¿Ha tenido alguna vez perdida o aumento repentino de peso adquirido sin intención?

Psychiatric

Do you have problems with depression?	¿Tiene usted problemas de depresión?
(If yes, see "Screening Questions for Depression" in Chapter 7, "Comprehensive Adult History.")	
Have you ever been treated for depression?	¿Ha sido tratado por depresión?
Do you have frequent mood changes?	¿Tiene usted cambios de humor con frecuencia?
	¿Tiene usted cambios **de su carácter** con frecuencia?
	¿Tiene usted cambios de **disposición** con frecuencia?
Do you have difficulty concentrating or completing a task from start to finish?	¿Tiene usted dificultad para concentrarse o para completar un trabajo de principio a fin?
	¿Tiene usted dificultad para concentrarse o para **terminar** un trabajo de principio a fin?
Are you able to remember most things well?	¿Puede usted recordar bien la mayor parte de las cosas?
	¿**Es capaz de** recordar bien la mayor parte de las cosas?
Do you sleep well?	¿Duerme usted bien?
Too much?	¿Demasiado?
Too little?	¿Muy poco?
How many hours a night do you sleep total?	¿Cuántas horas en total duerme cada noche?
Do you feel nervous most of the time?	¿Se siente usted nervioso/a la mayor parte del tiempo?
Do you feel anxious most of the time?	¿Se siente usted ansioso/a la mayor parte del tiempo?
Have you ever been treated for anxiety?	¿Alguna vez recibió tratamiento para la ansiedad?
Do you feel irritable frequently?	¿Se siente frecuentemente irritable?
Do you have thoughts of wanting to hurt or kill yourself or others?	¿Tiene usted pensamientos de herirse o matarse al igual que a otras personas?
	¿Tiene usted pensamientos de quererse **hacer daño** o matarse al igual que a otras personas?

Psychiatric

Do you have a plan?	¿Tiene usted un plan para hacer esto?
Do you have a way to carry out your plan?	¿Tiene alguna manera de llevar a cabo su plan?
Do you think you might try?	¿Piensa usted intentarlo?
Have you ever tried to kill yourself?	¿Ha tratado usted de matarse?

Chapter 9

Physical Exam

Unlike most of the other chapters, this chapter on physical exam contains mostly commands for body positioning, as well as instructions to patients for the purpose of specific testing and explanations as to what to expect with specific exams or maneuvers. This section will be quite useful to many people during the patient encounter, including the health care provider during the actual physical exam, nurses and medical assistants preparing patients for specific exams (e.g., gynecologic), and radiology technicians positioning patients for testing.

Each section is organized by body system and is fairly self-explanatory. In addition, several yes/no questions are included when the specific examination requires a patient response.

General

Please remove all your clothes (except your underwear) and put on this gown.	Por favor quítese toda su ropa (excepto su ropa interior) y póngase esta vata. Por favor quítese toda su ropa (**salvo** su ropa interior) y póngase esta vata.
Please remove your shoes and socks.	Por favor quítese sus medias y zapatos.
Sit down.	Siéntese.
Lie down.	Acuéstese.
Turn around.	Vírese. **Dese la vuelta.**
Sit up.	Siéntese derecho.
Stand up.	Párese.
Bend over.	Inclínese hacia el frente.

HEENT

Look straight ahead.	Mire hacia el frente.
Do not move your eyes.	No mueva sus ojos.
Open your eyes wide.	Habra bien sus ojos.
Do not move your head.	No mueva su cabeza.
Look up with your eyes only.	Mire hacia arriba solo con sus ojos.
Look down.	Mire hacia abajo.
Look side to side.	Mire de lado a lado.
Do not close your eyes.	No cierre sus ojos.
You will feel a puff of air. Try not to blink.	Usted va a sentir un soplido de aire en su ojo. Por favor trate de no pestañear. Usted va a sentir un soplido de aire en su ojo. Por favor trate de no **parpadear**.
Are you able to read?	Puede usted leer.

HEENT

Do you wear glasses?	¿Usted usa lentes? ¿Usted usa **espejuelos**? ¿Usted usa **anteojos**? ¿Usted usa **gafas**?
Do you have them with you?	¿Las/los tiene con usted?
Please put them on.	Por favor pongáselas/los.
Please read aloud this line of letters.	Por favor lea en alta voz las siguientes letras.
I am going to show you some letters.	Le voy a enseñar unas letras.
Please tell me which one is easier (clearer) to read.	Por favor dígame cuales de ellas son más fáciles para usted de leer o las ve más claras.
One or two?	¿Uno o dos?
Three or four?	¿Tres o cuatro?
Can you hear this?	¿Puede oír esto?
Repeat what you hear me whisper. One, two, three *(whispered)*.	Repita lo que yo le diga en voz baja. Uno, dos, tres.
Open your mouth.	Habra su boca.
Stick out your tongue.	Saque su lengua.
Say "Ah."	Diga "aaaaaaa."
Lift up your tongue.	Alce su lengua. **Suba** su lengua.
Swallow.	Trague.

Cardiorespiratory Exam

Breathe deeply. With your mouth open.	Respire hondo. Respire **profundamente**. Con su boca abierta.
Breathe softly.	Respire suave.
Inhale.	Inhale. **Aspire.**
Exhale.	Exhale. **Espire.**
Again.	Otra vez.
Hold your breath.	Aguante su respiracion.

Cardiorespiratory Exam

Cough.	Tosa.
Say "EEE."	Diga "iiii"
Say "99."	Diga "99"
Don't talk please.	Por favor, no hable.

Abdominal Exam

Lie on your back.	Recuéstese con la espalda hacia la cama.
Bend your knees.	Doble sus rodillas
Relax your stomach.	Relaje su estomago.
Does it hurt more when I press? Or when I let go?	¿Le duele más al presionarle? ¿O cuándo quito la mano y no presiono?
Take a deep breath.	Respire hondo.
Exhale.	Exhale. **Espire.**
Raise your head.	Levante su cabeza.
Keep your knees straight.	No doble sus rodillas, manténgalas derecha. No doble sus rodillas, manténgalas **rectas**.
Lie on your stomach. Turn over.	Virese boca abajo. Virese or dese la vuelta or voltease.
Turn on your side.	Virese de lado.
Face the wall.	Mire hacia la pared.
I need to do a rectal exam.	Necesito hacerle un examen rectal. Necesito hacerle **una prueba** rectal.
I'm going to insert one finger in your rectum.	Le voy a introducir un dedo en su recto. Le voy a **poner** un dedo en su **ano**.
Please relax as much as possible.	Por favor relajese lo más que pueda (**lo más posible**). Por favor relajese lo más posible.
Bear down like you are straining to defecate.	Empuje como si estuviera defecando. Empuje como si estuviera **ensuciando**.

Neurologic Exam

Cranial Nerves

Look straight ahead.	Mire hacia el frente.
Do not move your eyes.	No mueva sus ojos.
Say "Yes" when you see my finger.	Díga "Si" cuando vea mi dedo.
Follow my finger with just your eyes. Do not move your head.	Siga mi dedo solamente con sus ojos no con su cabeza. Por favor no mueva su cabeza.
Look up and to the right/left.	Mire hacia arriba y a su derecha/izquierda.
Can you feel this?	Puede sentir esto?
Tell me if this feels sharp or dull.	Dígame si esto se siente agudo o sordo. Dígame si esto se siente **cortante** o **mate**.
Open your mouth wide.	Habra su boca lo más posible.
Clench your teeth.	Apriete sus dientes.
Raise your eyebrows like this.	Suba sus cejas de esta forma. Suba sus **pestañas así**.
Close your eyes tightly.	Cierre y apriete sus ojos.
Do not let me open them.	No me deje abrirselos.
Open your eyes wide.	Habra bien sus ojos.
Do not move your head.	No mueva su cabeza.
Look up with your eyes only.	Mire hacia arriba solo con sus ojos.
Look down.	Mire hacia abajo.
Look side to side.	Mire de lado a lado.
Roll your eyes around in a circle.	Déle vuelta a sus ojos en la forma de un círculo.
Smile.	Ríase.
Puff out your cheeks like this.	Sople sus mejillas de esta forma. Sople sus mejillas **así**.
Frown.	Frunza el ceño.
Show me your teeth.	Enséñeme sus dientes.
Stick out your tongue.	Saque la lengua.
Point to the ear in which you hear me rubbing my fingers.	Enséñeme el oído por el cual oye el sonido al friccionar mis dedos. Enséñeme el oído por el cual oye el sonido al **frotar** mis dedos.

Neurologic Exam

I'm going to place this (tuning fork) on your forehead.	Le voy a poner esto en su frente.
You will hear some buzzing.	Usted va a oír un zumbido.
Can you hear it?	¿Puede oírlo?
Point to where you hear the buzzing come from.	Enséñeme por donde usted oye el zumbido.
Can you hear buzzing now?	¿Puede oír el zumbido ahora?
Tell me when you no longer hear the buzzing.	¿Dígame cuando ya no pueda oír mas el zumbido?
Can you still hear it?	¿Puede todavia oírlo?
Tell me when you no longer hear the buzzing.	¿Dígame cuando ya no pueda oír mas el zumbido?
Open your mouth.	Habra su boca.
Stick out your tongue.	Saque su lengua.
Say "Ah."	Diga "aaaaaaa."
Lift up your tongue.	Alce su lengua.
Swallow.	Trague.
Cough.	Tosa.
Lift your shoulders, like this.	Alce sus hombros de esta forma. Alce sus hombres **así**.
Turn your head to the right/left.	Voltee su cabeza hacia su derecha/izquierda.
Push against my hand.	Empuje contra mi mano.
Make a fist.	Hago un puño.
Squeeze my fingers in your hand. Harder.	Apriete mis dedos con su mano. Mas fuerte.
Can you feel this? Does it feel sharp or soft or like a vibration? Hot or cold? Say "Yes" every time you feel it. Say "Sharp" or "Soft" or "Hot" or "Cold" every time you feel it. Say "None" when you can't feel it anymore.	¿Puede sentir esto? ¿Lo siente agudo, suave o como si vibrase? ¿Caliente o frio? Diga "Si" cada vez que lo sienta. Diga "Agudo" o "Suave" o "Caliente" o "Frio" cada vez que lo sienta. Diga "Ya no" cuando ya no lo sienta mas. Diga "**No mas**" cuando ya no lo sienta mas.

Neurologic Exam

Push your foot/toe up/down.	Empuje su pie/dedos del pie hacia arriba/hacia abajo.
Do this.	Haga esto.
Faster. Slower.	Rápido, despacio.
Lift your leg/arm.	Alce su pierna/brazo.
Resist me.	Hágame resistencia.
I'm going to move your toe. Tell me if your toe is pointing up or down.	Voy a moverle el dedo del pie. Dígame si el dedo de su pie está apuntando hacia arriba o hacia abajo.
Stand up.	Párese.
Close your eyes.	Cierre sus ojos.
I am going to push you. Resist my push.	Voy a empujarlo. No deje que lo empuje, ponga resistencia al empujarlo.
Hold your arms out in front of you with your palms facing up.	Extienda sus brazos al frente de usted con las palmas de sus manos hacia arriba.
Close your eyes.	Cierre sus ojos.

Musculoskeletal

Walk forward in a straight line.	Camine hacia el frente en una linea recta.
Walk like this.	Camine de esta forma. Camine **así**.
Bend down to touch your toes.	Inclínese y tóquese los dedos de sus pies.
Don't bend your knees.	No doble sus rodillas.
Do this.	Haga esto.
Lift your leg/arm.	Levante su pierna/brazo.
Resist me.	Hágame resistencia.
Relax and let me move your . . . hands. feet. arms. legs. fingers. toes.	Relaje y dejeme mover sus . . . manos. pies. brazos. piernas. dedos de la mano. dedos del pie.

Musculoskeletal

Don't let me move your [insert body part].	No deje que yo le mueva su (insert body part).
Put your hand behind your back.	Ponga su mano atrás de su espalda.
Lift your hand off your back and push my hand away (like this).	Alce sus manos en su espalda y empuje mis manos hacia fuera (de esta forma).
Does this hurt where I touch?	¿Le duele aquí donde yo lo/la estoy tocando?
Point to where it hurts.	Enséñame al lugar donde le duele. **Muéstreme** al lugar donde le duele. **Apúnteme** al lugar donde le duele.
Hold it.	Agárrelo.

Breast Exam

Please lie down.	Por favor acuéstese.
I am going to examine your breasts.	Le voy a examinar sus senos. Le voy a examinar **su pecho**.

(See "Breast Self-Exam" in Chapter 12, "Special Patient Instructions.")

GYN Exam

Please remove your underwear.	Por favor quítese sus **bragas**. Por favor quítese sus **pantaletas**. Por favor quítese sus **pantalones cortos íntimos de mujer**.
Move down to the end of the table and put your feet in the stirrups.	Muevase hacia el final de la mesa y ponga sus pies en los estribos.
A little farther.	Muevase un poco mas hacia abajo.
That's enough.	Ya es suficiente.
Let your knees fall to the side.	Deje que sus rodillas caigan hacia los lados. **Relaje** sus rodillas **hacia** los lados.
I'm going to insert the speculum in your vagina.	Le voy a insertar el espéculo vaginal en su vagina. Le voy a **entrar** el espéculo vaginal en su vagina.

GYN Exam

Try to relax as much as possible.	Trate de relajarse lo más posible.
You will feel some pressure.	Usted va a sentir un poco de presión.
Tell me if you are feeling too much pain.	Dígame si siente demasiada presión.
I'm going to insert 2 fingers inside your vagina and press down to check your ovaries.	Voy a insertar dos dedos dentro de su vagina y voy a presionar su abdomen para poder inspeccionar sus ovarios. Voy a **poner** dos dedos dentro de su vagina y voy a presionar su abdomen para poder **sentir** sus ovarios.
Push (bear down).	Empuje como si estuviera defecando. Empuje como si estuviera **ensuciando**.
I'm going to put one finger inside your rectum to check for any masses.	Voy a insertar un dedo dentro de su recto para poder inspeccionar si hay masas. Voy a **poner** un dedo dentro de su **ano** para poder inspeccionar si hay masas.
I'm done with the exam.	Ya termine con el examén.

Prostate Exam

I need to examine your prostate.	Necesito examinarle su prostata.
Please pull down your pants and underwear.	Por favor bájese sus pantalones al igual que su ropa interior.
Bend over the exam table with your elbows on the table.	Inclínese sobre la mesa de examén con sus codos sobre la mesa.
I'm going to insert one finger in your rectum to check your prostate.	Voy a insertar un dedo en su recto para inspeccionar su prostata. Voy a **poner** un dedo en su **ano** para inspeccionar su prostata.
I'm done with the exam.	Ya terminé con el examen.

Testicular Exam

I am going to examine your testicles.	Le voy a examinar sus testículos.
Please stand up and face me.	Por favor parece y mire hacia mi.
Please pull down your pants and underwear.	Por favor bájese sus pantelones al igual que su ropa interior.
Turn your head to the side and cough.	Vire su cabeza hacia al lado y tosa.
You should periodically examine your testicles at home.	Usted debe examinarse en su casa periódicamente sus testículos.
Your testicle should feel like a hard-boiled egg that has been peeled.	Su testículo debe de sentirse como un huevo cocinado después de ser pelado.
If it feels hard or you feel other masses, you need to come in to be checked.	Si se siente duro, o siente algún tipo de masa, usted necesita venir aquí para que lo examinen.

Chapter 10

Questions for Special Populations

This chapter contains questions for those patients who fall outside the 18–65-year-old age range. Pediatric, geriatric, and obstetric patients all have special needs and issues that must be addressed.

Taking a pediatric history is often somewhat of a challenge since the clinician must ask the caregiver the questions. Special issues such as developmental milestones, home environment, and screening for certain symptoms are crucial for assessing a child's or infant's overall health status.

Geriatric medicine is now considered to be a subspecialty of internal medicine for the very reason that older patients have specific needs and risks that should be assessed and reassessed on a regular basis. For example, eyesight, hearing, and the ability to perform the activities of daily living all tend to decline as the patient ages, whereas fall risk and cognitive decline tend to increase.

And finally, evaluating an obstetric patient must include questions on obstetric history, risk factors, and specific symptoms to ensure a healthy delivery.

Use the questions in these sections as needed as an adjunct to the other chapters.

Pediatric Patient / Paciente Pediátrica

Age Dependent	Dependiendo en la Edad
Birth	*Al nacer*
How many weeks were you pregnant?	¿Cuántas semanas estuvo usted embarazada? ¿Cuántas semanas estuvo usted **encinta**?
Did you smoke during pregnancy?	¿Usted fumó durante su embarazo?
Use illegal drugs?	¿Usted utilizó drogas ilegales? ¿Usted **usó** drogas ilegales
Use alcohol?	¿Tomó bebidas alcohólicas?
Was the delivery natural?	¿Su parto fue natural?
Was the delivery induced?	¿Su parto fue inducido?
Were there any complications with the delivery? Was it a breech birth (feet first)? Did you have a cesarean? Did they use forceps?	¿Tuvo usted alguna complicación con su parto? ¿Salió el bebe de pie? ¿Tuvo usted una cesárea? ¿Utilizaron fórceps? ¿**Usaron pinzas**?
Was the baby normal at birth?	¿El niño/a salió normal?
How much did the baby weigh at birth? Pounds and ounces?	¿Cuanto pesó el niño/a al nacer? ¿Libras y onzas?
Neonatal	*Neonatal*
Was the baby's color good after birth?	¿El color del niño/a estaba bien después de nacer?
Did she/he need oxygen?	¿Ella/el necesitó oxígeno al nacer?
Did she/he have problems with breathing?	¿Él/ella tuvo problemas respirando al nacer?
Did she/he have a strong cry?	¿Él/ella lloró fuerte al nacer?
Did she/he have a weak cry?	¿Él/ella lloró débil al nacer?

Pediatric Patient

Did she/he have any illnesses at birth?	¿Él/ella tuvo alguna enfermedad al nacer?
Did she/he have jaundice (yellow skin)?	¿Ella/él tuvieron ictericia?
	¿Él/ella tuvieron **piel amarilla**?
How many days/weeks/months was the baby in the hospital after birth?	¿Cuánto tiempo estuvo el niño/a en el hospital después de nacer?

Feeding

Is the baby breast-fed?	¿Le están dando el pecho al bebe?
Is the baby bottle-fed?	¿Le están dando la leche en botella?
How often does the baby feed (every hour, every 2 hours)?	¿Qué tan a menudo el bebé toma el pecho (cada hora, cada dos horas)?
How many ounces (minutes) each time?	¿Cuántas onzas (cuántos minutos) cada vez que le da el pecho?
Is the baby gaining weight?	¿Está el bebe ganando peso?
	¿Está el bebe **aumentando** peso?
How much (pounds and ounces)?	¿Cuánto (en libras y onzas)?
Does she/he have a good appetite?	¿Tiene buen apetito?
How old was the child when he/she stopped bottle-feeding, breast-feeding?	¿Qué edad tenía el bebé cuando pararon de darle leche en pomo o de pecho?
Does your baby eat baby food from jars?	¿Come su bebe comida en botellitas?
	¿Come su bebe comida en **jaritas**?
Cereals?	¿Cereales?
Fruits?	¿Frutas?
Vegetables?	¿Vegetales?
Meats?	¿Carnes?
Solid food (table food)?	¿Comida solida (comida de mesa)?
Can the child feed himself/herself?	¿Puede el bebe darse de comer solo/a?
	¿Puede el bebe darse de comer **sin ayuda**?
What kinds of foods does she/he eat regularly?	¿Qué tipo de comidas el bebe come regularmente?
Cereals?	¿Cereales?
Breads?	¿Pan?
Fruits?	¿Frutas?
Vegetables?	¿Vegétales?

Pediatric Patient

Meats?	¿Carnes?
Eggs?	¿Huevos?
Chicken?	¿Pollo?
Do you give your baby vitamins?	¿Le dan vitaminas a su bebe?
You need to give your baby vitamins.	¿Usted necesita darle vitaminas a su bebe?
Do not feed the baby while she/he is lying down.	No le den de comer al bebe cuando ella/él esté acostado.

Developmental Milestones

How old was the child when he/she could . . .	¿Qué edad tenía el niño/a cuando él/ella pudo . . .
roll over?	darse la vuelta?
hold his/her head up?	mantener su cabeza derecha?
	mantener su cabeza **hacia arriba**?
sit up with support?	sentarse con apoyo?
	sentarse con **soporte**?
sit up without support?	sentarse sin apoyo?
	sentarse sin **soporte**?
stand up with support?	pararse con apoyo?
	pararse con **soporte**?
stand up without support?	pararse sin apoyo?
	pararse sin **soporte**?
take his/her first steps?	tomar sus primeros pasos?
walk without help?	caminar sin ayuda?
say his/her first word?	hablar las primeras palabras?
say a few words together?	hablar las primeras palabras juntas?
say his/her first sentence?	hablar la primera oración?
dress himself/herself?	vestirse solo/a?
tie his/her shoes?	amarrarse los zapatos?
Is he/she toilet trained?	¿Ya él/ella está entrenado/a a ir al baño?
	¿Ya él/ella **no necesita pañales**?
For his/her bladder?	¿Para orinar?
For his/her bowels?	¿Para defecar?
How old was he/she when he/she was toilet trained?	¿Qué edad tenía cuando empezó a ir al baño solo/a?
	¿Qué edad tenía cuando empezó a ir al baño **sin necesidad de pañales**?

Pediatric Patient

Illnesses

Are his/her immunizations current?	¿Están las vacunas de sus hijos al día?
Is he/she vaccinated against . . .	¿Están vacunados con la siguientes vacunas . . .
hepatitis B?	hepatitis B?
DPT?	DPT (difteria, tos ferina, and tétano)?
H flu?	Hflu (Haemophilus influenzae)?
influenza?	gripe (influenza)?
pneumonia?	pulmonía?
polio?	polio?
measles?	sarampión?
mumps?	paperas?
rubella?	rubéola?
chicken pox?	varicela?
Has she/he ever had . . .	¿Él/ella ha tenido . . .
measles?	sarampión?
mumps?	paperas?
chicken pox?	varicela?
diphtheria?	difteria?
tuberculosis?	tuberculosis?
Has she/he had any accidents or injuries?	¿Él/ella ha tenido algún accidente o lesión?
	¿Él/ella ha tenido algún accidente o **herida**?
Broken bones?	¿Huesos rotos?
Has she/he been in the hospital?	¿Él/ella ha estado en el hospital?
When?	¿Cuándo?
For illness or injury?	¿Por enfermedad o por lesión?
	¿Por enfermedad o por **trauma**?
	¿Por enfermedad o por **herida**?
	¿Por enfermedad o por **daño**?
Has she/he had any surgeries?	¿Ella/él ha tenido algún tipo de cirugía?
Does he/she have any allergies to food/animals/insects?	¿Tiene él/ella algún tipo de alergia a comidas/animales/insectos?

Pediatric Patient

Social History

Do both parents live at home?	¿Los dos, madre y padre viven en la casa?
Does one or both parents work outside the home?	¿Uno de los dos o ambos trabajan fuera de la casa?
How many brothers and sisters does he/she have? How old are they?	¿Cuántos hermanos y hermanas él/ella tiene? ¿Qué edad tienen? ¿**Cuántos años** tienen?
How many people live at home?	¿Cuánta gente vive en la casa?
Do you live in a house?	¿Vive usted en una casa?
Apartment?	¿En un apartamento?
Shelter? Do you live on the streets?	¿En un refugio? ¿En un **asilo**? ¿Vive usted en la calle?
How many bedrooms at home?	¿Cuántos cuartos tiene la casa donde usted vive?
Does she/he sleep alone? Does she/he share a bedroom? With how many other people?	¿Él/ella duerme sola/o? ¿Ella/él comparte un cuarto? ¿Con cuánta otra gente comparte el cuarto?
Do you live in a safe neighborhood?	¿Vive usted en un vecindario seguro? ¿Vive usted en un vecindario **fuera de peligro**?
Do you get financial aid, like welfare, food stamps, or Medicaid?	¿Usted tiene ayuda financiara como asistencia social, cupones de alimento, o Medicaid? ¿Usted tiene ayuda financiara como asistencia **de welfare**, cupones de alimento, o **seguro médico para personas con bajos recursos que necesitan asistencia médica**? ¿Usted tiene ayuda financiara como asistencia **de welfare**, cupones de alimento, o **ayuda médica federal/estatal**?
Who usually takes care of the child when not in school?	¿Usualmente quién se ocupa del niño cuando él/ella no está en la escuela?

Pediatric Patient

Mother?	¿Madre?
Father?	¿Padre?
Sister?	¿Hermana?
Brother?	¿Hermano?
Grandparents?	¿Abuelos?
Friend?	¿Amigos?
Neighbor?	¿Vecinos?
Does the child go to day care?	Su niño va a una guarderia infantil/ **day care?**
Does the child get good grades in school?	Tiene su niño buenas cualificaciones/**notas** en la escuela?
Does she/he have problems with . . .	¿Ella/él tiene problemas . . .
bed wetting?	orinandose en la cama?
temper tantrums?	con pataletas? **con berrinches?**
thumb sucking?	chupandose el dedo?
nail biting?	mordiendose las uñas?
adjusting to school?	adaptándose a la escuela?
starting fires?	iniciando fuegos? **empezando** fuegos?
controlling his/her bowels or bladder?	controlando su intestino y vejiga? **no defecándose ni orinándose en la ropa?**
sleeping?	durmiendo?
nightmares?	con pesadillas?
sleepwalking?	caminando dormido(a)?
Does the child have good relationships with their family, friends or teachers?	Tiene el niño una buena relacion con su familia, amistades, or maestros?

Screening

When was she/he last tested for . . .	¿Cuándo fue ella/él examinado/a . . .
hearing?	en los oídos?
vision?	en la vista?
tuberculosis?	por tuberculosis?

Pediatric Patient

When was his/her last dental examination?	¿Cuándo fue su último examen dental?
Does she/he ride in a car seat?	¿Él/ella usa una butaca de seguridad en el carro? ¿Él/ella usa una butaca de seguridad en el **auto**? ¿Él/ella usa una butaca de seguridad en el **automobil**? ¿Él/ella usa una butaca de seguridad en el **vehículo**?
He/she must ride in a car seat!	¡Él/ella tiene que utilizar la butaca de seguridad en el carro! ¡Él/ella tiene que utilizar la butaca de seguridad en el **auto**! ¡Él/ella tiene que utilizar la butaca de seguridad en el **automobil**! ¡Él/ella tiene que utilizar la butaca de seguridad en el **vehículo**!
Does she/he use seat belts?	¿Él/ella utiliza el cinturón de seguridad? ¿Él/ella **usa** el cinturón de seguridad?
Does he/she ride in the front or back seat?	¿El/ella se monta en el asiento del frente o de atrás?
Do you have a smoke detector in the house?	¿Tiene usted un detector de humo en su casa?

General Questions

Does she/he sleep well at night?	¿Él/ella duerme bien por la noche?
How many hours?	¿Cuántas horas?
Take a nap in the day?	¿Toma una siesta durante el día?
How many hours a day?	¿Cuántas horas durante el día?
Does she/he cry all the time?	¿Él/ella llora todo el tiempo? ¿Él/ella llora **en todo momento**?
Is she/he generally happy?	¿Generalmente ella/él es feliz?
Is she/he generally fussy?	¿Generalmente ella/él es exigente? ¿Generalmente ella/él es **un poco malcriado/a**? ¿Generalmente ella/él es **quisquilloso/a**? ¿Generalmente ella/él es **noño/a**?
Is she/he generally colicky?	¿Generalmente ella/él tiene cólicos?

Pediatric Patient

Symptoms

Does she/he have a fever/chills?	¿Él/ella tiene fiebre/escalofríos?
Do you check her/his temperature?	¿Le ha revisado la temperatura?
How high is it?	¿Qué tan alta es?
Do the fevers come and go?	¿La fiebre viene y se va?
Is she/he gaining weight normally?	¿Está él/ella ganando peso normalmente?
Is her/his appetite normal?	¿El apetito de él/ella es normal?
Decreased?	¿Reducido? **¿Bajo?** **¿Disminuido?** **¿Pobre?**
Increased?	¿Aumentado?
Does she/he get frequent infections?	¿A él/ella frecuentemente le dan infecciones? ¿Él/ella **seguidamente se enferman con infecciones**?
Rashes?	¿erupciónes? **¿salpullidos?** **¿pintas rojas en su piel?**
Diaper rash?	¿erupciónes por el pañal? ¿**salpullidos** por el pañal? ¿**pintas rojas** por el pañal?
Scaly/crusty/greasy scalp?	¿Él/ella tiene el cuero cabelludo/escamoso/grasoso? ¿Él/ella tiene el cuero cabelludo/escamoso/**con costras**?
Does she/he have allergies to . . .	¿Él/ella tiene alergias a . . .
foods?	comidas?
pets?	animales domésticos?
medicines?	medicamentos?
dust?	polvo?
pollens?	polen?
Do others in the family have allergies?	¿Algunas otras personas en la familia tienen alergias?
Are his/her eyes ever crossed?	¿Los ojos de ella/él alguna vez estuvieron cruzados?

Pediatric Patient

Do both eyes move together?	¿Los dos ojos de ella/él se mueven a la misma vez?
Does she/he frequently sit too close to the television?	¿Él/ella frecuentemente se sienta muy cerca de la televisión?
Does she/he pull or rub her/his ear?	¿Él/ella se hala o frota sus oídos?
	¿Él/ella se hala o **restriega** sus oídos?
Does she/he respond to loud noises?	¿Él/ella responde a ruidos fuertes?
Has she/he had many ear infections?	¿Él/ella ha tenido muchas infecciones de oído?
How many in the past year?	¿Cuántas a tenido en el pasado año?
Does she/he have a runny nose?	¿Él/ella tiene flujo nasal?
What color?	¿De qué color?
Stuffy nose?	¿Tiene la nariz congestionada?
Does she/he sneeze frequently?	¿Él/ella estornuda frecuentemente?
Does she/he cough/wheeze?	¿Él/ella tose/resolla?
	¿Él/ella tose/**silba al respirar**?
Does she/he frequently cough at night?	¿Ella/él frecuentemente tose por la noche?
Does she/he have difficulty breathing?	¿Él/ella tiene dificultad respirando?
At rest or with activity?	¿Él/ella tiene dificultad descansando o cuando está activa/o?
Does she/he turn blue when crying?	¿Él/ella se vuelve/**pone** azul cuando llora?
Is she/he active?	¿Él/ella es activa/o?
	¿Él/ella **no es sedentaria/o**?
Does she/he get tired quickly when playing?	¿Él/ella se cansa rápido al jugar algo?
	¿Él/ella se cansa rápido al jugar **algún deporte**?
Does she/he have vomiting?	¿El vomito de él/ella...
Is it sudden and very forceful?	¿es de repente y con mucha fuerza?
Or is it weak with little vomit?	¿es débil con poco vómitos?
Is he/she constipated?	¿Él/ella está constipado/a?
	¿Él/ella está **estreñido/a**?
Are the stools hard or soft?	¿Las heces de él/ella están duras o suaves?

Pediatric Patient

	¿Los **excrementos** de él/ella están duros o suaves?
	¿Sus **excretas** de él/ella están duras o suaves?
Diarrhea?	¿Él/ella tiene diarrea?
Loose/watery stools?	¿Tiene las heces sueltas?
	¿Tiene la **excreta** suelta?
	¿Tiene el **excremento aguado**?
What color?	¿De qué color?
How many stools a day?	¿Cuántas veces defeca al día?
	¿Cuántas veces **ensucia** al día?
	¿Cuántas veces **va al baño** al día?
For how many days/weeks/months?	¿Por cuantos días/semanas/meses?
How many diapers does she/he use each day?	¿Cuántos pañales él/ella utiliza al día?
	¿Cuántos pañales él/ella **usa cada** día?
Does she/he have . . .	¿Él/ella tiene . . .
yellow skin?	piel amarilla?
convulsions?	convulsiones?
Does she/he cry when urinating?	¿Él/ella llora cuando orina?
Has she/he lost control of her/his bladder recently?	¿Él/ella ha perdido recientemente el control de su vejiga?
Does she/he have normal coordination?	¿Él/ella tiene coordinación normal?
Does she/he have normal strength?	¿Él/ella tiene fuerza normal?
Has she/he lost coordination recently?	¿Él/ella ha perdido recientemente la coordinación?
Has she/he ever broken a bone?	¿Él/ella se ha roto alguna vez un hueso?
Show me where.	Enséñeme adonde.
	Muéstreme adonde.
Does she/he have excessive thirst?	¿Ella/él tiene sed excesiva?
Does she/he have excessive hunger?	¿Ella/él tiene hambre excesiva?
Does she/he have excessive urination?	¿Ella/él orina excesivamente?
Is anyone else sick at home?	¿Hay alguna otra persona enferma en la casa?
With these same symptoms?	¿Con los mismos síntomas?

Geriatric Patient

Functional Level

Can you feed yourself without help?	¿Necesita usted ayuda para comer?
	¿Puede usted comer sin ayuda?
Do you need help with every meal?	¿Necesita usted ayuda con cada una de sus comidas?
Can you bathe yourself without help?	¿Necesita usted ayuda para bañarse?
	¿Puede usted bañarse sin ayuda?
Do you need help getting in and out of the bathtub or shower?	¿Necesita usted ayuda para salir y entrar de la bañera o ducha?
	¿Necesita usted ayuda para salir y entrar de la **tina** o ducha?
Do you have railings in the bath?	¿Tiene usted barandillas protectoras en su baño?
Can you dress yourself without help?	¿Puede usted vestirse sin ayuda?
Can you get out of bed or stand up from a chair without help?	¿Puede usted levantarse de la cama o de una silla sin ayuda?
Do you have problems controlling your bladder?	¿Tiene usted problemas controlando su vejiga?
Do you have problems controlling your bowels?	¿Tiene usted problemas controlando su intestino?
	¿Tiene usted problemas controlando sus **entrañas**?
Can you go to the bathroom without help?	¿Necesita usted ayuda para ir al baño?
	¿Puede usted ir al baño sin ayuda?
Can you comb your hair/brush your teeth without help?	¿Puede usted peinarse y cepillarse sus dientes sin ayuda?
Are you able to walk without help?	¿Puede usted caminar sin ayuda?
	¿Es capaz de caminar sin ayuda?
Do you use a . . .	¿Utiliza usted un . . .
	¿Usa usted...?
Cane?	¿Bastón?
Walker?	¿andador?
Wheelchair?	¿silla de ruedas?
Can you use the telephone without help?	¿Puede usted utilizar el teléfono sin ayuda?

Geriatric Patient

	¿Puede usted **usar** el teléfono sin ayuda?
Can you use the answering machine without help?	¿Puede usted utilizar el contestador automático sin ayuda? ¿Puede usted **usar la máquina de contestar el teléfono** sin ayuda?
Do you do your own grocery shopping?	¿Compra usted sus propios comestibles? ¿Compra usted sus propias **provisiones**? ¿Hace usted sus **compras de supermercado**? ¿Hace usted sus **mandados**?
Do you need help with buying groceries?	¿Necesita usted ayuda con sus comestibles? ¿Necesita usted ayuda con sus **proviciones**? ¿Necesita usted ayuda con sus **compras de supermercado**? ¿Necesita usted ayuda con sus **mandados**?
Can you prepare your meals without help?	¿Puede usted prepararse sus comidas sin ayuda?
Can you use the stove, microwave, oven without help?	¿Puede usted utilizar su fogón, microonda, horno sin ayuda? ¿Puede usted **usar** su **estufa**, microonda, horno sin ayuda?
Can you do your housecleaning without help?	¿Puede usted limpiar su casa sin ayuda?
Can you dust?	¿Puede usted quitar el polvo?
Can you mop?	¿Puede usted trapear? ¿Puede usted **fregar**? ¿Puede usted **mapear**?
Can you vacuum?	¿Puede usted pasar la aspiradora?
Can you wash dishes?	¿Puede usted lavar los platos? ¿Puede usted **fregar** los platos?
Can you change the beds?	¿Puede usted hacer su cama?

Geriatric Patient

Can you do the laundry without help?	¿Puede usted lavar su ropa sin ayuda?
	¿Puede usted **hacer la lavandería** sin ayuda?
Do you take the bus/train?	¿Toma usted el autobús/tren?
Without help?	¿Sin ayuda?
Can you take all your medicines as they are prescribed without help?	¿Puede usted tomar todos sus medicamentos recetados sin ayuda?
Do you pay your bills without help?	¿Paga usted todos sus cuentas sin ayuda?
	¿Paga usted todas sus **facturas** sin ayuda?
Can you manage a bank account without help?	¿Puede usted administrar su cuenta de banco sin ayuda?

Social History

Do you live with someone?	¿Vive usted con alguien?
Who?	¿Con quién?
Spouse?	¿Con su esposo/a?
Partner?	¿Con un compañero/a?
Son?	¿Con su hijo?
Daughter?	¿Con su hija?
Relative?	¿Con un familiar?
	¿Con un pariente?
Friend?	¿Con un amigo/a?
Do you have someone who helps take care of you?	¿Tiene usted alguna persona que se ocupa de usted?
Is it a relative/friend?	¿Es familia/amigo/a?
	¿Es **pariente**/amigo/a?
Is it a home health nurse or aid?	¿Es una enfermera de ayuda para la casa o una ayudante en general?
Do they live with you?	¿Viven con usted?
How many times a week do they come to your house?	¿Cuántas veces a la semana viene a la casa?
Do they help you with . . .	¿Le ayudan con . . .
housecleaning?	la limpieza de la casa?
cooking?	la cocina o a cocinar?
laundry?	la lavandería?
bathing?	el proceso de bañarse?
shopping?	las compras de supermacado u otras tiendas?

dressing?	el proceso de vestirse?
medications?	con sus medicamentos o medicinas?
paying your bills?	sus cuentas o facturas?
	las factures?
Do you feel you are well cared for?	¿Se siente usted bien atendida?
Has anyone tried to hurt you at home? (If yes, see "Screening Questions for Domestic Violence," Chapter 7, "Comprehensive Adult History.")	¿Ha tratado alguien de lastimarle en la casa?
	¿Ha tratado alguien de **hacerle daño** en la casa?
Additional Review of Symptoms	**Revisión Adicional de Síntomas**
	Estudio Adicional de Síntomas
Do you have pain or burning when urinating?	¿Tiene usted dolor o quemazón al orinar?
Do you have vaginal dryness or itching?	¿Tiene usted sequedad o picazón en su vagina?
	¿Tiene usted **aridez** o picazón en su vagina?
Do you have pain with intercourse?	¿Tiene usted dolor al tener sexo?
	¿Tiene usted dolor al tener **relaciones sexuales**?
	¿Tiene usted dolor al tener **coito**?
	¿Tiene usted dolor al **hacer el sexo**?
Do you have hot flashes?	¿Tiene usted cambios de temperatura repentinos?
	¿Tiene usted cambios **de calor** repentinos?
For how many years?	¿Por cuántos años?
Are they getting less frequent?	¿La frecuencia de estos a bajado?
Do you take hormones?	¿Toma usted hormonas?
How many years have you been taking hormones?	¿Cuántos años hace que usted está tomando hormonas?
Have you fallen recently?	¿Se ha caido recientemente?
How many times in the past year?	¿Cuántas veces en el pasado año?
Do you have problems with hearing?	¿Tiene usted problemas escuchando?
	¿Tiene usted problemas **oyendo**?

Has your hearing gotten worse lately?	¿Ha empeorado su audición últimamente?
Do you wear a hearing aid?	¿Usa usted una prótesis auditiva?
	¿Usa usted **una ayuda auditiva**?
	¿Usa usted **un aparato de corrección auditiva**?
	¿Usa usted **una prótesis auditiva acústica**?
	¿Usa usted **un audífono**?
	¿Usa usted **un dispositivo de comunicación (inalámbrico) de deficiencia auditiva**?
Do you have trouble remembering things?	¿Tiene usted trabajo acordándose de las cosas?
Do you drive?	¿Usted maneja?
Alone?	¿Solo/a?
Do you wear seat belts?	¿Usa usted cinturón de seguridad?
All the time?	¿En todo momento?
Sometimes?	¿De vez en cuando?
	¿**Algunas veces**?
	¿**A veces**?
Have you had a traffic accident in the past year?	¿Ha tenido usted algún accidente automovilístico en el pasado año?
	¿Ha tenido usted algún accidente **de carro** en el pasado año?
Have you had a traffic ticket in the past year?	¿Le han dado a usted alguna multa de tráfico?
Do you have problems driving at night?	¿Tiene usted problemas manejando por la noche?
Do you have problems with your vision?	¿Tiene usted problemas con su visión?
	¿Tiene usted problemas con sus **ojos**?
Do you feel depressed or anxious most of the time? (If yes, see "Screening Questions for Depression" in Chapter 7, "Comprehensive Adult History.")	¿Se siente usted deprimido/a o ansioso/a la mayoría del tiempo?
	¿Se siente usted deprimido/a o **preocupado/a** la mayoría del tiempo?

Obstetric Patient

Obstetric History

How many times have you been pregnant?	¿Cuántas veces ha usted estado embarazada? ¿Cuántas veces ha usted estado **encinta**?
How many times have you delivered?	¿Cuántas veces ha dado usted a luz? ¿Cuántas veces ha **concebido un bebe**? ¿Cuántas veces ha **concebido un niño**?
How many miscarriages have you had?	¿Cuántos abortos naturales ha tenido? ¿Cuántas **veces usted ha perdido un niño/a**?
How many abortions?	¿Cuántos abortos?
How many stillbirths?	¿Cuántos han nacido muertos?
How many of your children are living?	¿Cuántos de sus hijos todavía viven?
How many pregnancies were forty weeks?	¿Cuántos de sus partos llegaron a las cuarenta semanas?
How many pregnancies were less than 37 weeks?	¿Cuántos de sus partos fueron menos de treinta y siete semanas?
Did you have a cesarean or vaginal delivery?	¿Usted los tuvo por cesaría o vaginal?
How many hours were you in labor during each pregnancy?	¿Cuántas horas duró cada uno de sus partos?
Did you have any complications during your pregnancies? High blood pressure? Diabetes? Seizures? Bleeding?	¿Tuvo usted alguna complicación durante sus partos? ¿Alta presión? ¿Diabetes? ¿Convulsiones? ¿Pérdida de sangre?
Did you have any complications during or after labor? Bleeding? Infections? Seizures?	¿Tuvo usted algunas complicaciones durante o después del parto? ¿Pérdida de sangre? ¿Infecciones? ¿Convulsiones?

Risk Factors

Do you smoke?	¿Usted fuma?

Do you drink any alcohol?	¿Toma usted bebidas alcohólicas?
	¿**Consume** usted bebidas alcohólicas?
	¿**Bebe** usted bebidas alcohólicas?
Do you drink coffee/tea/ soda with caffeine?	¿Toma usted café/té/ soda con cafeína?
	¿**Consume** usted café/té/ soda con cafeína?
	¿**Bebe** usted café/té/soda con cafeína?
How many cups/glasses each day?	¿Cuántas tazas/vasos por día?
Do you use any drugs like cocaine, heroine, methamphetamine, or marijuana?	¿Utiliza usted drogas como cocaína, heroína, metanfetaminas (desoxiefedrina), o marihuana?
	¿**Usa** usted drogas como cocaína, heroína, metanfetaminas (desoxiefedrina), o marihuana?
Did you ever use these drugs?	¿Ha usted utilizado alguna vez este tipo de drogas ya mencionados?
Which ones?	¿Cuáles?
For how many months/years?	¿Por cuántos meses/años?
How many days/weeks/months/ years ago was the last time?	¿Cuántos días/semanas/meses/años fue la última vez que las utilizó?
	¿Cuántos días/semanas/meses/años fue la última vez que las **usó**?
How many months or years ago did you quit?	¿Cuántos meses o años hace que usted dejó de utilizarlas?
	¿Cuántos meses o años hace que usted dejó de **usarlas**?
Do you share needles?	¿Usted comparte agujas?
Have you ever been tested for HIV?	¿Ha sido usted alguna vez examinada por VIH (virus de inmunodeficiencia humana)?
	¿Ha sido usted alguna vez **chequeada** por VIH (virus de inmunodeficiencia humana)?
Was it positive or negative?	¿Fue positivo o negativo?
How long ago were you tested?	¿Cuánto tiempo hace que usted fue examinada?

Obstetric Patient

Do you have sexual intercourse with more than one partner?	¿Tiene usted sexo con más de un/una compañero/a?
Is your partner male or female?	¿Su compañero/a es hombre o mujer?
Do you use condoms?	¿Utiliza preservativos?
	¿Usa **condones**?
Always or sometimes?	¿Siempre o algunas veces?
How many sexual partners have you had in your lifetime?	¿Cuántos compañeros sexuales ha tenido usted en su vida?
More than 10?	¿Más de diez?
More than 50?	¿Más de cincuenta?
More than 100?	¿Más de cien?
Have they been male, female, or both?	¿Han sido todos hombres, mujeres o ambos?
	¿Todos han sido hombres, mujeres o **de los dos**?
Have you ever had diabetes during pregnancy?	¿Ha usted tenido diabetes durante su embarazo?
Did any of your children weigh more than ten pounds at birth?	¿Alguno de sus hijos pesó más de diez libras?

Pregnancy History	**Historial de su Embarazo**
How many days/weeks/months ago was your last menstrual period?	¿Cuántos días/semanas/meses atrás fue su última menstruación?
	¿Cuántos días/semanas/meses atrás **tuvo** su último **período**?
What was the date of your first day?	¿Cuándo fue el primer día de su menstruación?
	¿Cuándo fue el primer día de su **período**?
When are you due?	¿Cuándo va a ser el día de su parto/**alumbramiento**?
Are you working?	¿Está usted trabajando?
Manual labor?	¿Labor manual?
	¿**Trabajo** manual?
Sedentary work?	¿Trabajo sedentario?
	¿**Labor** sedentario?
How many hours a day?	¿Cuántas horas al día?
Do you travel a lot with your job?	¿Viaja usted mucho en su trabajo?

Obstetric Patient

In a car?	¿En carro?
	¿En **auto**?
	¿En **automobil**?
	¿En **vehículo**?
In an airplane?	¿En avión?
In [month] you need to stop traveling.	En [mes] usted necesita parar de viajar.
Do you have problems with bleeding?	¿Tiene usted problemas de pérdida de sangre?
How much?	¿Qué cantidad?
A teaspoon?	¿Una cucharadita?
A half cup?	¿Media taza?
More than a cup?	¿Más de una taza?
Is the blood clotted?	¿La sangre está coagulada?
Do you have . . .	¿Tiene usted . . .
nausea?	nausea?
vomiting?	vómitos?
diarrhea?	diarrea?
constipation?	constipación?
	estreñimiento?
Do you have burning or pain when urinating?	¿Tiene usted quemazón o dolor al orinar?
Do you have difficulty breathing?	¿Tiene usted dificultad respirando?
Do you have problems with your vision?	¿Tiene usted problemas con su vista?
Do you have swelling in your feet?	¿Tiene usted hinchazón en sus pies?
	¿Tiene usted **inflamación** en sus pies?
Hands?	¿En sus manos?
Face?	¿En su cara?
How many days/weeks/months have you had swelling?	¿Cuántos días/semanas/meses hace que tiene inflamación?
Have you had any severe headaches?	¿Ha usted tenido dolores de cabeza severos?
Have you had any seizures?	¿Ha tenido usted convulsiones?
Are you very fatigued?	¿Está usted muy fatigada?
Are you taking vitamins?	¿Está usted tomando vitaminas?
Show me.	Enséñemelas.
	Muéstremelas.

Obstetric Patient

Are you exercising?	¿Está usted haciendo ejercicios?
What kind?	¿Qué tipo/s de ejercicio/s?
Walking?	¿de caminar?
Jogging?	¿de correr?
Swimming?	¿de nadar?
Cycling?	¿de montar en bicicleta?
	¿Montando bicicleta?
Aerobics classes?	¿Clases de aeróbicos?
You may continue walking, jogging, swimming, cycling, doing aerobics.	Usted puede seguir caminando, corriendo despacio, nadando, ciclismo, o haciendo aeróbicos.
	Usted puede seguir caminando, corriendo despacio, nadando, **montando bicicleta**, o haciendo aeróbicos.
You should not swim on your back.	Usted no debe nadar en su espalda.
You should/should not jog or do aerobics.	Usted debe/no debe de correr despacio o hacer aeróbicos.
You should not exercise at all at this time.	Usted no debe de hacer ningún tipo de ejercicios en este tiempo.
	Usted no debe de hacer ningún tipo de ejercicios en este **momento**.
	Usted no debe de hacer ningún tipo de ejercicios en este **periódo de tiempo**.
You need bed rest.	Usted necesita guardar cama.
	Usted necesita **más reposo**.
You should not do any walking except around the house.	Usted no debe de caminar excepto en la casa.
	Usted no debe de caminar **a menos que sea** en la casa.
No lifting, bending, or cleaning.	No debe alzar nada pesado, agacharse, o hacer trabajo de limpieza.
No standing for longer than a few minutes.	No debe de estar parado/a por más de unos minutos.
Do you feel dizzy with activity?	¿Se siente usted mareado/a?
Do you plan to breastfeed?	¿Planea usted darle el pecho a su hijo/a?
	¿**Tiene pensado** usted darle el pecho a su hijo/a?

Chapter 11

Health Behaviors History and Education

This chapter was designed with the primary care health provider in mind. However, in certain situations most health care providers and nurses may find this chapter useful. In caring for patients, we find that unhealthy lifestyle behaviors are becoming increasingly important as a preventable cause of disease and disability and should be addressed on a regular basis.

Under the nutrition section, you will find not only questions on nutrition behaviors, but patient teaching on various commonly prescribed diets as well (low sodium, low fat, diabetic, etc.). Often, as a consequence of language barriers, patients come away from an encounter with their health care provider with an incomplete understanding of what foods are appropriate for their particular medical condition.

Exercise is also an often neglected topic, for any population. But even just a small increase in exercise can have major impacts on health and disease.

Again, in this section, you will find questions on exercise behaviors as well as patient teaching on exercise prescriptions.

Prevention covers the questions on health promotion and disease prevention. This section also covers basic screening tests for the general population, as well as gender-specific screening questions.

Nutrition History

Do you drink coffee?	¿Toma usted café?
	¿**Consume** usted café?
	¿**Bebe** usted café?
Regular?	¿Café con cafeína (regular)?
Decaf?	¿Descafeinado?
How many cups a day?	¿Cuántas tazas al día?
Do you drink tea?	¿Toma usted te?
	¿**Consume** usted te?
	¿**Bebe** usted te?
Do you drink alcohol?	¿Toma usted alcohol?
	¿**Consume** usted alcohol?
	¿**Bebe** usted alcohol?
Beer?	¿Cerveza?
Wine?	¿Vino?
Hard liquor?	¿Licores fuertes?
How much in a day/week/month (ounces/cans/bottles/glasses)?	¿Cuánto toma al día/semana/mes (onzas/latas/botellas/copas)?
Do you drink sodas?	¿Toma usted refrescos?
	¿**Bebe** usted **sodas**?
	¿**Consume** usted **sodas**?
Regular?	¿Regular?
Diet?	¿De dieta?
Caffeinated?	¿Con cafeína?
Caffeine free?	¿Sin cafeína?
How many a day?	¿Cuántos por día?
How many glasses of water do you drink each day?	¿Cuántos vasos de agua usted toma por día?
	¿Cuántos vasos de agua usted **consume** por día?
	¿Cuántos vasos de agua usted **bebe** por día?

Nutrition History

How many times a week do you eat . . .	¿Cuántas veces a la semana usted come . . .
fast food?	comida rápida?
fried food?	comida frita?
red meat?	carne roja?
fish?	pescado?
chicken?	pollo?
bacon?	tocino?
sausage?	embutidos?
	chorizo?
	salchichas?
Do you fry your foods?	¿Usted generalmente fríe su comida?
How many times a day do you eat . . .	¿Cuántas veces al día usted come . . .
fruit?	frutas?
vegetables?	vegetales?
How many meals a week do you eat out?	¿Cuántas comidas por semana usted consume fuera de su casa o en un restaurante?
	¿Cuántas comidas por semana usted **come** fuera de su casa o en un restaurante?
Do you order . . .	¿Usted ordena . . .
hamburgers?	hamburguesas?
fries?	papas fritas?
	patatas fritas?
burritos?	burritos?
tacos?	tacos?
fried chicken?	pollo frito?
fried fish?	pescado frito?
Do you eat three meals each day?	¿Usted come por lo general tres comidas por día?
Do you eat snacks?	¿Usted come meriendas entre comidas?
	¿Usted come **bocadillos** entre comidas?
	¿Usted come **entremeses**?
How many times a day?	¿Cuántas veces al día?

Nutrition History

Do you feel like you eat too much?	¿Usted siente que come demasiado?
Do you feel like you eat too little?	¿Usted siente que come muy poco?
Do you cook at home with . . . butter? shortening? lard?	¿Usted cocina en su casa con . . . mantequilla? grasas? manteca?

Nutritional Counseling

Low Sodium

You need to eat a low-salt (sodium) diet.	Usted necesita comer una dieta baja en sal (sodio).
Too much can increase your blood pressure and can cause swelling and fluid build-up.	¿Demasiada sal le puede aumentar su presión sanguínea y también hinchazón por medio de acumulación de líquido en su cuerpo? ¿Demasiada sal le puede aumentar su presión sanguínea y también **inflamación** por medio de acumulación de líquido en su cuerpo?
Do not add salt to your food.	No le añada sal a su comida.
Do not use flavored peppers like lemon pepper or garlic pepper.	No utilice pimienta condimentada como, por ejemplo, pimienta con limón o ajo. No **use** pimienta condimentada como, por ejemplo, pimienta con limón o ajo.
They have too much salt.	Estas contienen demasiada sal.
You can flavor foods with salt-free seasonings, herbs, spices, and lemon juice.	Usted puede sazonar sus comidas con sazones, hierbas, especias, y jugo de limón sin sal.
Avoid eating packaged and canned foods.	Evite comer comidas empacadas o en lata.
Look for food labels that say “no salt added” or “low sodium.”	Busque en las etiquetas de comestibles que digan “sin sal” o “baja en sal o sodio.” Busque en las etiquetas de comestibles que digan **“no sal agregada”** o “baja en sal o sodio.”

Nutritional Counseling

Try to eat mostly fresh fruits and vegetables.	Trate generalmente de comer frutas frescas y vegetales.
Frozen is okay as long as there is no sauce.	No importa si están congeladas, después que no contengan salsa.
	No importa si están **frisadas**, después que no contengan salsa.
Canned vegetables are very salty.	Los vegetales en lata contienen mucha sal.
If you have to eat canned vegetables, drain the vegetables and rinse them with water.	Si tiene o quiere comer vegetales en lata, saque los vegetales de la lata y enjuáguelos en agua.
Foods to avoid include . . .	Comidas que usted debe de evitar son . . .
fast foods.	comida rápida.
junk foods (chips, salted nuts, French fries).	comida chatarra (frituras, nueces sazonadas en sal, papas fritas).
	comida chatarra (frituras, nueces sazonadas en sal, **patatas** fritas).
	comida **de poco valor nutricional** (frituras, nueces sazonadas en sal, patatas fritas).
canned or dried soups.	sopa enlatada o seca.
	sopa **en conserva** o seca.
	sopa de **lata** o **en polvo**.
ramen noodles	fideos.
	tallarines ramen.
	fideos ramen.
packaged or canned gravies or sauces.	salsas empacadas o enlatadas.
	salsas empacadas o **en conserva**.
canned, cured, or smoked meats.	carnes curadas, ahumadas o enlatadas.
	carnes curadas, ahumadas o **en conserva**.
frozen dinners, unless they say "low sodium."	comidas congeladas, a menos que digan "baja en sal (sodio)."
	comidas **frisadas**, a menos que digan "baja en sal (sodio)."
bacon, sausage, hot dogs, and jerky.	tocino, embutidos, perros calientes o carne seca.

	tocino, **chorizo**, perros calientes o carne cecina.
	tocino, **salchichas**, perros calientes o carne seca.
pickles and pickled vegetables.	pepinillos y verduras encurtidas.
tomato juice.	jugo de tomate.
processed cheeses like American, Velveeta®, cottage cheese, and pimento cheese.	quesos procesados como American, Velveeta®, queso fresco/cottage, y queso de pimiento.
foods that are very salty, and you should limit . . .	comidas muy saladas, y usted debe limitar . . .
olives.	aceitunas.
cheese.	queso.
lunch meats and ham.	carne para sándwiches y jamón.
	carne para **emparedados** y jamón.
Try not to eat at restaurants very often because the food is very salty.	Trate de no ir a comer en restaurantes tan a menudo ya que la comida es más alta en sal.

Low Fat

You need to decrease the fat in your diet.	Usted necesita bajar el nivel de grasas en su dieta.
A low-fat diet will help lower your risk for heart disease and stroke.	Una dieta baja en grasas lo ayudará a reducir su riesgo de un ataque al corazón o de un derrame cerebral.
	Una dieta baja en grasas lo ayudará a reducir su riesgo de un ataque al corazón o de **una apoplejía**.
You should grill, bake, roast, broil, or boil your meats.	Usted debe de cocinar mas a la parrilla, hornear, o hervir su carne.
Because they are very high in fat, you should not eat . . .	Porque son altos en grasas, usted no debería de comer . . .
fried foods.	comidas fritas.
fast foods.	comidas rápidas.
junk foods (chips, French fries, pork rinds).	comida chatarra (frituras, papas fritas, chicharrones).
	comida **de poco valor nutricional** (frituras, **patatas** fritas, chicharrones).

Nutritional Counseling

sausage or bacon.	embutidos o tocino. **chorizos** o tocino. **salchichas** o tocino.
whole milk or cream.	leche entera y crema.
whole-fat cheeses.	quesos regulares. quesos **no bajo en calorías.**
butter, lard, or shortening.	mantequilla, manteca de cerdo, y otros tipos de manteca.
whole-fat ice cream.	helado regular. **nieve no baja en calorías.**
Try to buy foods that say "no trans fats."	Trate de comprar comidas que digan "no grasas transaturadas."
You should limit the number of eggs you eat to [insert number] a week.	Debería de limitar el número de huevos que come a [insert number] por semana.
Try not to eat at restaurants very often because the food generally has a lot of fat.	Trate de no comer en restaurantes muy seguido porque la comida regularmente contiene más grasa.
When you eat at restaurants, ask them to prepare your food with no sauce, no butter, no oil. You can ask for the sauce or dressing on the side.	Cuando coma en restaurantes pídales que cocinen su comida sin salsa, mantequilla, y sin aceite. Pida que le den la salsa o el aderezo en un platillo separado.
You can/cannot cook poultry with the skin on.	Usted puede/no puede cocinar el pollo con su pellejo. Usted puede/no puede cocinar **el ave** con su pellejo.
Do not eat the skin.	No se coma el pellejo.
Cut off the fat from meats before cooking.	Córtele la grasa a las carnes antes de cocinarlas.
Foods that are better to eat include . . .	Comidas que son mejores para comer incluyen . . .
egg whites.	la clara del huevo.
nonfat or low-fat milk.	leche sin o baja en grasa.
nonfat or low-fat yogurt.	yogurt sin o bajo en grasa.
nonfat cottage cheese and sour cream.	queso cottage sin grasa.
low-fat or fat-free cheese.	queso sin o bajo en grasas.
nonfat ice cream.	helado sin grasa. **nieve** sin grasa.

spray butter.	mantequilla en espray. mantequilla **en aerosol**.
oil sprays like Pam®.	aceite en espray como Pam®. aceite **en aerosol**.
low-cholesterol margarine.	margarina baja en colesterol.
especially brands like Promise® or Heart Smart®.	especialmente marcas como Promise® o Heart Smart®.
white meat.	carne blanca.
fish.	pescado.
Do not eat . . . (see "Foods" in Chapter 3, "Vocabulary")	No coma . . .
You need to eat more . . . (see "Foods" in Chapter 3, "Vocabulary")	Necesita comer mas . . .
You should eat at least [insert number] servings of fruits and vegetables each day.	Usted debería de comer por lo menos [insert number] porciones de frutas y vegetales al día.
You should eat [insert food] no more than [insert number] times a day/week.	Debería de comer [insert food] no más de [insert number] veces al día/semana.

Healthy Eating

I am going to give you some advice on healthy eating habits.	Le voy a dar unos consejos en hábitos alimenticios saludables.
Drink at least 8 glasses of water a day.	Tome por lo menos ocho vasos de agua al día. **Consuma** por lo menos ocho vasos de agua al día. **Beba** por lo menos ocho vasos de agua al día.
Eat at least [insert number] servings of fruits and vegetables each day.	Coma por lo menos [insert number] porciones de frutas y vegetales al día.
Choose a variety of fruits and vegetables.	Escoja una variedad de frutas y vegetales.
Choose a variety of colors.	Escoja también una variedad de frutas y vegetales de diferentes colores.
Brightly colored fruits and vegetables have a lot of healthy nutrients.	Frutas y vegetales de color brillante tienen muchos nutrientes saludables.
Eat more servings of vegetables than of fruit each day.	Coma más porciones de vegetales que de frutas al día.

Nutritional Counseling

Choose whole-grain bread, cereal, pasta, rice, tortillas.	Escoja pan, cereal, pastas, arroz, y tortillas de trigo.
Choose whole-wheat breads and pastas instead of white.	Escoja pan y pastas de trigo en vez de blanco.
Choose whole-wheat tortillas instead of flour.	Escoja tortillas de trigo en vez de arina.
Choose brown rice instead of white rice.	Escoja arroz café en vez de blanco.
	Escoja arroz **marrón** en vez de blanco.
	Escoja arroz **brown** en vez de blanco.
Choose low-fat or nonfat cheese, milk and yogurt.	Escoja queso, leche y yogurt bajo en grasas o sin grasas.
Eat low-fat meats, poultry, and fish.	Coma carnes, aves, y pescado bajos en grasas.
White meat has less fat and fewer calories than dark meat.	La carne blanca tiene menos grasa y menos calorías que la carne roja.
Avoid eating processed meats (canned, smoked, cured).	Evite comer comidas procesadas (enlatadas, ahumadas, o curadas).
	Evite comer comidas procesadas (**en preserva**, ahumadas, curadas).
Try to eat fish at least [insert number] times a week.	Trate de comer pescado por lo menos [insert number] veces a la semana.
Limit eating out at restaurants.	Limite las comidas en restaurantes.
The food you order is high in calories, fat, and salt.	La comida que usted ordena es alta en calorías, grasa y sal.
Usually the portion sizes are too big.	Usualmente los tamaños de las porciones son mucho más grandes.
Avoid eating junk food and fast food.	Evite comer comida chatarra y rápida.
Avoid highly processed foods (packaged, canned).	Evite comer comidas altamente procesadas (en paquete, enlatadas).
	Evite comer comidas altamente procesadas (en paquete, **en preserva**).
Whole, fresh foods are always healthier.	Comidas enteras y frescas siempre son más saludables.

Exercise History and Counseling

Do you participate in regular activity or exercise like . . .	¿Usted participa en una actividad regular o se ejercita . . .
walking?	caminando?
jogging?	corriendo?
swimming?	nadando?
cycling?	montando bicicleta?
aerobics?	haciendo aeróbicos?
water exercise?	haciendo ejercicios acuáticos?
classes?	en clases de ejercicios?
	en **cursos** de ejercicios?
Do you exercise outside or inside?	¿Hace usted ejercicio adentro o afuera?
	¿Hace usted ejercicio adentro o **al aire libre**?
Have you been exercising for a long time?	¿Ha estado ejercitándose por mucho tiempo?
Months, years?	¿Meses, años?
How many times a week?	¿Cuántas veces a la semana?
How many minutes each time?	¿Cuántos minutos por sesión?
Do you feel good when you exercise regularly?	¿Se siente bien cuando hace ejercicio regularmente?
Do you go to a gym or senior center?	¿Va al gimnasio o centro para personas mayores de edad?
Can you go to a senior center or recreation center that has equipment you can use?	¿Puede ir a un centro de recreación o centro de personas mayores de edad que tenga equipo que usted pueda utilizar?
	¿Puede ir a un centro de recreación o centro de personas mayores de edad que tenga equipo que usted pueda **usar**?
Do you do any exercise with weights?	¿Hace usted ejercicios que incluye el uso de pesas?
Free weights?	¿Pesas libres?
Weight machines?	¿Máquinas de pesas?
With resistance bands?	¿Con bandas de resistencia?
With your arms?	¿Con sus brazos?

Exercise History and Counseling

With your legs?	¿Con sus piernas?
Do you do any exercises like push-ups or sit- ups?	¿Hace ejercicio como planchas o abdominales? ¿Hace ejercicio como **push up** o **sentadillas**?
Do you have any exercise equipment at home, like a treadmill or stationary bicycle?	¿Tiene equipo de ejercicio en su casa como una cinta rodante o bicicleta estacionaria? ¿Tiene equipo de ejercicio en su casa como **una cinta de caminar** o **bicicleta inmóvil**? ¿Tiene equipo de ejercicio en su casa como **máquina de andar o correr estática** o **bicicleta inmóvil**?
The best kind of exercise for your health is . . .	El mejor tipo de ejercicio para su salud es . . .
Exercise is very good for your health.	El ejercicio es muy bueno para su salud.
You need to increase your activity level.	Necesita incrementar su nivel de actividad. Necesita **aumentar** su nivel de actividad.
I want you to increase the time you exercise to [insert number] minutes each day.	Quiero que aumente el tiempo en el cual usted hace ejercicio a [insert number] minutos al día.
You can do all [insert number] minutes in one session.	Usted puede hacer [insert number] minutos en una sesión.
Or you can do [insert number] minutes [insert number] times a day.	O puede hacer [insert number] minutos [insert number] de veces al día.
I want you to exercise [insert number] times each week.	Quiero que haga ejercicio [insert number] veces al día.
Keep a log of what days you exercise and for how many minutes each time.	Mantenga una lista de que días hizo ejercicio y por cuantos minutos al día.
Bring this log with you to your appointments.	Traiga esta lista la próxima vez que venga a su cita.

Exercise History and Counseling

Start increasing your exertion or speed gradually.	Empiece a incrementar su intensidad y velocidad gradualmente. Empiece a **aumentar** su intensidad y velocidad **despacio**.
You should be able to talk most of the time while exercising.	Debería de poder mantener una conversación mientras se está ejercitando.
If you can't finish a sentence, you should slow down a little.	Si no puede terminar una oración mientras habla, entonces debería de bajar la intensidad un poco. Si no puede terminar una oración mientras habla, entonces debería de bajar **la cantidad** un poco.
If you are able to sing a song, you are not exercising hard enough.	Si puede cantar una canción, entonces no está ejercitando tan intensamente como debería. Si puede cantar una canción, entonces no está ejercitando tan **duro** como debería.
Make sure you start out slowly and build up your speed over 5–10 minutes.	Asegúrese de comenzar despacio y poco a poco incremente su velocidad en los siguientes 5–10 minutos. Asegúrese de comenzar despacio y poco a poco **aumente** su velocidad en los **próximos** 5–10 minutos.
Make sure you gradually slow your speed down at the end over 5–10 minutes.	Asegúrese de bajar su intensidad y velocidad gradualmente en los últimos 5–10 minutos. Asegúrese de bajar su intensidad y velocidad **despacio** en los últimos 5–10 minutos.
Make sure you drink plenty of water during and after your exercise.	Asegúrese de tomar suficiente agua durante y después de su ejercicio. Asegúrese de **consumir** suficiente agua durante y después de su ejercicio. Asegúrese de **beber** suficiente agua durante y después de su ejercicio.

Exercise History and Counseling

If you have chest pain or feel like you are going to faint while exercising, you need to stop and get help immediately.	Si tiene dolor de pecho o se siente como que se va a desmayar mientras hace el ejercicio, necesita parar y pedir ayuda inmediatamente.

Health Promotion/ Disease Prevention

General

Have you ever had a colonoscopy or other test for colon cancer?	¿Le han hecho alguna vez una colonoscopia o algún otro tipo de examen para el cáncer del colon?
How many years ago?	¿Hace cuántos años?
Was it normal?	¿Fue normal?
Did you have any polyps?	¿Tuvo usted pólipos?
How many months ago was the last time you had your cholesterol checked?	¿Hace cuántos meses fue la última vez que le revisaron su colesterol?
	¿Hace cuántos meses fue la última vez que le **chequearon** su colesterol?
How many years ago was your last tetanus shot?	¿Hace cuántos años fue su última vacuna para: el tétano?
Flu shot?	¿La influenza?
	¿La **gripe**?
Pneumonia shot?	¿La pulmonía?
Measles/mumps/rubella immunization?	¿La inmunización de sarampión/paperas/rubeola?
Hepatitis immunization?	¿La inmunización de hepatitis?
How many years ago was your last TB test?	¿Hace cuántos años fue su último examen para la tuberculosis?
Was it positive?	¿Fue positivo?
Was it negative?	¿Fue negativo?
Were you treated for TB?	¿Lo trataron por tuberculosis?
How many months ago was your last vision test?	¿Hace cuántos meses fue su último examen de la vista?
	¿Hace cuántos meses fue su último examen de la **visión**?

How many months ago was your last dental exam?	¿Hace cuántos meses fue su último examen dental?
	¿Hace cuántos meses fue su último examen **dentario**?
	¿Hace cuántos meses fue su última **visita al dentista**?
Have you had a hearing test?	¿Le han hecho un examen auditivo?
	¿Ha tenido un examen **para la audición**?
Do you . . .	¿Usted . . .
drive a car/motorcycle?	maneja un carro/motocicleta?
	maneja **un auto**/motocicleta?
	maneja **un automobil**/motocicleta?
	maneja **un vehículo**/moto?
wear seatbelts?	utiliza cinturón?
	usa cinturón?
ride a bicycle?	monta bicicleta?
Do you wear a helmet?	¿Usa un casco?
Do you wear sunscreen when outdoors?	¿Usa bloqueador del sol cuando está afuera?

Women's Health

Have you ever had a Pap smear?	¿Ha tenido un Papanicolaou?
	¿Ha tenido **una citología vaginal**?
	¿Ha tenido **un frotis vaginal**?
How many months/years ago was your Pap smear?	¿Hace cuántos meses/años fue su último Papanicolaou?
	¿Hace cuántos meses/años fue **su último citología vaginal**?
	¿Hace cuántos meses/anos fue **su último frotis vaginal**?
Was it normal?	¿Fue normal?
Was it abnormal?	¿Fue atípico?
	¿Fue **irregular**?
	¿Fue **anormal**?

Health Promotion/Disease Prevention

Do you have a history of abnormal Pap smears?	¿Tiene usted una historia médica de algún Papanicolaou atípico?
	¿Ha tenido alguna citología vaginal irregular?
	¿Ha sufrido de frotis vaginal anormales?
How many months/years ago was your last mammogram?	¿Hace cuántos meses/años fue su última mamografía?
Do you examine your breasts?	¿Usted se examina sus senos?
	¿Usted se examina **su pecho**?
Once a month?	¿Una vez al mes?
More often?	¿Más a menudo?
Do you take hormones?	¿Toma hormonas?
How many years have you taken hormones?	¿Por cuántos años ha tomado hormonas?

Men's Health

How many months ago was your last prostate exam?	¿Cuántos meses atrás fue su último examen de la próstata?
Was it normal?	¿Fue normal?
Was it abnormal?	¿Fue atípico?
	¿Fue **irregular**?
	¿Fue **anormal**?
Do you do examine your testicles?	¿Usted se examina sus testículos?

Chapter 12

Special Patient Instructions

Frequently during a visit, patients will require instructions on self-examinations, laboratory testing, or tests that they are expected to complete at home and turn in at a later date. Several different people may be involved in patient teaching, including the health care provider, nurses, medical assistants, and laboratory technicians.

In this chapter, we include instructions on some of the more common testing encountered in a primary care setting. Each section includes simple, direct phrases to guide the patient through the instructions or teaching. Since instructions for certain tests are quite specific, at the end of each section there is a chance to ask if the patient has further questions, which may necessitate an interpreter.

Breast Self-Exam

You should examine your breasts once a month at the same time each month.	Usted debe examinarse sus senos una vez por mes un día en específico todos los meses.
The best time to examine your breasts is one week after your period.	El mejor momento para examinarse sus senos es una semana después de su menstruación. El mejor momento para examinarse sus senos es una semana después de su **período**.
If you do not have periods, then do it on the first day of each month.	Si usted ya no tiene menstruación, entonces examínese sus senos el primero de cada mes. Si usted ya no tiene **períodos**, entonces examínese sus senos el primero de cada mes.
You can do this in the shower, standing in front of a mirror, or lying on the bed.	Usted puede examinarse en la ducha, parada al frente de un espejo, o acostada en la cama. Usted puede examinarse en la ducha, parada **delante** de un espejo o acostada en la cama.
It is best to use all three methods to examine your breasts.	Es mejor/**más óptimo** utilizar los tres métodos mencionados para examinarse sus senos. Es mejor **usar** los tres métodos mencionados para examinarse sus senos.
Face the mirror, turn to the side, lift your arms over your head, and do one side and then the other.	Mirando hacia el espejo, vírese de lado, levante sus brazos sobre su cabeza **empiece con** un lado y después vaya al otro.

Breast Self-Exam

You should look for . . .	Al mirar usted debe buscar lo siguiente . . .
changes in the size, shape, or color of your breasts,	cambios de tamaño, forma y color de sus senos,
dimples in your breasts,	hoyuelos en sus senos,
changes in the size shape or color of the nipples	cambios en el tamaño, forma o color del pezón,
discharge from the nipples	**descargas por su pezón**.
In the shower, with soapy hands, check both breasts for any lumps or masses.	En la ducha, con sus manos enjabonadas, examínese ambos senos buscando algún tipo de masa o nudo en sus senos.
Use the pads of your three middle fingers, not the fingertips, to feel your breasts.	Utilice la almohadilla de sus tres dedos centrales, no utilice la yema del dedo para examinar sus senos. **Use** la almohadilla de sus tres dedos **del medio**, no utilice la yema del dedo para examinar sus senos.
Check each breast by pressing down firmly over the breast in a circle.	Examine cada seno oprimiendo firmemente hacia abajo siguiendo su seno en forma circular.
Feel for lumps under your armpit.	Busque masas y nudos en su axila. Busque masas y nudos en su **sobaco**.
Lying on the bed, put a small towel under the breast you are checking.	Acostada en su cama ponga una pequeña toalla debajo del seno que usted esté examinando.
If you are checking your right breast, then put your right hand behind your head.	Si usted está examinando su seno derecho, entonces ponga su mano derecha debajo de su cabeza.
With your other hand, press your fingers firmly in a circle over all parts of your breast to feel for any lumps.	Con su otra mano, presione sus dedos firmemente en forma circular sobre todas las partes del seno en busca de nódulos. Con su otra mano, presione sus dedos firmemente sobre todas las partes del seno en busca de **masas**. Con su otra mano, presione sus dedos firmemente sobre todas las partes del seno en busca de **chichones**.

Breast Self-Exam

Do the same for the left side.	Haga lo mismo con el seno izquierdo.
If you feel anything abnormal or worrisome, call as soon as possible to make an appointment.	Si usted siente algo atípico o que le preocupase, llame lo más pronto posible y haga una cita. Si usted siente algo **irregular** o que le preocupase, llame lo más pronto posible y haga una cita. Si usted siente algo **anormal** o que le preocupase, llame lo más pronto posible y haga una cita.
Most lumps are not cancer but must be examined by a provider as soon as possible.	La mayoría de los nódulos no son cancerosos, pero deben ser examinados por su doctor lo más pronto posible. La mayoría de las **masas** no son cancerosas, pero deben ser examinados por su doctor lo más pronto posible. La mayoría de los **chichones** no son cancerosos, pero deben ser examinados por su doctor lo más pronto posible.
Do you understand the instructions?	¿Entiende usted estas instrucciones?
Do you need me to call a translator?	¿Usted necesita que yo llame a un traductor?

Diabetic Teaching

Diabetic Diet

Do you have a glucometer?	¿Usted tiene un glucómetro? ¿Usted tiene un **medidor de azúcar de sangre**?
Do you check your glucose (sugar)?	¿Usted se revisa su azúcar? ¿Usted se **inspecciona** su **glucosa**? ¿Usted se **chequea** su **glucosa**?
Every day?	¿Todos los días?
Each time before you use insulin?	¿Cada vez, antes de utilizar insulina? ¿Cada vez, antes de **usar** insulina?
Before breakfast?	¿Antes del desayuno?

Diabetic Teaching

Before lunch?	¿Antes del almuerzo?
Before dinner?	¿Antes de la comida?
Before going to bed?	¿Antes de acostarse?
You must check your glucose level before each time you use insulin.	Antes de utilizar insulina, usted siempre tiene que examinarse sus niveles de azúcar. Antes de **usar** insulina, usted siempre tiene que examinarse sus niveles de **glucosa**.
If your glucose is less than 80 before breakfast or dinner, you need to eat or drink something then check your glucose again.	Si sus niveles de azúcar son menos de ochenta antes del desayuno o la comida, usted necesita comer o tomar algo, y después, examínese su azúcar otra vez. Si sus niveles de **glucosa** son menos de ochenta antes del desayuno o la comida, usted necesita comer o **consumir** algo, y después, examínese su **glucosa** otra vez. Si sus niveles de **glucosa** son menos de ochenta antes del desayuno o la comida, usted necesita comer o **beber** algo, y después, examínese su **glucosa** otra vez.
Once your glucose is 100 or more, you can use the insulin and eat your meal.	Cuando su azúcar esté en cien o más, usted debe de utilizar su insulina primero y entonces comer su comida. Cuando su **glucosa** esté en cien o más, usted debe de **usar** su insulina primero y entonces comer su comida.
You need to eat 3 meals a day.	Usted necesita comer tres comidas al día.
Do not skip meals.	No salte/**brinque** ninguna comida.
Do not eat large meals.	No coma una gran cantidad de comida en ningún momento dado. **No consuma** una gran cantidad de comida en **una sentada**.
Try to eat your meals at the same time each day.	Trate de comer sus comidas a la misma hora todos los días.

Diabetic Teaching

You need to eat a snack . . .	Necesita usted comer una merienda . . . Necesita usted comer **un bocadillo** . . . Necesita usted comer **un entremés** . . .
between breakfast and lunch.	entre el desayuno y el almuerzo.
between lunch and dinner.	entre el almuerzo y la comida.
at bedtime.	al acostarse.
Snacks can be . . .	Ejemplos de meriendas pueden ser . . . Ejemplos de **bocadillos** pueden ser . . . Ejemplos de **entremeses** pueden ser . . .
one piece of fruit and one slice of low-fat cheese.	un pedazo de fruta y una tajada de queso bajo en grasas. un pedazo de fruta y una **rebanada** de queso bajo en grasas.
one piece of bread with 2 teaspoons of peanut butter.	un pedazo de pan con dos cucharaditas de mantequilla de maní. **una tajada** de pan con dos cucharaditas de mantequilla de maní. **una rebanada** de pan con dos cucharaditas de mantequilla de maní.
graham crackers with a glass of nonfat milk.	galletas graham con un vaso de leche bajo en grasas.
half a tuna sandwich.	la mitad de un emparedado de tuna. la mitad de un **bocadillo** de tuna. la mitad de un **sándwich** de tuna.
Do not eat fruit at bedtime.	No coma frutas antes de acostarse.
Avoid sugar and sweets like candy, soda, cake, ice cream, jam, and syrup.	Evite azúcar o cosas dulces como dulces, refrescos, torta, helado, mermelada, y almíbar. Evite azúcar o cosas dulces como **golosinas**, **sodas**, **pastel**, **nieve**, mermelada, y **jarabes**.
You can eat sugar-free foods or diet drinks.	Usted puede comer comidas libres de o sin azúcar, como refrescos de dietas. Usted puede comer comidas libres de o sin azúcar, como **sodas** de dietas.

Diabetic Teaching

Do not eat high-fat foods like fried foods, chips, or fast foods.	No coma comidas altas en grasas como comidas fritas, frituras, o comidas rápidas.
Do not cook with fat, butter, oil, or lard.	No cocine con grasa, mantequilla, aceite o manteca de cerdo.
Bake, broil, boil, roast, or grill all meats.	Cocine al horno, hierva, ase, o hágalo a la parrilla. Cocine al horno, hierva, ase, o hágalo a la **plancha**.
Cut off the fat from meats.	Córtele la grasa a todas las carnes. **Quítele** la grasa a todas las carnes. **Sáquele** la grasa a todas las carnes. **Remuévale** la grasa a todas las carnes.
Do not eat the skin on poultry.	No se coma el pellejo del pollo.
Your protein (meat, chicken, or fish) at each meal should be no bigger than the palm of your hand or a deck of cards.	La cantidad de proteínas (carne, pollo, o pescado) que usted consume en cada comida no debe de ser mas gran de que la palma de su mano o que un conjunto de cartas. La cantidad de proteínas (carne, pollo, o pescado) que usted consume en cada comida no debe de ser mas grande que la palma de su mano o que un **grupo** de **barajas**.
Try to eat whole-grain breads, cereals, tortillas*, rice, and pasta.	Trate de comer pan de trigo integral, cereales, tortillas*, arroz o pasta.
Limit your bread or tortillas* to one or two per meal.	Limite la cantidad de pan o tortillas* a uno o dos por comida.
Limit your pasta and rice to one-half cup per meal.	Limite la cantidad de pastas y arroz a media taza por comida.
You should eat no more than six servings of bread, tortillas*, rice, or pasta each day.	Usted no debe de comer más de seis porciones de pan, tortillas*, arroz o pastas por día.
It is better to eat fresh fruits and vegetables.	Es mejor comer frutas frescas y vegetales.
You can buy canned fruit packed in water or juice, not syrup.	Usted puede comer frutas enlatadas en agua o jugo pero no en almíbar. Usted puede comer frutas enlatadas en agua o jugo pero no en **jarabes**.

Diabetic Teaching

Do you understand the instructions?	¿Entiende usted estas instrucciones?
Do you need me to call a translator?	¿Usted necesita que yo llame a un traductor?

***Here, "tortilla" refers to the thin bread made of wheat or corn flour commonly eaten in Latin America, not to the Spanish tortillas that are made of eggs and potatoes.**

Hypoglycemia (Low Blood Sugar)

With diabetes, you may occasionally have low blood sugar levels.	Con diabetes, usted ocasionalmente puede tener bajos niveles de azúcar. Con diabetes, usted ocasionalmente puede tener bajos niveles de **glucosa**.
This happens when your blood sugar drops so low that it can't provide enough energy for your body.	Esto sucede debido a que sus niveles de azúcar le han bajado tanto que ya usted no puede proveer suficiente energía para su cuerpo. Esto sucede debido a que sus niveles de **glucosa** le han bajado tanto que ya usted no puede proveer suficiente energía para su cuerpo.
Low blood sugar can be very dangerous.	Niveles bajos de azúcar pueden ser muy peligrosos. Niveles bajos de **glucosa** pueden ser muy peligrosos.
If your sugar drops too low, you can faint or even fall into a diabetic coma.	Si su azúcar le bajase demasiado, usted puede desmayarse, o peor, entrar en una coma debido a su diabetes. Si su **glucosa** le bajase **mucho**, usted pudiese desmayarse, o peor, **caer** en una coma debido a su diabetes.
Ways that your sugar can drop too low can include: taking too much insulin or diabetes medicine.	Maneras en las cuales su diabetes pudiese bajarle demasiado: **Formas** en las cuales su diabetes pudiese bajarle **mucho**: tomando demasiada insulina. **poniéndose mucha insulina**.
eating too little food.	comiendo muy poca comida.
delayed or skipped meals	retrasando o saltando comidas.

Diabetic Teaching

drinking too much alcohol.	tomando demasiado alcohol. **consumiendo mucho** alcohol. **bebiendo mucho** alcohol.
increased activity or exercise without proper pre-exercise snack.	aumentando sus actividades o ejercicios sin meriendas antes de sus actividades o ejercicios. aumentando sus actividades o ejercicios sin **bocadillos** antes de sus actividades o ejercicios. aumentando sus actividades o ejercicios sin **entremeses** antes de sus actividades o ejercicios.
When your blood sugar drops below 70, you may have some or all of these symptoms:	Cuando sus niveles de azúcar bajen por debajo de setenta (70), usted podría tener algunos o todos estos síntomas: Cuando sus niveles de **glucosa** bajen por debajo de setenta (70), usted podría tener algunos o todos estos síntomas:
sleepiness	somnolencia
weakness	debilidad
confusion	confusión
dizziness	vértigo **mareo**
headache	dolor de cabeza
irritability	irritabilidad
shakiness	inestabilidad
nervousness	nerviosismo
blurry vision	visión borrosa
sudden cold sweats	sudores fríos repentinos sudores fríos **de momentos**
sudden hunger	hambres repentinos hambres **de momentos**
fainting	desmayos

Sometimes, when your body is used to a very high level of blood sugar and you now get your blood sugar to normal levels, you may experience symptoms of low blood sugar, even though it is in the normal range.	De vez en cuando, cuando su cuerpo se acostumbra a niveles altos de azúcar en la sangre, y de repente usted se encuentra con niveles normales, usted podría sentir síntomas de azúcar baja en la sangre, aun cuando está se encuentra en niveles normales. **Algunas veces**, cuando su cuerpo se acostumbra a niveles altos de **glucosa** en la sangre, y de repente usted se encuentra con niveles normales, usted podría **experimentar** síntomas de **glucosa** baja en la sangre, aun cuando está se encuentra en niveles normales. **A veces**, cuando su cuerpo se acostumbra a niveles altos de azúcar en la sangre, y de repente usted se encuentra con niveles normales, usted podría sentir síntomas de azúcar baja en la sangre, aun cuando está se encuentra en niveles normales.
You should be prepared for occasional episodes of low blood sugar.	Usted debería estar preparado/a a bajas ocasionales de azúcar en su sangre. Usted debería estar preparado/a a **bajones** ocasionales de **glucosa** en su sangre.
If you think your blood sugar is too low, it is always best to check your level with a glucometer.	Si usted cree que sus niveles de azúcar en su sangre están muy bajos, es siempre mejor revisar sus niveles con un glucómetro. Si usted **piensa** que sus niveles de **glucosa** en su sangre están muy bajos, es siempre mejor **inspeccionar** sus niveles con un **medidor de azúcar en la sangre**. Si usted cree que sus niveles de azúcar en su sangre están muy bajos, es siempre mejor **chequear** sus niveles con un glucómetro.

Diabetic Teaching

When you find that your sugar is too low, there are certain things you can do to bring it back up to normal:	Cuando usted se dé cuenta que sus niveles de azúcar están muy bajos, hay ciertas cosas que usted puede hacer para subir sus niveles a un nivel más apropiado: Cuando usted se dé cuenta que sus niveles de **glucosa** están muy bajos, hay ciertas cosas que usted puede hacer para subir sus niveles a un nivel normal:
Immediately eat or drink something with sugar in it:	Coma o tome algo que contenga azúcar inmediatamente: Coma o **consuma** algo que contenga azúcar inmediatamente: Coma o **beba** algo que contenga azúcar inmediatamente:
1/2 cup of fruit juice or regular soda (not diet)	Media taza de jugo de frutas o de refresco regular (no de dieta) Media taza de jugo de frutas o de **soda** regular (no de dieta)
1 cup of milk and 2 graham crackers	Una taza de leche y dos galletas graham
hard candy	Dulce duro
1–2 glucose tablets	Una o dos tabletas de glucosa
1–2 teaspoons of sugar or honey	Una o dos cucharadas de azúcar o miel
Wait 15 minutes and check your blood sugar again.	Espere quince minutos y revise después sus niveles de azúcar en la sangre. Espere quince minutos e **inspeccione** sus niveles sanguíneos de **glucosa**. Espere quince minutos y **chequee** después sus niveles sanguíneos de azúcar.
If it is still low, have another serving of the above.	Si todavía están bajos, tome o coma otro servicio de lo ya mencionado.

Diabetic Teaching

Wait another 15 minutes and check again. You want to repeat these steps until your blood sugar is at least 70.	Espere otros quince minutes y revise sus niveles otra vez. Usted necesita repetir todos estos pasos ya mencionados hasta que sus niveles de azúcar en la sangre estén por lo menos en setenta.
	Espere otros quince minutes e **inspeccione** sus niveles otra vez. Usted necesita repetir todos estos pasos ya mencionados hasta que sus niveles de **glucosa** en la sangre estén por lo menos en setenta.
	Espere otros quince minutes e **chequee** sus niveles otra vez. Usted necesita repetir todos estos pasos ya mencionados hasta que sus niveles sanguíneos de azúcar estén por lo menos en setenta.
If it is more than 2 hours or so before your next meal, eat a snack like:	Si han pasado, más o menos dos horas antes de su próxima comida, coma una merienda como:
	Si han pasado, más o menos dos horas antes de su próxima comida, coma un **bocadillo** como:
	Si han pasado, más o menos dos horas antes de su próxima comida, coma un **entremés** como:
half a sandwich and a glass of milk	medio emparedado y un vaso de leche
	medio **bocadillo** y un vaso de leche
	medio **sándwich** y un vaso de leche
peanut butter and crackers	mantequilla de maní con galletas
cheese and crackers	queso con galletas
fruit and cheese	frutas y queso
Always carry something with sugar in it with you, like hard candies, packets of honey or sugar, or glucose tablets, in case your blood sugar levels drop when you are away from home.	Siempre cargue con sigo algo que contenga azúcar, como un caramelo, pequeños sobres de miel o azúcar, tabletas de glucosa, en caso que sus niveles sanguíneos de azúcar bajen cuando usted no se encuentre en su casa.

Diabetic Teaching

	Siempre **lleve con usted** algo que contenga azúcar, como un **dulce duro**, pequeños sobres de miel o azúcar, tabletas de **azúcar**, en caso que **sus niveles de azúcar en su sangre** bajen cuando usted no se encuentre en su casa.
Always check your blood sugar level before you start to exercise.	Siempre revise sus niveles de azúcar antes de empezar sus ejercicios. Siempre **inspeccione** sus niveles de **glucosa** antes de empezar sus ejercicios. Siempre **chequee** sus niveles de azúcar antes de empezar sus ejercicios.
It is always a good idea to wear a medical identification bracelet so that others will know you are a diabetic.	Es una buena idea tener siempre puesto un brazalete con su información médica ya que así otras personas sabrán que usted es diabético/a. Es una buena idea tener siempre puesto **una pulsera** con su información médica ya que así otras personas sabrán que usted es diabético/a.

Diabetic Foot Care

Because of your diabetes, you may lose some feeling in your feet.	Debido a su diabetes, usted puede perder sensación en sus pies.
It is very important to check your feet every day.	Es muy importante que usted se examine sus pies a diario.
It is important to prevent infections and amputation.	Es muy importante prevenir infecciones y hasta una amputación.
Look at the soles and between the toes.	Mire la planta de sus pies y entre sus dedos. **Revísese** la planta de sus pies y entre sus dedos.
Look for rashes, blisters, ulcers.	Mire por erupciones, ampollas, o úlceras. Mire por **salpullidos**, ampollas, o úlceras. **Revise** por **pintas rojas en su piel**, ampollas, o úlceras.

Diabetic Teaching

Always wear shoes or slippers.	Siempre ande con zapatos o alpargatas. Siempre ande con zapatos o **zapatillas**. Siempre ande con zapatos o **sandalias**. Siempre ande con zapatos o **chancletas**. Siempre ande con zapatos o **pantuflas**. Siempre ande con zapatos o **chinelas**.
Do not walk barefoot inside or outside.	No camine sin zapatos adentro o afuera de su casa.
Look inside your shoes and socks for holes or places that might cause blisters.	Busque dentro de sus zapatos y medias por imperfecciones y huecos o lugares que puedan causar ampollas. Busque dentro de sus zapatos y medias por imperfecciones y huecos o **aéreas** que puedan causar ampollas.
Wash your feet when you bathe.	Límpiese sus pies al bañarse. **Lavase** sus pies al bañarse.
Check the water temperature with your elbow before you put your feet in the water.	Examine la temperatura del agua con su codo antes de poner sus pies dentro del agua.
Do not soak your feet.	No remoje sus pies. No **emerja** sus pies. **No deje sus pies en agua por mucho tiempo.** **No ponga sus pies en agua por mucho tiempo.**
Make sure you dry your feet well.	Asegurase bien de secarse sus pies.
Use lotion on the top and bottom of your feet.	Utilice loción en la parte de arriba y de debajo de sus pies. **Use** loción en la parte de arriba y de debajo de sus pies.
Do not use lotion or oil between your toes.	No utilice loción o aceite entre los dedos de sus pies. No **use** loción o aceite entre los dedos de sus pies.
Cut your toenails straight across.	Corte sus uñas rectas.
Do not cut them shorter than the ends of your toes.	No se las corte más atrás de la yema de los dedos sus pies.

Diabetic Teaching

You can sand down calluses and toenails with an emery board, pumice stone, or fine sand paper.	Usted se puede limar sus callos y uñas de los pies con una tabla de emery, piedra pone o papel de lija fino.
Wear shoes that are made of soft leather, have a low heel, and have deep, wide toes.	Use zapatos que estén hechos de cuero suave, que tengan un tacón pequeño y que tengan amplio espacio para los dedos del pie.
Do not wear open-toed shoes or sandals.	No use zapatos o alpargatas abiertas al frente o sin protección para los dedos del pie. No use zapatos o **zapatillas** abiertas al frente o sin protección para los dedos del pie. No use zapatos o **chancletas** abiertas al frente o sin protección para los dedos del pie. No use zapatos o **sandalias** abiertas al frente o sin protección para los dedos del pie. No use zapatos o **chinelas** abiertas al frente o sin protección para los dedos del pie.
Do not buy shoes with a high heel or narrow toe.	No compre zapatos de tacón alto o muy apretados en el área de los dedos del pie. No compre zapatos de tacón alto o **de poco espacio** para los dedos del pie.
If you find an ulcer or rash, call and make an appointment as soon as possible.	Si encuentra una úlcera o una erupción, llame y haga una cita en la clínica. Si encuentra una úlcera o **salpullido**, llame y haga una cita **con su doctor lo más pronto posible**. Si encuentra una úlcera o **pintas rojas en su piel**, llame y haga una cita **con su doctor lo más pronto posible**.
Do you understand the instructions?	¿Entiende usted estas instrucciones?
Do you need me to call a translator?	¿Usted necesita que yo llame a un traductor?

Nursing Instructions

24-Hour Urine Collection

On [insert name of day] when you get out of bed, urinate in the toilet and flush.	En [insert name of day], cuando usted se levante de su cama, orine en el inodoro y después descargue. En [insert name of day], cuando usted **salga** de su cama, orine en el **excusado** y después descargue. En [insert name of day], cuando usted **salga** de su cama, orine en el **retrete** y después descargue. En [insert name of day], cuando usted **salga** de su cama, orine en el **toilet** y después descargue.
Look at the time and write it down.	Mire la hora y escríbala.
From then until exactly the same time on [insert name of day], save all your urine in this jug.	Desde ese momento hasta, exactamente la misma hora, el próximo [insert name of day] guarde su orine en esta jarra que le vamos a dar. Desde ese momento hasta, exactamente la misma hora, el próximo [insert name of day] **coleccione** su orine en esta **botija** que le vamos a **entregar**.
It is important to save all your urine.	Es muy importante que usted guarde todo su orine. Es muy importante que usted **coleccione** todo su orine.
Do not flush any of it away.	No bote o descargue el inodoro con el orine guardado durante todo el día. No bote o descargue el inodoro con el orine **coleccionado** durante todo el día.
You do/do not need to keep the jug on ice (in an ice chest with ice, or in the refrigerator).	Usted necesita/no necesita mantener la jarra con orine en hielo (en una hielera portátil o dentro del refrigerador). Usted necesita/no necesita mantener la **botija** con orine en hielo (en una **neverita** portátil o dentro de la **nevera**).

Nursing Instructions

When the ice melts, put in fresh ice.	Cuando el hielo se derrita, póngala en hielo fresco. Cuando el hielo se derrita, **cámbiele el hielo y póngala en hielo nuevo**.
Return the jug to this clinic on [insert name of day].	Regrese la jarra con el orine a esta clínica el [insert name of day]. Regrese la **botija** con el orine a esta clínica el [insert name of day].
Return it by 10:00 am.	Regrésela a las diez de la mañana.
You must bring the jug back in an ice chest.	Usted tiene que traer la jarra con el orine dentro de la hielera portátil. Usted tiene que traer la **botija** con el orine dentro de la **neverita** portátil.
It is very important to always keep the urine on ice.	Es muy importante que usted mantenga siempre el orine en hielo.
Do you understand the instructions?	¿Entiende usted estas instrucciones?
Do you need me to call an interpreter?	¿Usted necesita que yo llame a un intérprete?

Fecal Occult Blood Cards

Your doctor/provider has ordered a test to look for blood in your stools.	Su doctor/proveedor de servicios médicos ha ordenado una prueba para ver si usted tiene sangre en las heces. Su doctor/ proveedor de servicios médicos ha ordenado **un examen** para ver si usted tiene sangre en la **excreta**. Su doctor/ proveedor de servicios médicos ha ordenado una prueba para ver si usted tiene sangre en el **excremento**.
Blood in your stools can be a sign of gastrointestinal bleeding or colon polyps or an early sign of colon cancer.	Sangre en sus heces puede ser un signo de sangrado gastrointestinal, de pólipos en su colon o un signo temprano de cáncer en el colon. Sangre en su **excreta** puede ser un signo de sangrado gastrointestinal, de pólipos en su **intestino grueso** o un signo **precoz** de cáncer en el colon.

	Sangre en su **excremento** puede ser un signo de sangrado gastrointestinal, de pólipos en su **intestino grueso** o un signo **prematuro** de cáncer en el colon.
This is one way to screen for colon cancer.	Esto es una forma de investigar la presencia de cáncer del colon. Esto es una forma de analizar la presencia de cáncer del colon.
If caught early, colon cancer can be curable.	Si se detecta temprano, el cáncer del colon puede ser curado. Si se detecta temprano, el cáncer del **intestino grueso** puede ser curado.
You may follow your regular diet and take your medicines as usual during this test.	Usted puede seguir su dieta regular y seguir tomando sus medicamentos de la forma usual. Usted puede seguir su dieta regular y seguir tomando sus **medicinas** de la forma usual.
This test involves collecting a sample of your stool each day for 3 days in a row.	Este examen envuelve la colección de una muestra de sus heces cada día por tres días. Esta **prueba** envuelve la colección de un espécimen de su **excreta** cada día por tres días. Esta **prueba** envuelve la colección de una prueba de su **excremento** cada día por tres días.
You may want to eat a bowl of bran every day.	Usted debe de pensar en comer un tazón de salvado cada día. Usted debe de pensar en comer un **cereal alto en fibra** de **plato todos los días**. Usted debe de pensar en comer una **vasija** de **bran todos los días**.
This is important to help you have a bowel movement every day.	Esto es importante para ayudarle diariamente a tener un buen ritmo evacuatorio.
You may drink what you like during this test.	Puede tomar lo que usted desee durante este examen.

Nursing Instructions

	Puede **consumir** lo que usted desee durante esta **prueba**. Puede **beber** lo que usted desee durante esta **prueba**.
Do not start to collect stool samples until at least 3 days after your period ends.	No coleccione sus muestras de heces hasta por lo menos tres días después de terminarse le su menstruación. No recoja sus muestras de **excreta** hasta por lo menos tres días después de terminarse le su período. No recoja sus muestras de **excremento** hasta por lo menos tres días después de terminarse le su período.
Do not collect stool samples if you have bleeding hemorrhoids or blood in your urine.	No coleccione muestras de heces si usted tiene hemorroides que le están sangrando o sangre en la orina. No coleccione muestras de **excreta** si usted tiene hemorroides que le están sangrando o sangre en la orina. No coleccione muestras de **excremento** si usted tiene hemorroides que le están sangrando o sangre en la orina.
You have three cards and three sticks.	Usted tiene tres tarjetas y tres palitos.
Put the cards and sticks in the bathroom so they will be ready.	Ponga las tarjetas y los palitos en el baño, de esta forma estarán listos para cuando los necesite.
Make sure you write your name and medical record number or birth date on each card.	Esté seguro de escribir su nombre, el número de su archivo médico o de su nacimiento en cada tarjeta.
On the first day, start collecting the samples.	Empiece a coleccionar las muestras en el primer día. Empiece a **recoger** las muestras en el primer día.
Before you have a bowel movement, put a large plastic bag or plastic wrap under the toilet seat to catch the stool.	Antes de defecar, ponga una bolsa plástica grande o papel plástico debajo del asiento del inodoro para así atrapar las heces. Antes de **ensuciar**, ponga una bolsa plástica grande o papel plástico debajo del asiento del inodoro para así **agarrar** el **excremento**.

	Antes de **ir al baño**, ponga una bolsa plástica grande o papel plástico debajo del asiento del inodoro para así **apresar** la **excreta**.
Or catch the stool in a clean container like a margarine tub or clean milk carton with the top cut off.	Usted también puede atrapar las heces en un recipiente limpio, como los que se utilizan para la mantequilla o la leche con la parte de arriba cortada. Usted también puede **agarrar** la **excreta** en un **envase** limpio, como los que se **usan** para la mantequilla o la leche con la parte de arriba cortada. Usted también puede **apresar** el **excremento** en un **envase** limpio, como los que se utilizan para la mantequilla o la leche con la parte de arriba cortada.
Use the stick to get a small amount of stool and wipe it on one of the windows on the card.	Utilice el palito para atrapar una pequeña cantidad de heces y aplíquela en una de las ventanas en la tarjeta. Utilice el palito para atrapar una pequeña **porción** de **excreta** y aplíquela en una de las ventanas en la tarjeta. **Use** el palito para atrapar una pequeña cantidad de **excremento** y **úntela** en una de las ventanas en la tarjeta.
Take another sample from a different area of stool and wipe it on the other window of the card.	Tome otra muestra de un área diferente de las heces y aplíquela en la otra ventana en la tarjeta. Tome otro **espécimen** de **una parte** diferente de la **excreta** y aplíquela en la otra ventana en la tarjeta. Tome otra muestra de una sección diferente del **excremento** y **úntela** en la otra ventana en la tarjeta.
Close the cover of the card.	Cierre la cubierta de la tarjeta
Store the card with the samples in a plastic bag.	Guarde la tarjeta con la muestra en una bolsa plástica. Guarde la tarjeta con el **espécimen** en una bolsa plástica.

Nursing Instructions

Flush away the rest of the stool.	Descargue en su inodoro el resto de sus heces. Descargue en su inodoro el resto de su **excreta**. Descargue en su inodoro el resto de su **excremento**.
On the second day, collect more samples on another card. Store the card in the plastic bag.	En el segundo día, coleccione más muestras en otra tarjeta y después guarde la tarjeta en la bolsa plástica. En el segundo día, **guarde** más **especímenes** en otra tarjeta y después guarde la tarjeta en la bolsa plástica.
On the third day, collect more samples on another card. Store the card in the plastic bag.	En el tercer día, coleccione más muestras en la última tarjeta, y después guarde la tarjeta en la bolsa plástica. En el tercer día, **guarde** más **especímenes** en la última tarjeta, y después guarde la tarjeta en la bolsa plástica.
Bring the three stool cards in the plastic bag to the clinic.	Traiga a la clínica las tres tarjetas que contienen las heces en la bolsa plástica. Traiga a la clínica las tres tarjetas que contienen la **excreta** en la bolsa plástica. Traiga a la clínica las tres tarjetas que contienen el **excremento** en la bolsa plástica.
Or mail the cards to the laboratory in this envelope.	Usted también puede mandar por correo las muestras para el laboratorio en este sobre. Usted también puede **enviar** por correo los **especímenes** para el laboratorio en este sobre. Usted también puede **poner en el buzón** las muestras para el laboratorio en este sobre. Usted también puede **echar** por correo las muestras para el laboratorio en este sobre.

Nursing Instructions

Even if you are able to complete only 1 or 2 days, return the cards	Mande las muestras, no importa si usted solo haya completado uno o dos días. **Envíe los especímenes** no importa si usted solo haya completado uno o dos días.
Do you understand the instructions?	¿Entiende usted estas instrucciones?
Do you need me to call a translator?	¿Usted necesita que yo llame a un traductor?

Laboratory Tests

Urinalysis Collection

We need for you to collect some urine.	Necesitamos que usted coleccione un poco de su orina. Necesitamos que usted **recoja** un poco de su orina.
If you are unable to urinate right now, please drink plenty of water and wait until you are able.	Si usted no puede orinar en este momento, por favor tome suficiente agua y espere hasta que pueda orinar. Si usted no puede orinar en este momento, por favor **consuma** suficiente agua y espere hasta que pueda orinar. Si usted no puede orinar en este momento, por favor **beba** suficiente agua y espere hasta que pueda orinar.
Before you start to urinate, please wipe the outside of your genitals with this towelette so the sample will be free of outside contamination.	Antes de que usted empiece a orinar, por favor limpie la parte de afuera de sus órganos genitales con esta toallita, de esta forma la muestra estará libre de contaminación.
Urinate directly into the toilet for the first few drops.	Orine en el **inodoro** las primeras gotas de orine. Orine en el **escusado** las primeras gotas de orine. Orine en el **retrete** las primeras gotas de orine.

Laboratory Tests

	Orine en el **váter** las primeras gotas de orine. Orine en el **toilet** las primeras gotas de orine.
Then place the cup so that you are able to collect the rest of the urine directly in the cup.	Entonces, ponga el vaso plástico pequeño cerca de sus órganos genitales para así poder coleccionar el resto de su orine. Entonces, ponga la **vasijita** plástica cerca de sus órganos genitales para así poder **recorger** el resto de su orine.
When you are done, please put the cap on the cup and wash your hands.	Cuando termine, por favor póngale la tapa al vaso plástico pequeño y lávese sus manos. Cuando termine, por favor póngale la tapa a la **vasijita** plástica y lávese sus manos.
When you have finished, please leave the urine sample . . . with me. in the lab. on the counter.	Cuando termine, por favor deje la muestra de orine . . . conmigo. en el laboratorio. en el mostrador. en **la ventanilla**.
Do you understand the instructions?	¿Entiende usted estas instrucciones?
Do you need me to call an interpreter?	¿Usted necesita que yo llame a un intérprete?

Blood Collection

We need to draw some blood from you.	Necesitamos sacarle sangre. Necesitamos **extraerle** sangre.
Please have a seat here.	Por favor siéntese aquí.
Please remove your jacket and roll up your sleeve on this arm.	Por favor remueva su chaqueta y enrolle las mangas de su camisa en este brazo. Por favor **quítese** su **chamarra** y **córrase** las mangas de su camisa en este brazo.

Laboratory Tests

Hold your arm out straight, like this.	Mantenga su brazo en una manera recta, de esta forma. **Ponga** su brazo en una manera recta, de esta forma.
Relax your arm.	Relaje su brazo. Descanse su brazo.
Please make a fist.	Por favor cierre su mano en forma de puño. Por favor cierre su mano y **haga un puño**.
Open and close your fist several times, like this.	Abra y cierre su puño varias veces, de esta forma. Abra y cierre su puño **muchas** veces, de esta forma.
You will feel a stick.	Usted va a sentir una hincada. Usted va a sentir una **punzada**.
Relax your hand.	Relaje su mano. **Descanse** su mano.
You can remove the bandage after about an hour or so.	Usted puede quitarse su vendaje en más o menos una hora. Usted puede **removerse** su **apósito** en más o menos una hora.
We're done.	Ya terminamos. Ya **acabamos**.
You are free to go.	Ya usted puede irse. Ya usted puede **retirarse**.
Please follow me.	Por favor sígame.
Have a seat here until your name is called.	Tome asiento aquí, hasta que su nombre sea llamado. **Tenga** asiento aquí, hasta que su nombre sea llamado. **Siéntase aquí**, hasta que su nombre sea llamado.

Chapter 13

End-of-Visit Instructions

Many different people in various roles may be involved in the discharge of a patient—whether from the emergency department, an office, or a hospital environment—from the nurse or medical assistant reviewing with the patient the medical condition treated, medications, or test results, to the clerical staff making future appointments or scheduling procedures. This chapter covers the basics required for end-of-visit instructions given to the patient. And in cases where the discharge instructions may be lengthier or more complicated, there is an opportunity at the end to offer the use of interpretation services, if needed.

In particular, social workers deal with a variety of emotionally and culturally sensitive issues involving many psychosocial nuances. As such, social services would be an example of when you should utilize interpretation services. However, particularly in hospital settings, time is often spent waiting for interpretation services to become available. We have supplied questions and phrases in this chapter that you can use as a quick initial needs assessment until you can accomplish a more detailed interview through an interpreter.

Review of Condition

You have . . .	Usted tiene . . .
an infection.	una infección.
a broken bone.	un hueso roto.
a concussion.	una concusión.
muscle strain.	una lastimadura muscular.
a sprained [body part].	una torcedura muscular [body part].
	distención muscular.
	esguince muscular.
congestive heart failure.	insuficiencia cardiáca congestiva
high/low blood glucose.	azúcar alta/baja.
high/low blood pressure.	presión alta/baja.
diabetes.	diabetes.
a tumor.	tumor.
You had a/an . . .	Usted tuvo un/a . . .
heart attack.	ataque al corazón.
	ataque cardiáco.
stroke.	accidente cerebro vascular.
asthma exacerbation.	exacerbación asmática.
heart failure exacerbation.	exacerbación de la insuficiencia cardiáca congestiva.
infection.	infección.
drug overdose.	sobredosis de droga ilegal/ilícita.
Your [body part] [see "Anatomy," in Chapter 3, "Vocabulary"] is/are . . .	Su [body part] esta/están . . .
infected.	infectado/s.
	contaminado/s.
bruised.	magullado.
not functioning correctly.	funcionando incorrectamente.
too high.	muy alto.

Review of Condition

too low.	muy bajo.
overactive.	sobre activo.
underactive.	poco activo.
broken.	roto.
You have a serious condition that requires . . .	Usted tiene una condición seria que requiere . . .
treatment.	tratamiento.
medications.	medicamentos. **medicinas.**
follow-up visits.	visitas de seguimiento.
hospitalization.	hospitalización.
emergency treatment.	tratamiento de emergencia.
You are doing fine.	Usted está bien.
Your condition requires follow-up visits.	Su condición requiere vistas de seguimiento.
You should be fine once the required treatment is complete.	Usted mejorará después que el tratamiento sea completado.
You will be able to go home . . .	Usted podrá irse para su casa . . .
without medicine.	sin medicamentos. sin **medicinas.**
once the treatment is complete.	cuando el tratamiento sea terminado.
You are/are not contagious.	Usted está/no está contagioso/a.
You must always wear a mask.	Debe de siempre usar/**utilizar** una máscara
You must wear a mask only when you go out in public.	Cuando usted salga afuera y crea que va a estar en contacto con gente, debe de siempre ponerse/**utilizar** una máscara.
We don't know what causes this.	Nosotros no sabemos qué es lo que lo causa.
We need to do more tests to find out what is wrong.	Necesitamos hacer más exámenes para encontrar el problema. Necesitamos hacer más **pruebas** para encontrar el problema.
We were not able to find anything wrong with you.	No pudimos encontrar nada malo en usted.
Your tests were normal.	Sus exámenes resultaron normales. Sus **pruebas** resultaron normales.

Review of Condition

Your tests were abnormal.	Sus exámenes resultaron anormales. Sus **pruebas** resultaron **anómalas**. Sus **pruebas** resultaron **atípicas**. Sus **pruebas** resultaron **irregulares**.
We need to order further tests.	Necesitamos ordenar más exámenes. Necesitamos ordenar más **pruebas**.
These must be done right away.	Estos ya mencionados, necesitan ser ordenados en este momento
These can be done as an outpatient.	Estos ya mencionados pueden ser hechos/**obtenidos** como paciente ambulatorio. Estos ya mencionados pueden ser hechos/**obtenidos** como **paciente externo**.
To treat this . . .	Para tratar esto . . .
you need to drink plenty of water and get some rest.	necesita tomar suficiente agua y descansar.
you need to limit your water to no more than [insert number] liters each day.	necesita limitar su cantidad de agua a no más de [insert number] litros al día.
you need to change your diet [see "Nutrition History," in Chapter 10, "Health Behaviors History and Education"].	usted tiene que cambiar su dieta.
you need exercise therapy [see "Exercise History and Counseling," in Chapter 10, "Health Behaviors History and Education"].	usted necesita terapia de ejercicio.
you need medication.	necesita medicamentos. necesita **medicinas**.
you need a cast/splint/brace.	necesita un yeso/muletas/un refuerzo ortopédico.
you need physical therapy.	necesita terapia física.
you need occupational therapy.	necesita terapia ocupacional.
you need speech therapy.	necesita terapia de lenguaje.
you need hydrotherapy.	necesita hidroterapia.

Review of Condition

you need a special procedure [see "Special Procedures," in Chapter 3, "Vocabulary"].	necesita un procedimiento especial.
You need to be admitted to the hospital.	Necesita ser admitido al hospital.
You need to have surgery.	Necesita tener una operación. Necesita a rugía.
You need to go to the emergency room.	Necesita ir a la sala de emergencia.
We are calling an ambulance for you.	Le estamos llamando una ambulancia para usted.
Is there someone here with you? What is his or her name? Does he or she speak English?	¿Vino alguien aquí con usted? ¿Cuál es el nombre de la persona? ¿Como se llama esta persona? ¿Él o ella habla inglés?
Do you need to call someone?	¿Necesita llamar a alguien?
Would you like us to call someone for you?	¿Quiere que le llamemos a alguien?

Medicines

This is the medicine your doctor has prescribed for you.	Este es el medicamento que su doctor le recetó. Este es la **medicina** que su doctor le recetó.
This medicine is for your . . . blood pressure. diabetes. heart. cholesterol. stomach. breathing. thyroid.	Este medicamento es para su . . . Esta **medicina** es para su . . . presión sanguinea. diabetes. corazón. colesterol. estómago. respiración. tiroides.
Call, come back, or go to the ER if you have any serious side effects from this medicine (like chest pain, difficulty breathing, rash, or swelling).	Llame, regrese o vaya a la sala de emergencias si tiene algún efecto secundario serio al medicamento (como dolor de pecho, dificultad al respirar, salpullido o inflamación).

	Llame, regrese o vaya a la sala de emergencias si tiene algún efecto secundario serio a **la medicina** (como dolor de pecho, dificultad al respirar, **erupción** o inflamación).
	Llame, regrese o vaya a la sala de emergencias si tiene algún efecto secundario serio a **la medicina** (como dolor de pecho, dificultad al respirar, salpullido **pintas rojas en su piel** o inflamación).
You do not need any new medication.	Usted no necesita ningún medicamento.
	Usted no necesita **medicina**.
Your doctor/medical provider has changed your medicines.	Su doctor/proveedor médico le ha cambiado sus medicamentos.
	Su doctor/proveedor médico le ha cambiado sus **medicinas**.
This is the new medicine.	Este es su nuevo medicamento.
	Esta es su nueva **medicina**.
Take this medicine . . .	Tome este medicamento . . .
	Tome esta **medicina** . . .
once a day.	una vez por día.
two/three/four times a day.	dos/tres/cuatro veces por día.
in the morning.	en la mañana.
in the evening.	al anochecer.
at bedtime.	al acostarse.
with food.	con comida.
before meals.	antes de las comidas.
after meals.	después de las comidas.
only as needed.	solamente si la necesita.
Take this medicine thirty/sixty minutes before/after your other medicines.	Tome este medicamento treinta/sesenta minutos antes/después de sus otros medicamentos.
	Tome esta **medicina** treinta/sesenta minutos antes/después de sus otras **medicinas**.

Medicines

Do not take more than [insert number] a day.	No tome más de [insert number] por día.
Take this medicine until all the pills are gone.	Tome este medicamento hasta que todas las píldoras se le hayan acabado.
	Tome este medicamento hasta que todas las **pastillas** se le hayan acabado.
	Tome esta **medicina** hasta que todas las **tabletas** se le hayan **terminado**.
Do not stop taking this medicine suddenly.	No deje repentinamente de tomar este medicamento.
	No se **detenga de repente** de tomar **esta medicina**.
	No se **pare de repente** de tomar **esta medicina**.
If you need to stop taking this medicine, you will need to taper off slowly.	Si usted va a dejar de tomarse este medicamento usted necesita de pararlo lentamente a través de días.
	Si usted va a **parar** de tomarse **esta medicina usted va a tener que hacerlo despacio a través de días.**
If you feel you need to stop taking this medicine, please call us.	Si usted siente que quiere dejar de tomar este medicamento, por favor llámenos.
	Si usted piensa que quiere **parar** de tomar esta **medicina**, por favor llámenos.
If you think you are experiencing any side effects from this medicine, please call us or come in for an evaluation.	Si usted cree que está teniendo efectos secundarios a este medicamento, por favor llámenos o venga acá para hacerle una evaluación.
	Si usted cree que está teniendo efectos secundarios a esta **medicina**, por favor llámenos o **pásese** por acá para hacerle una evaluación.

Medicines

For safety reasons . . .	Por razones de seguridad . . .
do not chew or crush this medicine.	no masque o comprima este medicamento. no masque o **triture** esta **medicina.** no masque o **apachurre** esta **medicina.**
do not cut this tablet.	no divida/**corte** esta tableta. no divida/**corte** esta **pastilla.**
remove the old patch before you apply a new one.	remueva el parche viejo antes de ponerse el nuevo. **quítese** el parche viejo antes de ponerse el nuevo.
This is a list of all the medicines you take.	Esta es la lista de todos los medicamentos que usted toma. Esta es la lista de todas las **medicinas** que usted toma.
Can you tell me if this list is correct?	¿Me puede usted decir si esta lista ya mencionada es correcta? ¿Me **podría** usted **indicar** si esta lista ya mencionada es correcta?
Do you take any other medicines that are not listed here?	¿Toma usted algún otro medicamento que no está en la lista ya mencionada? ¿**Está tomando** usted alguna otra **medicina** que no está en la lista ya mencionada?
You will need to show them to your provider next time so your list can be updated.	Usted necesita enseñarle esta lista a su proveedor médico la próxima vez, ya que así su lista podrá ser actualizada. Usted necesita enseñarle esta lista a su proveedor médico la próxima vez, de esta forma su lista podrá ser **puesta al día.** Usted necesita enseñarle esta lista a su proveedor médico la próxima vez, ya que así su lista podrá ser **puesta al corriente.**

Medicines

It is important that you keep a complete list of all your medicines with you.	Es muy importante que usted mantenga una lista completa de todos sus medicamentos con usted. Es muy importante que usted mantenga una lista completa de todas sus **medicinas** con usted.
The list should include any over-the-counter medicines or herbal supplements.	Esta lista ya mencionada también debe de incluir todos los medicamentos sin recetas o suplementos botánicos.
Anytime you seek medical care, show them the list of your medicines.	En cualquier momento que usted busque ayuda médica usted debe de mostrarles su lista de medicamentos. En cualquier momento que usted busca ayuda médica usted debe de mostrarles su lista de **medicinas**.
This will help prevent drug interactions and errors.	De esta forma usted evitará interacciones entre drogas al igual que errores.
You need to continue all your current medicines.	Usted necesita continuar con todos sus medicamentos actuales. Usted necesita continuar con todas sus **medicinas** actuales.
You need to stop taking this/these medicine(s).	Necesita dejar de tomar este/estos medicamento(s). Necesita dejar de tomar esta/estas **medicina(s)**.
You need to continue taking this/these medicine(s).	Necesita continuar tomando este/estos medicamento(s). Necesita continuar tomando esta/estas **medicina(s)**.

Tests/Diagnostics Ordered

Your doctor/provider has ordered a diagnostic test/procedure [see "Special Procedures," in Chapter 3, "Vocabulary"]. . .	Su doctor/proveedor médico ha ordenado un examen/procedimiento diagnóstico . . . Su doctor/proveedor médico ha ordenado una/un **prueba**/procedimiento diagnóstico . . .

Tests/Diagnostics Ordered

for your heart.	para su corazón.
for your stomach problems.	para sus problemas estomacales.
for your lungs.	para sus pulmones.
to screen for cancer.	para detectar. para analizar. para identificar.
to better evaluate your pain.	para evaluar mejor su dolor.
to further evaluate your symptoms.	para evaluar mas allá sus síntomas.
to help us determine the cause of your symptoms.	para ayudarnos a determinar la causa de sus síntomas.
We will schedule the test(s) for you.	Nosotros le vamos a hacer una cita para su examen. Nosotros le vamos a hacer una cita para su **prueba**.
Your appointment for your test is on [insert date] at [insert time]	La cita para su examen es el [insert date] a/a las (insert time). La cita para su **prueba** es el [insert date] a/las (insert time).
You need to call this number to schedule your test.	Usted necesita llamar a este número para hacer la cita de su examen. Usted necesita llamar a este número para hacer la cita de su **prueba**.
We need to have you come back for fasting blood work.	Necesitamos que regrese en ayunas para hacerle un examen de sangre.
Do not eat or drink anything after midnight on [insert day] until after your blood is drawn.	No coma o tome nada después de la media noche el [insert day] hasta que le saquen la sangre.
You can take your blood pressure medicines with water before the test.	Usted se puede tomar el medicamento para la presión de sangre con agua antes del examen. Usted se puede tomar la medicina para la presión de sangre con agua antes de la **prueba**.
Do not take your diabetes medicines until you can eat.	No tome su medicamento para la diabetes hasta que pueda comer. No tome su **medicina** para la diabetes hasta que pueda comer.

Same-Day Procedures

Your doctor/medical provider has ordered a [tetanus, pneumonia, flu, hepatitis, measles, mumps] vaccine for you today.	Su doctor/ proveedor médico ha ordenado una vacuna de [tétano, neumonía, influenza, hepatitis, viruela, paperas] para usted hoy.
We need to take blood from you today.	Necesitamos sacarle sangre hoy.
We need a urine sample.	Necesitamos una muestra de su orina.
We need to do a special test today [see "Special Procedures," in Chapter 3, "Vocabulary"] . . .	Necesitamos hacerle hoy un examen especial . . .
	Necesitamos hacerle hoy una **prueba** especial . . .
for your heart.	para su corazón.
for your stomach problems.	para sus problemas estomacales.
for your lungs.	para sus pulmones.
to screen for cancer.	para detectar.
	para analizar.
	para identificar.
to better evaluate your pain.	para evaluar mejor su dolor.
to further evaluate your symptoms.	para evaluar mas allá sus síntomas.
to help us determine the cause of your symptoms.	para ayudarnos a determinar la causa de sus síntomas.

Follow-Up Appointment

You should return or call if you have any problems or if your condition worsens.	Debe de regresar o llamar si tiene problemas o si su condición empeora.
Your next appointment is on [insert date] at [insert time].	Su siguiente cita es el [insert date] a/ las (insert time).
Your doctor wants to see you again in [insert number] days/weeks/months.	Su doctor lo quiere ver otra vez en [insert number] días/semanas/meses.
What day of the week is best for you?	¿Qué día de la semana es mejor para usted?
Morning?	¿Mañana?
Afternoon?	¿Tarde?

Follow-Up Appointment

You need to call your doctor/ medical provider for a follow-up appointment in [number] days/weeks.	Necesita llamar a su doctor/ proveedor médico para una cita en [numero] días/semanas.
Please bring a copy of your medical records with you.	Por favor traiga una copia de sus expedientes médicos cuando venga. Por favor traiga una copia de sus **archivos médicos** cuando venga.

Referrals

You are being referred to see a specialist in [insert specialty] [see "In the Hospital" in Chapter 3, "Vocabulary"].	Lo estamos refiriendo con un especialista en . . . [insert specialty].
You need to call this number to make the appointment.	Necesita llamar a este número para hacer una cita.
They will call you to set up an appointment.	Ellos lo llamaran para hacer la cita.
Please call us for a follow-up appointment after you have seen them.	Por favor llámenos después de a su cita con ellos.

Discharge

We are discharging you today.	Lo vamos a dar de alta hoy. Lo vamos a dar de **baja** hoy.
Do you have someone at home to help you? Is he or she over the age of 18? Will he or she be staying with you?	¿Tiene alguien en su casa que lo pueda ayudar? ¿Él/ella es mayor de 18 años? ¿Él/ella se va a quedar con usted? ¿Él/ella se va a **hospedar** con usted?
We will order home health care to come out to help with your care.	Nosotros le ordenaremos cuidado médico a su casa para que lo ayuden con su tratamiento.
Do you need to call for someone to pick you up?	¿Necesita llamar a alguien para que lo vengan a recoger?
Do you need a taxi to get home?	¿Necesita un taxi para que lo lleven a su casa?

Discharge

Who will be driving you home?	¿Quién lo va a llevar a su casa?
Is he or she here?	¿Él/ella está aquí?
Tell me when he or she arrives.	Avíseme cuando él/ella llegue.
I will call transportation to take you to the car.	Le voy a llamar a alguien de transportación para que lo lleven a su carro.
You can go home now.	Usted se puede ir a su casa ya.
Do you understand everything I've told you?	¿Entende do lo que le dije?
Do you need me to call a interpreter?	¿Necesita que le busque un traductor?
Do you have any questions?	¿Tiene alguna pregunta?
Goodbye.	Adiós.

Social Services

I am a social worker.	Yo soy un/a trabajador/a social.
Your provider has ordered . . .	Su proveedor médico ordenó . . .
home health care services.	servicios de atención sanitaria en el hogar.
	servicios de atención **de salud** en el hogar.
nursing-home placement.	que lo pongamos en una casa de convalecencia.
	que lo pongamos en una **residencia de ancianos.**
skilled nursing care placement.	que lo pongamos en una enfermería especializada.
rehabilitation services.	servicios de rehabilitación.
	que le ofrescan servicios de **readaptación**.
medical equipment.	equipo médico.
counseling services.	servicios consultivos.
	servicios **de asesoría**.
	servicios **consejería**.
in-home services.	servicios a su casa.
In-home services provides someone to assist you with household chores and/or transportation.	Servicios a su casa le proveená una persona para que lo ayuden con tareas caseras y/o transportación.

	Servicios a su casa le **facilitaná** una persona para que lo **atiendan** con **labores del hogar** y/o transportación. Servicios a su casa le **facilitana** una persona para que lo **atiendan** con **faenas del hogar** y/o transportación.
You need to call this phone number to apply for in-home services.	Usted necesita llamar a este teléfono para aplicar para este tipo de servicio a su casa.
I can help you find services in the community to assist you.	Yo le puedo ayudar a encontrar otros servicios en la comunidad que le pueden ayudar.
I have called an interpreter to help us.	Yo llame a un traductor para que nos ayude.
While we wait I am going to ask you questions to determine which services you might need.	En lo que esperamos yo le voy a preguntar varias preguntas para así determinar los servicios que usted pudiese necesitar.
Please answer yes, no, or I don't know.	Por favor conteste con sí, no, o no sé.
When I am done, I will call an interpreter to help us.	Cuando yo termine, llamaré a un intérprete para que nos ayude.
Do you have a permanent place to live?	¿Usted tiene un lugar permanente en el cual vive? **¿Usted vive en un lugar fijo?**
Do you live alone?	¿Usted vive solo/a?
Do you live with a friend or family member? Permanently or temporarily?	¿Usted vive con un/a amigo/a o con un familiar? ¿Permanentemente o por el momento? ¿Permanentemente o **temporalmente**? ¿Permanentemente o **provisionalmente**?
Do you stay in a shelter?	¿Usted se está quedando en un refugio? ¿Usted se está **hospedando** en un **albergue**?

Social Services

Do you know where the shelters are located?	¿Usted sabe donde los refugios están localizados? ¿Usted **conoce** donde los **albergues se encuentran**?
Do you live on the streets?	¿Usted vive en la calle?
Are you homeless?	¿Usted está sin hogar? ¿Usted está **sin casa**?
Do you need a place to live/stay?	¿Necesita usted un lugar para vivir/quedarse?
Do you need a place to spend the night?	¿Necesita usted un lugar para pasar la noche?
Do you need temporary housing?	¿Necesita usted un lugar provisional para hospedarse? ¿Necesita usted un lugar **temporal** para hospedarse?
Do you need permanent housing?	¿Necesita usted un lugar permanente para vivir?
Do you need financial assistance with paying your rent?	¿Necesita usted ayuda financiera para pagar su renta? ¿Necesita usted ayuda **económica** para pagar su renta? ¿Necesita usted ayuda **monetaria** para pagar su renta?
Do you need assistance with obtaining food?	¿Necesita usted asistencia para comprar comida? ¿Necesita usted asistencia para **obtener** comida? ¿Necesita usted asistencia para **adquirir** comida?
Do you receive food stamps?	¿Usted recibe cupones canjeables por alimentos? ¿Usted recibe cupones canjeables por medio de **estampillas de subsidio**? ¿Usted recibe cupones canjeables por **vales alimenticios**?
Do you get enough to eat?	¿Usted come lo suficiente?

Social Services

Do your children get enough to eat? Do you get three meals a day? Do you get at least two meals a day?	¿Sus hijos/a(s) comen lo suficiente? ¿Usted come tres comidas al día? ¿Usted come por lo menos dos comidas al día?
Do you eat at the shelters?	¿Usted come en los refugios? ¿Usted come en los **albergues**?
Do you need help with getting food stamps?	¿Usted necesita ayuda para conseguir cupones canjeables por alimentos? ¿Usted necesita ayuda para conseguir cupones canjeables por **estampillas de subsidio**? ¿Usted necesita ayuda para conseguir cupones canjeables por **vales alimenticios**?
Do you need help with fixing meals at home?	¿Usted necesita ayuda para cocinar comidas en su casa? ¿Usted necesita ayuda para **preparar** comidas en su casa?
Do you need help with receiving a hot meal during the day?	¿Usted necesita ayuda para recibir comida preparada durante el día?
Do you need help with paying your utilities?	¿Usted necesita ayuda para pagar sus servicios públicos?
Do you need help with child care or babysitting?	¿Usted necesita ayuda para el cuidado de su(s) niño(s)? ¿Usted necesita ayuda **con su cuidado infantil**?
Do your children stay with someone you know while you are away?	¿Sus niños se quedan con otra persona cuando usted no se encuentra en su casa? ¿Sus niños se quedan con otra persona cuando usted **no está en su casa**?
Do your children stay at home alone while you are away?	¿Sus niños se quedan solos en su casa cuando usted no se encuentra en su casa? ¿Sus niños se quedan solos en su casa cuando usted **no está en su casa**?

Social Services

Would you like to speak with a counselor or therapist about . . .	¿Quisiera usted hablar con un consejero/a o terapista acerca de . . .
	¿**Le gustaría** a usted hablar con un consejero/a o terapista acerca de . . .
drugs or alcohol?	drogas ilegales?
	drogas **ilícitas**?
family problems?	problemas familiares?
relationship problems?	problemas con su cónyuge?
	problemas con su **compañero/a**?
domestic violence?	violencia doméstica?
	abuso doméstico?
emotional or mental health problems?	problemas de salud mentale o emocionales?
Do you have problems with domestic violence?	¿Tiene usted problemas de violencia domestica?
	¿Tiene usted problemas de **abuso doméstico**?
With your spouse or partner?	¿Con su cónyuge o con su compañero/a?
	¿Con su **esposo/a** o con su compañero/a?
With your ex-husband, ex-wife, or ex- partner?	¿Con su ex cónyuge o ex compañero/a?
	¿Con su **ex esposo/a** o ex compañero/a?
With your boyfriend/girlfriend?	¿Con su novio/a?
With a family member?	¿Con un miembro de familia?
Have you called the police?	¿Ha llamado usted a la policía?
Have you filed a police report?	¿Ha presentado un reporte policíaco?
Would you like to talk with a police officer?	¿Usted quisiera hablar con un policía?
Do you feel safe living at home?	¿Se siente usted seguro/a viviendo en su casa?
Are your children safe at home?	¿Sus hijos están seguros en su casa?
Do you need assistance with filling out forms for . . .	¿Necesita usted ayuda para llenar las siguientes aplicaciones para . . .
	¿Necesita usted ayuda para llenar las siguientes **solicitudes** para . . .

Social Services

advance directives?	directivas anticipadas?
a living will?	testamento vital de vida? testamento de **voluntad** de vida?
medical power of attorney?	declaración referente al poder médico?
durable power of attorney? (This gives permission for someone to make legal and medical decisions for another person if that person becomes incapacitated either mentally or physically.)	poder durable (permiso o **autoridad** para actuar en nombre de otra persona en caso de que la otra persona pierda su aptitud judicial o **facultades mentales**)?
Do you want to speak with a pastor or with clergy?	¿Desea usted hablar con un pastor o con un clericó? ¿**Quiere** usted hablar con un pastor o con un clericó?
Catholic?	¿Católico?
Protestant?	¿Protestante?
Baptist?	¿Bautista?
This is a list of addresses for shelters in the community.	Esta es la lista de refugios en la comunidad. Esta es la lista de **albergues** en la comunidad.
They can provide hot meals, a place to sleep, and other services.	Ellos pueden proveerles una comida caliente, un lugar para dormir, u otros servicios.
This is the address and phone number of the food stamps office.	Esta es la dirección y número telefónico de la oficina de cupones canjeables por alimentos. Esta es la dirección y número telefónico de la oficina de **estampillas de subsidio**. Esta es la dirección y número telefónico de la oficina de **vales alimenticios**.
You can call or go in person to apply for the food stamps program.	Usted puede llamar o ir en persona para aplicar al programa de cupones canjeables por alimentos. Usted puede llamar o ir en persona para aplicar al programa de **estampillas de subsidio**.

Social Services

	Usted puede llamar o ir en persona para aplicar al programa de **vales alimenticios**.
This is the address of the local food bank.	Esta es la dirección para el banco local alimentario (es un lugar que almacena y distribuye donaciones de alimentos).
You can get nonperishable food items.	Usted puede conseguir alimentos no perecederos (alimentos que no se dañan o muy duraderos, como por ejemplo comidas en lata).
	Usted puede **obtener** alimentos no perecederos (alimentos que no se dañan o muy duraderos, como por ejemplo comidas en lata).
	Usted puede **adquirir** alimentos no perecederos (alimentos que no se dañan o muy duraderos, como por ejemplo comidas en lata).
This is a list of phone numbers for the crisis centers.	Esta es la lista de teléfonos para los centros de crisis.
You can call them twenty-four hours a day if you are having problems with abuse, thoughts of suicide, or other crises.	Usted los puede llamar veinticuatro horas al día en caso de problemas de abuso, pensamientos de suicidio, u otras crisis.
They have counselors available to talk with you at any time.	Ellos tiene consejeros disponibles para hablar con usted a cualquier momento.
This is a list of counseling services in the community.	Esta es la lista de los servicios de consejería en la comunidad.
You will need to call or go in to make an appointment for counseling services.	Usted necesita ir o llamarlos para hacer una cita y obtener este servicio de consejería.
This is a list of shelters or safe houses.	Esta es la lista de refugios.
	Esta es la lista de **albergues**.
A safe house can provide you and your children a safe place to stay.	Un refugio puede proveerle a usted y a sus hijo(s) un lugar seguro para quedarse.
	Un refugio puede proveerle a usted y a sus hijo(s) un lugar seguro para **alojarse**.

	Un refugio puede proveerle a usted y a sus hijo(s) un lugar seguro para **hospedarse**.
This is the phone number to call for in- home services.	Este es el teléfono para llamar si necesita servicios a su casa.
In-home services provides someone to assist you with household chores and/or transportation.	Servicios a su casa le pueden proveen una persona para que lo ayuden con sus tareas caseras y/o transportación.
	Servicios a su casa le **pueden facilitar** una persona para que lo **atiendan** con sus labores **del hogar** y/ o transportación.
	Servicios a su casa le **facilitan** una persona para que lo **atiendan** con sus **faenas del hogar** y/ o transportación.
You need to call this phone number to apply for these services.	Usted necesita llamar a este número para aplicar por estos servicios.
Do you want to apply for disability benefits?	¿Usted desea aplicar por beneficios de incapacidad?
	¿Usted desea aplicar por **asistencia para incapacidad**?
Have you already filed for disability?	¿Ya usted aplico por incapacidad?
This is the address and phone number of the Social Security office.	Esta es la dirección y número telefónico de la Oficina del Seguro Social.
You can call or go in person to apply for disability benefits.	Usted puede llamar o ir en persona para aplicar por beneficios de incapacidad.
	Usted puede llamar o ir en persona para aplicar por **asistencia para incapacidad**.
This is the phone number for the Meals On Wheels program.	Este es el número de teléfono de comidas gratis llevadas al hogar.
	Este es el número de teléfono de comidas **sin pago alguno** llevadas al hogar.
	Este es el número de teléfono de comidas **sin provecho económico** llevadas al hogar.

Social Services

They will deliver hot meals to your home.	Ellos le llevaran una comida caliente a su casa. Ellos le **entregaran** una comida caliente a su casa.
You need to call this phone number to apply for the Meals On Wheels program.	Usted necesita llamar a este número telefónico para aplicar por el programa de comidas gratis al hogar. Usted necesita llamar a este número telefónico para aplicar por el programa de comidas **sin pago alguno** al hogar. Usted necesita llamar a este número telefónico para aplicar por el programa de comidas **sin provecho económico** al hogar.

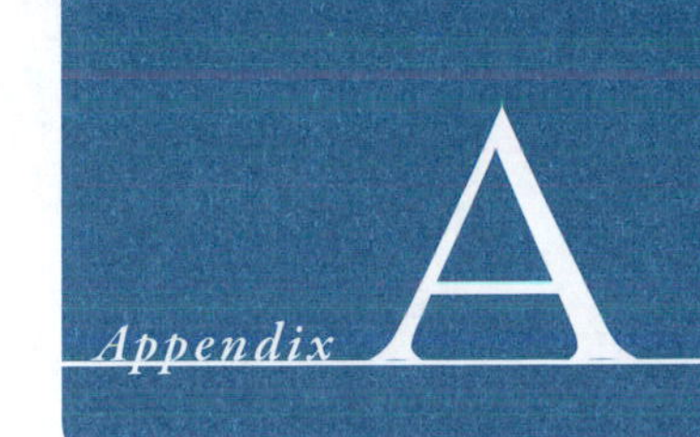

CAGE Questionnaire

The CAGE questionnaire is commonly used clinically as a screening tool for potential problems with alcohol use.[1] The questions should be asked as part of the general history or in the course of a routine visit and should not be preceded by any questions about alcohol use, as this may decrease sensitivity. [2]

Have you ever felt you should **C**ut down on your drinking?	¿Ha sentido alguna vez que debería **R**educir su consumo de alcohol?
Have people **A**nnoyed you by criticizing your drinking?	¿Se siente **M**olesto con la gente que le critican su consumo de alcohol?
Have you ever felt bad or **G**uilty about your drinking?	¿Se ha sentido mal o **C**ulpable alguna vez acerca de su consumo de alcohol?
Have you ever had a drink first thing in the morning to steady your nerves or to get rid of a hangover (**E**ye opener)?	¿Ha consumido usted alcohol al levantarse en la mañana para calmarse sus nervios o para quitarse una resaca (el primer trago en la mañana para abrirle los **O**jos)?
	¿Ha consumido usted alcohol al levantarse en la mañana para **estabilizarse** sus nervios o para quitarse una **tomadera** (el primer trago en la mañana para abrirle los **O**jos)?

A total score of 2 or greater is considered clinically significant for the identification of alcohol overuse.

1. Ewing, J.A. (1984). Detecting alcoholism: The CAGE questionnaire. *JAMA*, 252 (14),1905–1907.
2. Steinweg, D.L., Worth, H. (1993). Alcoholism: The keys to the CAGE. *Am J Med*, 94 (5), 520–523.

Appendix B

Geriatric Depression Scale (Short)

I am going to ask you a series of questions to assess your overall mood.	Le voy a preguntar una serie de preguntas para poder evaluar en general su humor o disposición.
Please answer yes or no only.	Por favor conteste solamente sí o no.
1. Are you basically satisfied with your life? Yes **No**	1. ¿Se encuentra usted satisfecho con su vida? Sí **No**
2. Have you dropped many of your activities and interests? **Yes** No	2. ¿Ha abandonado usted muchas de sus actividades e intereses? **Sí** No
3. Do you feel happy most of the time? Yes **No**	3. ¿Si siente usted feliz la mayoria del tiempo? Sí **No**
4. Do you prefer to stay at home rather than go out and do new things? **Yes** No	4. ¿Prefiere usted quedarse en la casa en vez de salir y tratar nuevas cosas? **Sí** No

If any of the answers to the above questions indicates depression (bold), continue with questions 5–15. Otherwise, stop here.

5. Do you feel that life is empty? **Yes** No	5. ¿Siente usted que su vida está vacia? **Sí** No
6. Do you often get bored? **Yes** No	6. ¿A menudo o con frecuencia, se siente usted aburrido (a)? **Sí** No
7. Are you in good spirits most of the time? Yes **No**	7. ¿Se siente usted alegre la mayoria del tiempo? Sí **No**
8. Are you afraid that something bad is going to happen to you? **Yes** No	8. ¿Tiene usted miedo de que algo malo le va a pasar? **Sí** No
9. Do you feel helpless? **Yes** No	9. ¿Se siente usted indefenso? ¿Se siente usted **desamparado**? ¿Se siente usted **incapaz**? **Sí** No

10. Do you feel that you have more problems with memory than most? **Yes** No	10. ¿Siente usted que tiene más problemas con la memoria que la mayoria? **Sí** No
11. Do you think it is wonderful to be alive? Yes **No**	11. ¿Cree usted que es una maravilla estar vivo? Sí **No**
12. Do you feel pretty worthless the way you are now? **Yes** No	12. ¿Siente usted que no vale nada basado en su forma de ser? **Sí** No
13. Do you feel full of energy? Yes **No**	13. ¿Se siente usted lleno de energía? Sí **No**
14. Do you feel that your situation is hopeless? **Yes** No	14. ¿Siente usted que su situación no tiene esperanza? **Sí** No
15. Do you think that most people are better off than you are? **Yes** No	15. ¿Cree usted que la mayoria de la gente se encuentran mejor que usted? **Sí** No

Scoring:

0–4: None;
5–10: Mild;
11+: Severe

Sources: Van-Marwijk, H.W., et al. (1995). Evaluation of the feasibility, reliability and diagnostic value of shortened versions of the geriatric depression scale. *Br J Gen Pract,* 45 (393), 195–199.

Neal, R.M., & Baldwin, R.C. (1994). Screening for anxiety and depression in elderly medical outpatients. *Age-Ageing,* 23(6), 461–464.

Appendix C

Dementia Screening

I am going to ask you some questions to test your memory.	Le voy a preguntar algunas preguntas para examinarle su memoria.
We may repeat these tests at a later date to evaluate any changes as you age.	Puede que le repitamos estos examenes en una fecha mas tarde para evaluarle cualquier tipo de cambios a medida que usted envejece.
Try to relax as you answer the questions.	Trate de relajarse al contester estas peguntas.
Are you ready?	¿Está listo?

The Short Portable Mental Status Questionnaire (SPMSQ) / Cuestionario Portátil Corto para el Estado Mental

The Short Portable Mental Status Questionnaire (SPMSQ)	Cuestionario Portátil Corto para el Estado Mental
1. What is the date, month, and year?	1. ¿En qué día, mes, y año estamos?
2. What is the day of the week?	2. ¿En qué día de la semana estamos?
3. What is the name of this place?	3. ¿Cuál es el nombre de este lugar donde nos encontramos?
4. What is your phone number?	4. ¿Cuál es su número de teléfono?
5. How old are you?	5. ¿Qué edad tiene usted?
6. When were you born?	6. ¿Cuándo nació usted?
7. Who is the current president?	7. ¿Cuál es el nombre de nuestro presidente actual?
8. Who was the president before him?	8. ¿Cuál es el nombre del presidente antes del actual?
9. What was your mother's maiden name?	9. ¿Cuál es su apellido materno?
10. Can you count backwards from twenty by threes?	10. ¿Puede usted contar de veinte hacia abajo de tres en tres, por ejemplo veinte, diez y siete, etcétera?
For example, start with 20 and subtract 3 each time.	Por ejemplo, empiece con veinte y quítele tres sucesivamente.

Scoring:

0–2 errors: normal mental functioning
3–4 errors: mild cognitive impairment
5–7 errors: moderate cognitive impairment
8 or more errors: severe cognitive impairment

One additional error is allowed in each level of scoring if a patient has had an 8th grade school education or less.
One less error is allowed at each scoring level if the patient has had education beyond the high school level.

Source:

Pfeiffer, E. (1975). A short portable mental status questionnaire for the assessment of organic brain deficit in elderly patients. *Journal of American Geriatrics Society,* 23, 433–441.

The Mini-Cog Assessment Instrument for Dementia

The Mini-Cog assessment instrument combines an uncued three-item recall test with a clock drawing test (CDT). The Mini-Cog is relatively uninfluenced by level of education or language variations.

Administration:

1. Instruct the patient to listen carefully to and remember three unrelated words and then to repeat the words.
2. Instruct the patient to draw the face of a clock, either on a blank sheet of paper or on a sheet with the clock circle already drawn on the page. After the patient puts the numbers on the clock face, ask him or her to draw the hands of the clock to read a specific time, such as 11:20. These instructions can be repeated, but no additional instructions may be given. Give the patient as much time as needed to complete the task. The CDT serves as the memory distracter.
3. Ask the patient to repeat the three previously presented words.

Scoring:

Give 1 point for each word recalled after the CDT distracter. Score 1–3.

A score of 0 indicates positive screen for dementia.

A score of 1 or 2 with an abnormal CDT indicates positive screen for dementia.

A score of 1 or 2 with a normal CDT indicates negative screen for dementia.

A score of 3 indicates negative screen for dementia.

The CDT is considered normal if all numbers are present in the correct sequence and position, and the hands correctly display the requested time.

Source:

Borson, S., Scanian, J., Brush, M., Vitaliano, P., & Dokmak, A. (2000). The mini-cog: A cognitive "vital signs" measure for dementia screening in multi-lingual elderly. *Int J Geriatr Psychiatry,* 15(11), 1021–1027.

Instructions to Patient	Instrucciones para el paciente
I am going to say three words. I want you to listen carefully, remember the three words, and then repeat the three words out loud when I am done telling them to you.	Voy a decir tres palabras. Quiero que usted escuche cuidadosamente y se acuerde de estas tres palabras, y despues quiero que me las repita en voz alta al terminar de decírselas.
I will ask you again in a few minutes to repeat these same words.	Le voy a preguntar en unos cuantos minutos que me repita las mismas tres palabras que yo le dije.
Are you ready?	¿Está listo/a?
Apple	Manzana
Television	Televisión
Dog	Perro
Can you repeat those words back to me?	¿Puede usted repetirme estas tres palabras?
I want you to draw the face of a clock with the numbers but with no hands on the clock yet.	Quiero que me dibuje la cara de un reloj con sus numeros, pero sin sus manesillas.
Now I want you to draw the hands of the clock to read 11:20.	Ahora en el reloj que usted dibujo, quiero que le coloque las manesillas en las once y veinte. Ahora en el reloj que usted dibujo, quiero que le **dibuje** las manesillas en las once y veinte.
Can you repeat the three words I asked you to remember before?	¿Podría usted repetirme las tres palabras que yo le indique que se acordara? ¿Podría usted repetirme las tres palabras que yo le **mencione** que se acordara?

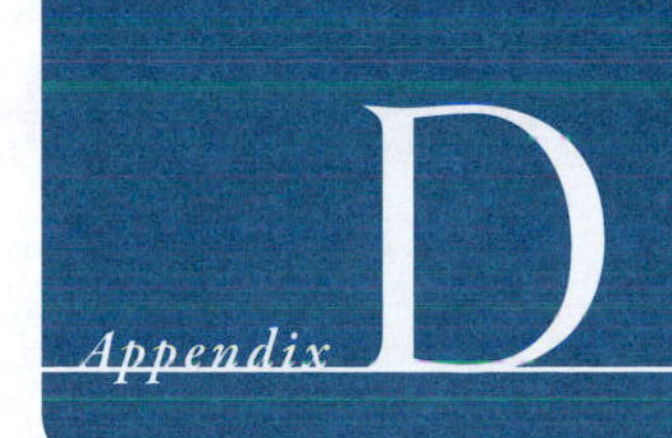

Functional Assessment Tools

For questions/terminology on disability, see "Legal/Disability Terminology" in Chapter 3, "Vocabulary."

Activities of Daily Living	Actividades del Diario Vivir
Do you use the bathroom without help?	¿Usted utiliza el baño sin necesidad alguna?
	¿Usted no necesita ayuda en el baño?
Can you do some of it alone?	¿Puede usted hacer la mayoría de sus necesidades en el baño solo/a?
	¿Puede usted hacer la mayoría de sus necesidades en el baño sin ayuda?
Are you able to completely control your bladder without accidents?	¿Puede usted completamente controlar su vejiga sin accidente alguno?
During the last week have you leaked urine?	¿En la pasada semana usted a goteado orina?
	¿En la pasada semana usted a **perdido** orina?
	¿En la pasada semana usted a **pasado** orina?
More than once a week?	¿Más de una vez por semana?
Do you need to be reminded to use the bathroom?	¿Necesita usted que alguien le acuerde de ir al baño?
Do you need help with wiping or cleaning yourself?	¿Necesita ayuda para limpiarse despues de ir al bano?
Are you able to completely control your bowels without accidents?	¿Puede usted completamente controlar sus intestinos sin accidente alguno?
During the last week have you leaked stool?	¿En la pasada semana usted a goteado heces?

Activities of Daily Living	*Actividades del Diario Vivir*
	¿En la pasada semana usted a **perdido** heces?
	¿En la pasada semana usted a **pasado** heces?
More than once a week?	¿Más de una vez por semana?
Do you feed yourself without help?	¿Puede usted comer sin ayuda?
Do you need help with cutting food?	¿Necesita usted ayuda para cortar su comida?
Do you prepare the meals?	¿Usted es el/la que prepara su comida?
Always?	¿Siempre?
Sometimes?	¿Algunas veces?
Do you clean up after the meals?	¿Limpia usted después de la comida?
Do you need a lot of help with eating each meal?	¿Necesita usted mucha ayuda para comer cada una de sus comidas?
Do you resist when someone else tries to feed you?	¿No le gusta cada vez que alguien trata de ayudarle a comer?
	¿No quiere que alguien trate de darle de comer?
Do you dress yourself without help?	¿Se viste usted sin ayuda?
Do you undress yourself without help?	¿Se puede usted quitar su ropa sin ayuda?
	¿Se puede usted **desvestir** sin ayuda?
	¿Se puede usted **desnudar** sin ayuda?
Do you pick out your clothes each day without help?	¿Escoge usted su ropa diariamente sin ayuda alguna?
Does someone help you with small things, like buttons, laces, or zippers?	¿Alguien le ayuda con pequeñas cosas como: a abotonarse su ropa, con los cordones de sus zapatos o con su cremallera?
	¿Alguien le ayuda con pequeñas cosas como: a abotonarse su ropa, con los cordones de sus zapatos o con su **zíperes**?
	¿Alguien le ayuda con pequeñas cosas como: a abotonarse su ropa, con los cordones de sus zapatos o con **cierres relámpagos**?
	¿Alguien le ayuda a abotonarse su ropa, con los cordones de sus zapatos o con **eclaires**?

Activities of Daily Living	*Actividades del Diario Vivir*
Does someone help you with most of the dressing and undressing?	¿Alguien le ayuda a usted a ponerse su ropa o quitarse su ropa la mayoría de las veces?
	¿Alguien le ayuda a usted a **vestirse** o **desvestirse** la mayoría de las veces?
Do you resist when someone else tries to dress you?	¿No le gusta que alguien trate de ayudarle a ponerse su ropa?
	¿Usted resiste cuando alguien trata de vestirlo/a?
Do you comb your hair without help?	¿Se peina usted sin ayuda?
Do you brush your teeth without help?	¿Se limpia (cepilla) usted sus dientes sin ayuda?
Do you shave yourself without help?	¿Se afeita usted sin ayuda?
Can you keep yourself well groomed throughout the day?	¿Se puede usted mantener bien arreglado/a durante el día?
	¿Se puede usted mantener bien **preparado/a a través del día**?
Do you resist when someone else tries to help groom you?	¿No le gusta que alguien trate de ayudarle a arreglarse?
	¿Usted resiste cuando alguien trata de ayudarle a asearse?
Do you walk without help?	¿Camina usted sin ayuda?
Are you able to walk around the house without help?	¿Puede usted caminar por su casa sin ayuda?
	¿Puede usted caminar **alrededor** de su casa sin ayuda?
Do you use a cane?	¿Utiliza usted bastón?
	¿**Usa** usted bastón?
Walker?	¿Andador?
Wheelchair?	¿Silla de ruedas?
Do you get in and out of the wheelchair without help?	¿Usted puede sentarse o salirse de su silla de ruedas sin ayuda alguna?
Do you use the wheelchair without help?	¿Usted utiliza su silla de ruedas sin ayuda?
	¿Usted **usa** su silla de ruedas sin ayuda?

Activities of Daily Living	*Actividades del Diario Vivir*
Does someone push the wheelchair for you?	¿Alguien le ayuda a empujar su silla de ruedas?
Do you sit up in a chair without support?	¿Puede usted levantarse de su silla sin tener que sostenerse?
Are you bedridden more than half the time?	¿Está usted encamado la mayoría del tiempo?
Do you bathe yourself completely without any help?	¿Puede usted bañarse completamente sin ayuda alguna?
Does someone help you get in or out of the tub or shower?	¿Alguien le ayuda a entrar o salir de la bañera o ducha?
	¿Alguien le ayuda a entrar o salir de la **tina** o ducha?
	¿Alguien le ayuda a entrar o salir de la **tarrima** o ducha?
	¿Alguien le ayuda a entrar o salir de la **bañadera**?
	¿Alguien le ayuda a entrar o salir de la **regadera**?
Do you wash your own face or hands?	¿Usted mismo se puede lavar su cara y manos?
Does someone else bathe you?	¿Alguien lo baña?
Do you resist when someone else tries to bathe you?	¿Pone usted resistencia o no le gusta cuando alguien lo/la baña?
Do you give yourself a sponge bath without help?	¿Puede usted darse un baño de esponja por si mismo(a)/**por si solo(a)**?
Are you able to walk up stairs without help?	¿Puede usted subir las escaleras sin ayuda alguna?
Can you walk up stairs if you hold on to a railing for support?	¿Puede usted subir las escaleras sin agarrarse de la reja de la escalera?
	¿Puede usted subir las escaleras sin agarrarse del **enrejado** de la escalera?
Can you walk up the stairs if someone helps you?	¿Puede usted subir las escaleras si alguien lo ayudase?
Are you able to walk down stairs without help?	¿Puede usted bajar las escaleras sin ayuda alguna?
Can you walk down stairs if you hold on to a railing for support?	¿Puede usted bajar las escaleras si usted se agarra de la verja de la escalera?

Activities of Daily Living	*Actividades del Diario Vivir*
	¿Puede usted bajar las escaleras si usted se agarra del **enrejado** de la escalera?
Can you walk down the stairs if someone helps you?	¿Puede usted bajar las escaleras si alguien lo ayudase?
Can you get in or out of the bathtub or shower if someone helps you?	¿Puede usted entrar o salir de la bañera o ducha sin alguien que lo ayudase?
	¿Puede usted entrar o salir de la **tina** o ducha sin que alguien lo ayude?
	¿Puede usted entrar o salir de la **bañadera** o **regadera** sin alguien que lo ayudase?

Source:

Lawton, M.P. & Brody, E.M. (1969). Assessment of older people: Self-maintaining and instrumental activities of daily living. *Gerontologist,* 9(3), 179–186.

Instrumental Activities of Daily Living	Actividades Inportantísimas del Diario Vivir
Do you use the telephone without help?	¿Puede usted utilizar el teléfono sin ayuda alguna?
	¿Puede usted **usar** el teléfono sin ayuda alguna?
Do you make phone calls without help?	¿Puede usted hacer llamadas telefónicas sin ayuda alguna?
Do you answer the phone without help?	¿Puede usted contestar el teléfono sin ayuda alguna?
Do you use the answering machine without help?	¿Puede usted utilizar la contestadora automática sin ayuda alguna?
	¿Puede usted utilizar la **máquina contestadora** sin ayuda alguna?
	¿Puede usted utilizar el **aparato de respuesta automático** sin ayuda alguna?
	¿Puede usted utilizar la **máquina de contestar mensajes** sin ayuda alguna?

Instrumental Activities of Daily Living	*Actividades Inportantísimas del Diario Vivir*
Do you buy your groceries without help?	¿Puede usted ir a la tienda de comestibles y hacer sus compras sin ayuda alguna? ¿Puede usted ir a la tienda **de compras** y hacer sus compras sin ayuda alguna? ¿Puede usted ir a la tienda **al comercio de comestibles** y hacer sus compras sin ayuda alguna? ¿Puede usted ir **al supermercado** y hacer sus compras sin ayuda alguna?
Do you buy small amounts of groceries yourself but need help with larger or bigger purchases?	¿Compra usted mismo(a) pequeñas cantidades de comestibles pero necesita ayuda con compras más grandes? ¿Compra usted mismo(a) pequeñas cantidades de comestibles pero necesita ayuda con las compras **abundantes**?
Do you need someone to accompany you to the store?	¿Necesita usted alguien que le acompañe a la tienda?
Do you plan, prepare, and serve meals without help?	¿Usted planifica, prepara, y sirve su comida sin ayuda alguna?
Do you cook a meal if someone else does the grocery shopping? Do you use the stove, microwave, or oven without needing help?	¿Puede usted cocinar si alguien le hiciese sus compras? ¿Puede usted usar la estufa, el microondas, o el horno sin ayuda alguna? ¿Puede usted usar el **fogón**, el microondas, o el horno sin ayuda alguna?
Do you do most of your housecleaning without help? Do you dust?	¿Puede usted hacer la limpieza de la casa sin ayuda alguna? ¿Puede usted quitarle el polvo a los muebles? ¿Puede usted **sacudir** los muebles?

Instrumental Activities of Daily Living	*Actividades Inportantísimas del Diario Vivir*
Do you mop?	¿Usted trapea? ¿Usted **limpia el piso**? ¿Usted **pasa la fregona**?
Do you vacuum?	¿Usted pasa la aspiradora?
Do you wash dishes?	¿Usted lava los platos? ¿Usted **limpia** los **trastes**?
Do you make the beds?	¿Tiende usted la cama? ¿Hace usted la cama?
Do you feel you are able to keep the house clean?	¿Usted cree que puede mantener su casa limpia?
Do you need help with all household chores?	¿Necesita usted ayuda con todas las areas del hogar? ¿Necesita usted ayuda con todas las areas de la **casa**?
Do you do any household chores?	¿Hace usted algún tipo de tarea casera?
Do you do all of your laundry without help?	¿Hace usted toda su lavandería sin ayuda alguna?
Do you wash small items, like socks or underwear, yourself?	¿Lava usted pequeñas cosas como medias o ropa interior sin ayuda alguna? ¿Lava usted pequeñas cosas como **calcetines** o ropa interior **sola**?
Do you drive?	¿Usted conduce? ¿Usted **maneja**? ¿Usted **guia**?
Do you take the bus/train without help?	¿Toma usted el autobús/tren sin ayuda alguna? ¿Toma usted el **camión**/tren sin ayuda alguna? ¿Toma usted el **colectivo**/tren sin ayuda alguna? ¿Toma usted el **ómnibus**/tren sin ayuda alguna? ¿Toma usted el **micro**/tren sin ayuda alguna? ¿Toma usted la **guagua**/tren sin ayuda alguna?

Instrumental Activities of Daily Living	*Actividades Inportantísimas del Diario Vivir*
Do you take the bus/ train if someone helps you?	¿Toma usted el autobús/tren si alguien le ayudase?
	¿Toma usted el **camión**/tren si alguien le ayudase?
	¿Toma usted el **colectivo**/tren si alguien le ayudase?
	¿Toma usted el **ómnibus**/tren si alguien le ayudase?
	¿Toma usted el **micro**/tren si alguien le ayudase?
	¿Toma usted la **guagua**/tren si alguien le ayudase?
Do you need someone else to drive you places?	¿Depende usted de alguien que la lleve a diferentes lugares?
Do you take all your medicines as they are prescribed, without help?	¿Toma usted sus medicamentos sin que nadie le ayude?
	¿Toma usted sus **medicinas** sin que nadie le ayude?
Do you need someone to remind you to take your medicines?	¿Necesita usted de alguien que le acuerde de tomar sus medicamentos?
	¿Necesita usted de alguien que le acuerde de tomar sus **medicinas**?
Can you take your medicines if they are prepared in advance, in a pill box?	¿Puede usted tomar sus medicamentos si alguien se las preparase en un estuche para píldoras?
	¿Puede usted tomar sus **medicinas** si alguien se las preparase en una **cajita** para píldoras?
Do you need someone to give you your medicines each time?	¿Necesita usted de alguien que le de sus medicamentos cada vez que las vaya a tomar?
	¿Necesita usted de alguien que le **provea** sus **medicinas** cada vez que las vaya a tomar?

Instrumental Activities of Daily Living	*Actividades Inportantísimas del Diario Vivir*
Do you manage your bank account without help?	¿Puede usted llevar su estado de banco sin ayuda alguna? ¿Puede usted llevar su estado de **cuentas** sin ayuda alguna?
Do you pay your bills without help?	¿Paga usted todas sus cuentas sin ayuda? ¿Paga usted todas sus **facturas** sin ayuda?
Do you manage most small purchases without help?	¿Puede usted administrar compras menores sin ayuda alguna? ¿Puede usted **manejar** compras **chicas** sin ayuda alguna?
Does someone help you with banking?	¿Alguien le ayuda con su cuenta bancaria?

Source:

Lawton, M.P. &, Brody, E.M. (1969). Assessment of older people: Self-maintaining and instrumental activities of daily living. *Gerontologist*, 9(3), 179–186.

Functional Assessment	Evaluación Funcional
Are you able to live independently?	¿Puede usted vivir independientemente?
Were you independent prior to this injury/illness?	¿Vivía usted solo/a sin ayuda alguna antes de su accidente/enfermedad?
Are you able to get around your house on your own?	¿Puede usted moverse a través de su casa por si solo/a? ¿Puede usted moverse **alrededor** de su casa por si solo/a?
How many stories does your house have?	¿Cuántos pisos tiene su casa?
How many steps must you climb to enter your house?	¿Cuántos escalones tiene usted que subir para entrar a su casa?
Are you able to walk up steps without help? Do you need a railing for assistance with stairs?	¿Puede usted subir escalones sin ayuda alguna? ¿Necesita usted ayuda de las barandas para subir las escaleras? ¿Necesita usted **apoyarse** de la **verja** para subir las escaleras?

Functional Assessment	Evaluación Funcional
	¿Necesita usted **apoyarse** del **enrejado** para subir las escaleras?
How many steps are you able to climb?	¿Cuántos escalones puede usted subir?
How many feet can you walk unassisted?	¿Cuántos pies puede usted caminar sin ayuda?
Can you walk one block unassisted?	¿Puede usted caminar una cuadra sin ayuda?
	¿Puede usted caminar una **manzana** sin ayuda?
	¿Puede usted caminar un **bloque** sin ayuda?
Two blocks?	¿Dos cuadras?
	¿Dos **manzana**?
	¿Dos **bloques**?
Do you use a cane at home?	¿Utiliza usted un bastón en su casa?
	¿**Usa** usted un bastón en su casa?
Do you use a walker at home?	¿Utiliza un andador en su casa?
	¿**Usa** un **burrito** en su casa?
Do you use a wheelchair at home?	¿Utiliza una silla de ruedas en su casa?
	¿**Usa** una silla de ruedas en su casa?
Can you get around the house without using the wheelchair?	¿Puede usted moverse a través de su casa sin la ayuda de su silla de ruedas?
	¿Puede usted **desenvolverse** a través de su casa sin la ayuda de sa silla de ruedas?
	¿Puede usted **desplazarse** a través de su casa sin la ayuda de su silla de ruedas?
	¿Puede usted **andar alrededor** de su casa sin la ayuda de su silla de ruedas?
Do you use a scooter at home?	¿Utiliza usted un escúter en su casa?
	¿**Usa** usted una **silla eléctrica** en su casa?
Can you get around the house without using the scooter?	¿Puede usted moverse a través de su casa sin la ayuda de su silla motorizada?

Functional Assessment	*Evaluación Funcional*
	¿Puede usted **desenvolverse** a través de su casa sin la ayuda de su silla motorizada? ¿Puede usted **desplazarse** a través de su casa sin la ayuda de su silla motorizada? ¿Puede caminar e **alrededor** de su casa sin la ayuda de su silla motorizada?
Have you fallen recently?	¿Se ha usted caído recientemente?
Can you get out of bed without help?	¿Puede usted levantarse de la cama sin ayuda?
Can you get out of bed if someone helps you?	¿Puede usted levantarse de su cama si alguien lo ayudase?
Can you stand up from a chair without help? Can you stand up from a chair if someone helps you?	¿Puede usted levantarse de una silla sin ayuda? ¿Puede usted levantarse de una silla si alguien lo ayudase?
Do you have railings in the bathroom for support?	¿Tiene usted barandillas protectoras en su baño?
How many minutes/hours are you able to stand?	¿Cuántos minutos/horas puede usted estar parado/a?
How many minutes/hours are you able to sit?	¿Cuántos minutos/horas puede usted estar sentado/a?
Are you able to carry a bag of groceries?	¿Puede usted calgar una bolsa de comestibles? ¿Puede usted calgar una bolsa de **compras**?
Are you able to do light housework, like dusting?	¿Puede usted hacer trabajo hogareño ligero como quitar el polvo? ¿Puede usted hacer trabajo hogareño ligero como **remover** el polvo?
Are you able to do heavy housework, like vacuuming?	¿Puede usted hacer trabajo hogareño mas pesado como pasar la aspiradora?
Are you able to bend down to pick up objects from the floor?	¿Puede usted doblarse y recoger objetos en el piso? ¿Puede usted **inclinarse** y recoger objetos en el piso? ¿Puede usted **agacharse** y recoger objetos en el piso?

Functional Assessment	*Evaluación Funcional*
Are you able to move furniture around the house?	¿Puede usted mover muebles a través de su casa? ¿Puede usted mover muebles a **alrededor** de su casa?
Do you drive?	¿Usted conduce? ¿Usted **maneja**? ¿Usted **guía**?
Is your level of functioning better, worse, or the same as before?	¿Usted encuentra su nivel de funcionamiento mejor, peor, o igual que antes?
Do you feel that your ability to function is improving?	¿Usted siente que su habilidad para funcionar está mejorando?
Do you feel that your ability to function is worsening?	¿Usted siente que su habilidad de funcionar está empeorando?
Are you going to physical therapy?	¿Esta usted hiendo a terapia física? **¿Se esta usted viendose con un/una terapista física?**
Have you ever been to physical therapy?	¿A ido alguna vez a terapia física?
How many months/years ago?	¿Cuántos meses/años atrás hace que fue?
Are you going to occupational therapy?	¿Esta usted hiendo a terapia ocupacional? **¿Se esta usted viendose con un/una terapista ocupacional?**
Are you going to speech therapy?	¿Está usted hiendo a la terapista de habla? **¿Se está usted viendo con un/una terapista de habla?**
Are you doing the exercises they taught you?	¿Está usted haciendo los ejercicios que le enseñaron? ¿Está usted **practicando** los ejercicios que le enseñaron?
Every day?	¿Todos los días?
How many times a week?	¿Cuántas veces a la semana?
Are you doing your home exercises?	¿Está usted practicando sus ejercicios en su casa?

Functional Assessment	*Evaluación Funcional*
	¿Está usted **haciendo** sus ejercicios **que le mandaron a hacer en su casa**?
Have you been discharged from therapy?	¿Ha sido usted dado de alta de su terapia?
Are you satisfied with your ability to function around the house?	¿Está usted satisfecha/o con su habilidad para funcionar a través de su casa? ¿Está usted satisfecha/o con su habilidad para funcionar **alrededor** de su casa?
Do you work? Full-time? Part-time?	¿Usted trabaja? ¿Trabaja tiempo completo? ¿Trabaja tiempo parcial?
Are you able to work?	¿Puede usted trabajar?
How many months/years ago did you last work?	¿Cuántos meses/años atrás hace que usted trabajó?
Do you want to return to work?	¿Quiere regresar a trabajar? ¿**Desea** regresar a trabajar?
Are you filing for disability?	¿Está usted aplicando para obtenere disabilidad?
Do you receive disability now?	¿Está usted recibiendo desabilidad en estos momentos? ¿Está usted **cogiendo** desabilidad en estos momentos?

Get-Up-and-Go Test

The following test is used as a screening tool to assess fall risk.

I am going to ask you to perform a series of actions.	Le voy a pedir que haga una serie de acciones. Le voy a **instruir** que haga una serie de **acciones**.
I want you to perform the actions as I say them.	Quiero que usted responda a estas acciones a la vez que se las vaya diciendo. Quiero que usted **ejecute** estas acciones a la vez que se las vaya diciendo.
Do you understand?	¿Usted me entiende?
1. Sit comfortably in a straight-backed chair.	1. Siéntese cómodamente en una silla de espaldar recto.
2. Stand up from the chair.	2. Párese de la silla.
3. Stand still momentarily.	3. Permanezca quieto/a por un momento.
4. Walk a short distance.	4. Cámine una corta distancia.
5. Stop.	5. Pare. **Deténgase.**
6. Turn around.	6. Vírese. **Dese la vuelta.**
7. Walk back to the chair.	7. Camine de regreso a la silla.
8. Turn around.	8. Vírese. **De se la vuelta.**
9. Sit down in the chair.	9. Siéntese en la silla.

Scoring:

1 = Normal
2 = Very slightly abnormal
3 = Mildly abnormal
4 = Moderately abnormal
5 = Severely abnormal

Instructions to reader: "Normal" indicates no evidence of fall risk at any time. "Moderately abnormal" reflects the possibility of falling, evidenced by exaggerated slowness, hesitancy, abnormal movements of trunk or upper limbs, staggering, or stumbling.
"Severely abnormal" indicates that the patient appeared at risk of falling throughout the test. A score of 3 or higher indicates a positive fall risk.

Source:

Mathias, S., Nayak, U.S.L., & Issacs, B. (1986). Balance in elderly patients: The "get-up and go" test. *Arch Phys Med Rehabil,* 67, 387–389.

Appendix E

English–Spanish and Spanish–English Dictionary

English	Español
abnormality *(n)*	abnormalidad
abortion *(n)*	aborto
abrasion *(n)*	abrasión
absorb *(v)*	absorber
abstain *(v)*	abstener
accept *(v)*	aceptar
accident *(n)*	accidente
ache *(v)*	doler
ache *(n)*	dolor
aching *(adj)*	dolorido
acid *(n)*	ácido
acne *(n)*	acné
activity *(n)*	actividad
acupuncture *(n)*	acupuntura
addicted *(adj)*	adicto
addiction *(n)*	adicción
addictive *(adj)*	adictivo
address *(n)*	dirección
adhesion *(n)*	adherencia
adhesive *(n)*	adhesivo
adjust *(v)*	ajustar
admission *(n)*	admisión
admission form *(n)*	formulario de admisión; impreso de admisión; forma de admisión
admit (to hospital) *(v)*	ingresar
adopt *(v)*	adoptar
adoption *(n)*	adopción
adolescence *(n)*	adolescencia
adolescent *(n)*	adolescente
adrenaline *(n)*	adrenalina
advanced *(adj)*	avanzado
adverse *(adj)*	adverso
advice *(n)*	consejo; consulta
aerobics *(n)*	aeróbicos
affect *(v)*	afectar
afflict *(v)*	afligir
afraid (to be ~) *(adj)*	tener miedo
after *(adv)*	después
afterbirth *(n)*	placenta
afternoon *(n)*	tarde
aftertaste *(n)*	regusto
again *(adv)*	otro véz; otra véz
against *(prep)*	contra
age *(n)*	edad

English	Español
agency *(n)*	agencia
agent *(n)*	agente
aggressive *(adj)*	agresivo; violento
agile *(adj)*	ágil
agnostic *(n)*	agnóstico
aid *(n)*	ayuda
air *(n)*	aire
air conditioning *(n)*	aire acondicionado
airplane*(n)*	avión
airsick *(adj)*	mareado: moreo de aire; mal de vuelo
airway *(n)*	vía respiratoria
alarm *(n)*	alarma
alcoholic *(n)*	alcohólico
alert *(adj)*	alerta
align *(v)*	alinear
alive *(adj)*	vivo
all *(adj)*	todo
allergic *(adj)*	alérgico
allergy *(n)*	alergia
almost *(adv)*	casi
alone *(adj)*	solo
already *(adv)*	ya
also *(adv)*	tambien
alternative *(adj)*	alternativa
altitude *(n)*	altitud
always *(adv)*	siempre
ambiguous *(adj)*	ambigüo
ambulance *(n)*	ambulancía
ambulatory*(adj)*	ambulatorio
amiable *(adj)*	amable
amnesia *(n)*	amnesia
amniocentesis *(n)*	amnioocentesis
amount *(n)*	cantidad
amphetamine *(n)*	anfetamina
amputate *(v)*	amputar
amputation *(n)*	amputación

English	Español
analgesia *(n)*	analgesía
analgesic *(n)*	analgésico
and *(conj)*	y
anesthesia *(n)*	anestesia
anesthesiologist *(n)*	anestesiólogo
anesthetic *(n)*	anestético
angel dust/ PCP *(n)*	polvo de ángel (PCP); fenilciclidina
angina *(n)*	angina
angiogram *(n)*	angiograma
angioplasty *(n)*	angioplastia
angle *(n)*	ángulo
angry *(adj)*	enfadado
animal *(n)*	animal
anniversary *(n)*	aniversario
annual *(adj)*	anual
another *(adj)*	otro
answer *(n)*	respuesta
answer *(v)*	contestar
ant *(n)*	hormiga
antacid *(n)*	antiácido
anthrax *(n)*	ántrax
antibiotic *(n)*	antibiótico
antibody *(n)*	anticuerpo
anticoagulant *(n)*	anticoagulante
antidepressant *(n)*	antidepresivo
antihistamine *(n)*	antihistamina
anti-inflammatory *(adj)*	antiinflamatorio
antipsychotic *(adj)*	antipsicotico
antispasmodic *(adj)*	antiespasmódico
anxiety *(n)*	ansiedad
anxious *(adj)*	ansioso; nervioso
any *(adj)*	algún
anytime *(adv)*	en cualquier momento
apparatus *(n)*	aparato

English	Español
appendectomy *(n)*	apendicéctomia
appendicitis *(n)*	apendicitis
appetite *(n)*	apetito
apply *(v)*	aplicar
appointment *(n)*	cita
appropriate *(adj)*	apropiado
approximately *(adv)*	aproximadamente
area *(n)*	área
around *(adv)*	alrededor
arouse *(v)*	despertar
~ sexually *(v)*	excitar
arrive *(v)*	llegar
artery *(n)*	arteria
arthritis *(n)*	artritis
rheumatoid ~ *(n)*	artritis reumatoidea
artificial *(adj)*	artificial
as *(adv)*	tan . . . como
as much *(adv)*	tanto
ask (for) *(v)*	perdir
ask (question) *(v)*	preguntar
asleep *(adj)*	dormido
aspirate *(v)*	aspirar
aspirin *(n)*	aspirina
assist *(v)*	ayudar
attack *(n)*	ataque
attention *(n)*	atención
atheist *(n)*	ateo
authorization *(n)*	autorización
authorize *(v)*	autoizar
available *(adj)*	disponible
average *(adj)*	medio; promedio
avoid *(v)*	evitar
awake *(adj)*	despierto
awaken *(v)*	Despierto
babble (baby) *(n)*	balbucear
baby *(n)*	bebé
babysitter *(n)*	niñera; canguro

English	Español
back (of a hand) *(n)*	dorso
back (of a person) *(n)*	espalda
backache *(n)*	dolor de espalda
backyard *(n)*	traspatio; patio trasero; jardin posterior; patio interior
bacterial *(adj)*	bacteriano
bad *(adj)*	malo
badly *(adv)*	mal
bag *(n)*	bolsa
balance (physical) *(n)*	equilibrio
bald *(adj)*	calvo
ball *(n)*	balón; pelota
bandage *(n)*	vendaje
bandage *(v)*	vendar
bare *(adj)*	desnudo
barefoot *(adj/adv)*	descalzo
basement *(n)*	sótano
basic *(adj)*	básico
bassinet *(n)*	moisés
bathe *(v)*	bañar
bathroom *(n)*	baño
bathtub *(n)*	bañera
battery *(n)*	bateria
beach *(n)*	playa
beaten *(adj)*	golpeado
~ up *(adj)*	apaleado; moler a golpes; aporreado
beautiful *(adj)*	bella
because *(conj)*	porque
bed *(n)*	cama
bedpan *(n)*	orinal; bacinilla
bedrail *(n)*	barandal
bedroom *(n)*	cuarto
bedsore *(n)*	llaga de cama

English	Español
bee *(n)*	abeja
begin *(v)*	comenzar
behind *(adj)*	atrás
Bell's palsy *(n)*	parálisis facial
below *(adj)*	abajo
bend *(v)*	doblar
beneficial *(adj)*	beneficioso
benefit *(n)*	benificio
beside *(adj)*	al lado
better *(adj)*	mejor
between *(prep)* in between *(adv)*	entre en medio
big *(adj)*	grande
bile *(n)*	biliar
biofeedback *(n)*	biorretroaliment-ación
biopsy *(n)*	biopsía
birth *(n)*	nacimiento
birth certificate *(n)*	certificado del nacimiento
birthday *(n)*	cumpleaños
birthday, happy	feliz cumpleaños
birthmark *(n)*	marca de nacimiento
bite (animal) *(n)*	mordedura
bite (insect) *(n)*	picadura
bitter *(adj)*	amargo
black eye *(n)*	ojo negro
blackhead *(n)*	espinilla
blackout *(n)*	desmayo; perdida de conocimiento
bland *(adj)*; bland food	suave; comida suave
blanket *(n)*	manta; cobija; colcha
bleach *(n)*	blanquear; aclarar
bleed *(v)*	sangrar
bleeding *(adj)*	sangrando
blind *(adj)*	ciego
blink *(v)*	parpadear
blockage *(n)*	obstrucción
blood *(n)*	sangre
blood count *(n)*	hemograma; recuento de globulos
blood pressure *(n)*	presión sanguínea
blood pressure monitor *(n)*	monitor de presión sanguínea; monitor de presión arterial
bloody *(adj)*	sangriento
bloody nose *(n)*	nariz sangrienta
blow *(v)*	sonar
blow (breathe out) *(v)*	soplar
blurred *(adj)*	borroso
body *(n)*	cuerpo
boil *(n)*	furunculo
bone marrow *(n)*	medula osea
both *(adj)*	ambas
bother *(v)*	molestar
bothersome *(adj)*	incómodo
bottle *(n)*	botella
botulism *(n)*	botulismo
bowel *(n)* large ~ *(n)* small ~ *(n)*	intestino intestino grueso intestino delgado
bowlegged *(adj)*	patizambo; patiestevado; zambo
boy *(n)*	chico; niño
braces (dental) *(n)*	aparatos ortodónticos
braces (orthopedic) *(n)*	aparatos ortopédicos
break (bone) *(v)*	fracturar
breast-feed *(v)*	dar de pecho; amamantar
breast pump *(n)*	bomba para el seno

English	Español
breath *(n)*	aliento
bad ~	mal aliento
breathe *(v)*	respirar
breathless *(adj)*	jadeante; falto de aire; sin aliento; sin resuello
breech (birth) *(n)*	presentación de nalgas
brief *(adj)*	breve
bring *(v)*	traer
brittle *(adj)*	fragil
broken *(adj)*	fracturado
bronchitis *(n)*	bronquitis
bruise *(n)*	moretón; morado; cardenal
bruised *(adj)*	golpeado
bulging *(adj)*	protuberante
bulimia *(n)*	bulimia
bump *(n)*	choque; golpe
burn *(n)*	quemadura
burn *(v)*	quemar
burning *(adj)*	quemante
burp *(v)*	eructo
bursa *(n)*	bolsa
bursitis *(n)*	bursitis
busy *(adj)*	ocupado
buy *(v)*	comprar
buzz *(n)*	zumbido
by *(prep)*	por
calamine *(n)*	calamina
calcium *(n)*	calcio
call *(v)*	llamar
callus *(n)*	callo
calm *(adj)*	tranquilo
calm *(v)*	calmar
can *(v)*	poder
can *(n)*	bote
cancel *(v)*	cancelar
cancerous *(adj)*	canceroso

English	Español
candidate *(n)*	candidato
cane *(n)*	bastón
capable *(adj)*	capaz
capacity *(n)*	capacidad
car *(n)*	carro
~ seat*(n)*	asiento de coche; asieñto de coche para niños
~ sickness *(n)*	mareo de coche/carro
cardiac *(adj)*	cardíaco
cardiologist *(n)*	cardiólogo
cardiomyopathy *(n)*	cardiomiopatía
care (for) *(v)*	cuidar
care *(n)*	cuidado; atención
careful *(adj)*	cuidadoso
caregiver *(n)*	cuidador; proveedor de cuidados
carpet *(n)*	alfombra
carrier (of disease) *(n)*	portador
carry *(v)*	llevar
cartilage *(n)*	cartilago
cash *(n)*	dinero en efectivo
cashier *(n)*	cajero
cast *(n)*	yeso
castrate *(v)*	castrar
castration *(n)*	castración
cataract *(n)*	catarata
catheter *(n)*	cateter
catheterization *(n)*	cateterismo
catheterize *(v)*	cateterizar
cause *(v)*	causar
cavity (dental) *(n)*	carie; cavidad
cellulitis *(n)*	celulitis
center *(n)*	centro

English	Español
centimeter *(n)*	centímetro
central *(adj)*	central
central nervous system *(n)*	sistema nervioso central
certain *(adj)*	cierto
certificate *(n)*	certificado
certification *(n)*	certificación
cerumen *(n)*	cera del oído
cesarean section *(n)*	cesárea
cessation *(n)*	cesación
chafing *(n)*	rozadura
chair *(n)*	silla
chance (probability) *(n)*	probabilidad
change *(v)*	cambiar
change *(n)*	cambio
change of life *(n)*	cambio de vida
changing room *(n)*	vestuario
chapped *(adj)*	agrietado/a
characteristic *(adj)*	característico
charge *(n)*	cobro
charge *(v)*	cobrar
cheap *(adj)*	barato
check *(v)*	revisar
check-up *(n)*	chequeo; revisión medica; reconocimiento médico
chemotherapy *(n)*	quimoterapía
chew *(v)*	mascar
chicken pox *(n)*	varicela
chigger *(n)*	garrapata; nigua (in Guatemala, a *nigua* is also a crybaby or coward)
child abuse *(n)*	maltrato infantil
childbirth *(n)*	parto
childproof *(adj)*	a prueba de niños

English	Español
chills *(n)*	calosfrios
chlamydia *(n)*	clamidia
chlorine *(n)*	cloro
choice *(n)*	opción
choke (on fumes) *(v)*	ahogar
choke (on food) *(v)*	atragantar
choking *(adj)*	ahogo
cholera *(n)*	cólera
choose *(v)*	elegir; escoger
Christian *(n)*	cristiano
Christmas *(n)*	Navidad
chronic *(adj)*	crónico
cigar *(n)*	cigarro
cigarette *(n)*	cigarillo
circle *(n)*	círculo
circulation *(n)*	circulación
circumcise *(v)*	cicuncidar
circumcision *(n)*	circumcisión
cirrhosis *(n)*	cirrosis
citizen *(n)*	cuidadano
citrate *(n)*	citrato
city *(n)*	ciudad
class *(n)*	clase
classroom *(n)*	sala de clase
claustrophobia *(n)*	claustrofobia
clay-colored stools *(n)*	heces color arcilla excreta color barro
clean *(v)*	limpiar
clean *(adj)*	limpio
clear *(adj)*	claro
cleft lip *(n)*	labio leporino
cleft palate *(n)*	hendidura palatina
clench (fist) *(v)*	apretar
clergy *(n)*	clero
clerk *(n)*	dependiente
click *(n)*	clic; oprimir; presionar

English	Español
climax (sexual) *(n)*	orgasmo
climb *(v)*	escalar
clinic *(n)*	clínica
clock *(n)*	reloj
close *(v)*	cerrar
close (proximity) *(adj)*	cercano
closed *(adj)*	cerrado
clot *(n)*	coágulo
clot *(v)*	coagular (verb); coagulo (noun); embolia (noun)
cloudy (liquid) *(adj)*	turbio
clubfoot *(n)*	pie deforme
clubfooted *(adj)*	talipédico
clumsy *(adj)*	torpe
coagulant *(n)*	coagulante
coagulate *(v)*	coagular
coagulation *(n)*	coagulación
coal tar shampoo *(n)*	champu de alquitrán
coarse *(adj)*	áspero
coated *(adj)*	cubierto
cocaine *(n)*	cocaina
cohabit *(v)*	cohabitar
cold (temperature) *(adj)*	frío
to be ~ *(v)*	tener frío
cold (illness) *(n)*	catarro; gripe; resfriado, gripa
colectomy *(n)*	colectomía
colic *(n)*	cólico
colitis, ulcerative *(n)*	colitis ulcerosa
collapse *(v)*	colapso; desmayo; caerse redondo
color *(n)*	color
~-blind *(adj)*	daltónico

English	Español
comatose *(adj)*	comatoso
combination *(n)*	combinación
come *(v)*	venir
come in *(v)*	pase usted
comfortable *(adj)*	cómodo
coming *(n)*	venida
committee *(n)*	comité
commode *(n)*	cómoda
common *(adj)*	común
common-law marriage *(n)*	union consensual; matrimonio de ley comun; concubinato; union libre
community *(n)*	comunidad
companion *(n)*	compañero
compassion *(n)*	compasión
competent *(adj)*	competente
complain (of/about) *(v)*	quejar
complaint *(n)*	queja
complete *(adj)*	completo
complex *(adj)*	complejo
complexion *(n)*	tez; cutis
complicated *(adj)*	complicado
complication *(n)*	complicación
component *(n)*	componente
compress *(n)*	compresa
compression *(n)*	compresión
compulsion *(n)*	compulsión
compulsive *(adj)*	compulsivo
concentrate *(v)*	concentrar
concentration *(n)*	concentración
conception *(n)*	concepción
concerned *(adj)*	preocupado
concussion *(n)*	concusión
condition *(n)*	condición
conditioned *(adj)*	condicionado; adaptado

English	Español
condom *(n)*	condón
cone-shaped *(adj)*	coniforme
conflict *(n)*	conflicto
conflicting *(adj)*	contradictorio
confused *(adj)*	confundido; confuso
confusion *(n)*	confusión
congenital *(adj)*	congénito
congested *(adj)*	congestionado
congestion *(n)*	congestión
congestive *(adj)*	congestivo
congratulations *(n)*	felicitaciónes
conscious *(adj)*	consciente
consent *(n)*	consentimiento
constant *(adj)*	constante
constipated *(adj)*	estreñido/a; constipado/a
constipation *(n)*	constipación; estreñimiento
consult *(v)*	consultar
contact *(n)*	contacto
~ lens *(n)*	lente de contacto
contagious *(adj)*	contagioso
contain *(v)*	contener
contaminate *(v)*	contaminar
content *(adj)*	contento
content *(n)*	contenido
continuous *(adj)*	continuado
continuously *(adj)*	continuamente
contraceptive *(n)*	contraceptivo
contraction (labor) *(n)*	contracción; pujo
control *(n)*	control
control *(v)*	controlar
convalescent *(n)*	convaleciente
convenient *(adj)*	conveniente
cool *(adj)*	fresco
cooperative *(adj)*	cooperativo
coordinate *(v)*	coordinar
coordination *(n)*	coordinación
copious *(adj)*	copioso
cord *(n)*	cordón
umbilical ~ *(n)*	cordón umbilical
coroner *(n)*	médico forense
correct *(adj)*	correcto
correctly *(adv)*	correctamente
cortisone *(n)*	cortisona
cosmetic *(adj)*	cosmético
cost *(n)*	coste; costo
couch *(n)*	diván; sofá; canapé; camilla
cough *(n)*	tos
cough *(v)*	toser
counselor *(n)*	consejero
country *(n)*	país
county *(n)*	condado
cover *(v)*	cubrir
cramp *(n)*	calambre
craving *(n)*	antojo
crawl *(v)*	gatear
crib (baby's) *(n)*	cuna
crippled *(adj)*	lisiado
critical *(adj)*	crítico
cross-eyed *(adj)*	bizco
crotch *(n)*	entrepierna
croup *(n)*	crup
crown *(n)*	corona
crush (pulverize) *(v)*	machacar
crushing *(adj)*	aplastante; opresivo
crust *(n)*	costra
crutch *(n)*	muleta
cry *(v)*	llorar
cup (drinking) *(n)*	copa
measuring ~ *(n)*	taza de medir
cure *(n)*	cura; remedio
cure *(v)*	curar
cut *(v)*	cortar
cyanide *(n)*	cianuro

English	Español
cycle *(n)*	ciclo
dab *(n)*	toque
daily *(adj)*	por día
dairy *(adj/n)*	lácteo
damp *(adj)*	húmedo
dandruff *(n)*	caspa
dangerous *(adj)*	peligroso
dazed *(adj)*	aturdido
dead *(adj/n)*	muerto
deaf *(adj)*	sordo
death *(n)*	defunción; muerte
~ certificate *(n)*	certificado de defunción
debride *(v)*	desbridar; remover el tejido dañado
deceased *(adj/n)*	difunto
decongestant *(adj/n)*	decongestivo
decrease *(v)*	disminuir
decrease *(n)*	disminución
deep *(adj)*	profundo
defecate *(v*	defecar
defect *(n)*	defecto
birth ~ *(n)*	defecto de nacimiente
defective *(adj)*	defectuoso
defense *(n)*	defensa
deficient *(adj)*	deficiente
definite *(adj)*	definitivo
deformed *(adj)*	deforme
deformity *(n)*	deformidad
dehydrated *(adj)*	deshidratado
delay *(n)*	demora
delicate *(adj)*	delicado; frágil
delirium *(n)*	delirio
delivery (parturition) *(n)*	parto
delusional *(adj)*	delusorio
demented *(adj)*	demente; dementado
dementia *(n)*	demencia
density *(n)*	densidad
dentist *(n)*	dentista
denture *(n)*	dentadura
deodorant *(n)*	desodorante
dependence *(n)*	dependencia
dependent *(adj)*	dependiente
depressed *(adj)*	deprimido
describe *(v)*	describir
desensitize *(v)*	desensibilizar
desire *(n)*	deseo
desperate *(adj)*	desesperado
despondent *(adj)*	desanimado
detached retina *(n)*	retina desprendida
detectable *(adj)*	perceptible
deteriorate *(v)*	empeorar
determination *(n)*	determinación
detoxication *(n)*	detoxicación
devastating *(adj)*	arrollador
development *(n)*	desarrollo
deviation *(n)*	desviación
device *(n)*	aparato
diagnose *(v)*	diagnosticar
diagnostic *(adj)*	diagnóstico
die *(v)*	morir
diet *(n)*	dieta
dietician *(n)*	dietético
digest *(v)*	digerir
dilute *(v)*	diluir
dim *(adj)*	oscuro
dirt *(n)*	suciedad; basura; mugre
disabled *(adj)*	incapacitado
disc *(n)*	disco
discharge *(v)*	dar de alta
disease *(n)*	enfermedad
dislocated *(adj)*	dislocado
disposable *(adj)*	disponible

English	Español
dissolve *(v)*	disolver
dizziness *(n)*	mareo
dizzy *(adj)*	mareado
dog *(n)*	perro
dominant *(adj)*	dominante
donate *(v)*	donar
dose *(n)*	dosis
double *(adj)*	doble
doubt *(v)*	dudar
douche *(n)*	ducha
Down's syndrome *(n)*	mal de Down; mongolismo
drain *(n)*	drenaje
drain *(v)*	drenar
drainage *(n)*	supuración; drenaje
draining *(adj)*	drenante
dream *(n)*	sueño
dress *(v)*	vestir
~ oneself *(v)*	vestirse
dressing (bandage) *(n)*	cura
dribble *(v)*	gotear
drip (postnasal) *(n)*	secreción; crónica mucosa postnasal
drive (impulse) *(n)*	impulso
drive *(v)*	manejar
drooling *(n)*	abeandose
drowsiness *(n)*	odormecimiento; amodorra miento; ganas de dormir; soñera; sopor
drowsy *(adj)*	somnoliento
drunk *(adj)*	borracho; bebido; ebrio; embriagado; tomado
dry *(adj)*	seco
dryness *(n)*	sequedad
dust *(n)*	polvo

English	Español
dwarf *(n)*	enano
dye *(n)*	colorante
dysentery *(n)*	disentería
easily *(adv)*	fácilmente
easy *(adj)*	fácil
eat *(v)*	comer
ECG/ electrocardiogram or EKG *(n)*	electrocardiograma
echocardiogram *(n)*	ecocardiograma
ecstasy *(n)*	éxtasis
ECT/electroconvul sive therapy *(n)*	terapia electroconvulsiva; terapia de electrochoques
eczema *(n)*	eccema
edge *(n)*	borde; margen
education *(n)*	educación
EEG/electroenceph-alogram *(n)*	electroencefal-ograma
effect *(n)*	efecto
effective *(adj)*	efectivo
effeminate *(adj)*	afeminado
effort *(n)*	esfuerzo
ejaculate *(v)*	eyacular
elasticity *(n)*	elasticidad
elective *(adj)*	electivo
elevate *(v)*	elevar
elevated *(adj)*	elevado
eliminate *(v)*	eliminar
employer *(n)*	empleador; empresario; patrón
employment *(n)*	empleo; trabajo
empty *(adj)*	vacío
empty *(v)*	vaciar
enamel *(n)*	esmalte
enema *(n)*	enema
energy *(n)*	energía
enough *(adj)*	suficiente

English	Español
entire *(adj)*	entero
entrance *(n)*	entrada
environment *(n)*	ambiente
environmental *(adj)*	ambiental
enzyme *(n)*	enzima
epidemic *(adj)*	epidémico
epilepsy *(n)*	epilepsia
episode *(n)*	episodio
Epsom salt *(n)*	sal de epsom
equilibrium *(n)*	balance; equilibrio
equipment *(n)*	aparato; equipo
erection *(n)*	erección
erode *(v)*	erosionar
erosion *(n)*	erosión
erratic *(adj)*	errático
eruption *(n)*	erupción
eruption (skin) *(n)*	sarpullido
escalator *(n)*	escalera mecánica
established *(adj)*	establecido
estimate *(n)*	cálculo; estimado; tasación; valoración
estrogen *(n)*	estrógeno
ethical *(adj)*	ético
ethics *(n)*	ética
medical ~	ética medica
ethnic *(adj)*	étnico
evaluate *(v)*	evaluar
evaluation *(n)*	evaluación
event *(n)*	episodio
eventually *(adv)*	con el tiempo
ever *(adv)*	alguna vez
every *(adj)*	cada
everywhere *(adv)*	en todas partes
evidence *(n)*	evidencia
evident *(adj)*	evidente
exacerbation *(n)*	exacerbación
examination *(n)*	exámen; prueba
examine *(v)*	examinar
example, for	por ejemplo
excessive *(adj)*	excesivo
exchangeable *(adj)*	intercambiable
excitement *(n)*	excitación
exciting *(adj)*	estimulante
excuse *(n)*	excusa; perdón
exercise *(n)*	ejercicio
exercise *(v)*	hacer ejercicio
exhale *(v)*	exhalar; respirar hacia afuera
exhausted *(adj)*	agotado
exit *(n)*	salida
expanding *(adj)*	expansivo; agrandar; ampliar; dilatar; extender
expect *(v)*	esperar
expecting (pregnant) *(adj)*	esperando un bebé; en estado; en cinto
expectorant *(n)*	expectorante
expensive *(adj)*	costoso
experience *(n)*	experiencia
experience *(v)*	experimentar
experienced *(adj)*	experto
experimental *(adj)*	experimental
explain *(v)*	explicar
explanation *(n)*	explicación
explore *(v)*	explorar
expose *(v)*	exponer
extensive *(adj)*	extenso
extreme *(adj)*	extremo
extremity *(n)*	extremidad
eyeglasses *(n)*	lentes
failure (organ) *(n)*	insuficiencia
faint *(adj)*	desmayo
fair (complexion) *(adj)*	blanco
faith *(n)*	confianza
fall *(v)*	caer

English	Español
fall *(n)*	caída
familiar *(adj)*	conocido
farsighted *(adj)*	hipermetrope
fast *(v)*	ayunar
fast *(adv)*	rápido
fasting *(adj)*	ayuno
~ glucose	glucosa en aynunas
fat (obese) *(adj)*	gordo
fatal *(adj)*	mortal; fatal
fatigue *(n)*	cansancio; fatiga
unexplained ~	fatiga sin causa
fatigue *(v)*	cansar
fatty *(adj)*	grasoso
fear *(n)*	miedo
feces *(n)*	excremento; heces
fee *(n)*	honorarios; tarifa; cuota; factura
feel *(v)*	sentir
feeling (sensation) *(n)*	sensación
female *(adj/n)*	hembra; mujer
fertile *(adj)*	fértil
fetus *(n)*	feto
fever *(n)*	fiebre
fiber *(n)*	fibra
fibrocystic *(adj)*	fibrocístico
fibroid *(n)*	fibroide
fight *(n)*	lucha
file (archive) *(n)*	archivo
fill *(v)*	llenar; rellenar
filling (tooth) *(n)*	empaste
fire *(n)*	incendio; fuego
fissure *(n)*	fisura
fist *(n)*	puño
fitness (good health) *(n)*	bien de salud
fixative *(n)*	fíjador
flaccid *(adj)*	flacido

English	Español
flaky *(adj)*	escamoso
flammable *(adj)*	inflamable
flat *(adj)*	llano; mate
flatulence *(n)*	flatulencia
flavor *(n)*	sabor
flea *(n)*	pulga
fleabite *(n)*	salpullido
fleeting *(adj)*	fugaz; de corta duración; pasajero; transitorio
flexible *(adj)*	flexible
floater (eye) *(n)*	flotador dentro de lojo; depositos o manchas flotando en el campo de visión
floor (of building) *(n)*	piso
floor (flooring) *(n)*	suelo; piso
flower *(n)*	flor
flu *(n)*	gripa; gripe; influenza
fluently *(adv)*	con soltura
fluid *(n)*	fluido
flushed *(adj)*	enrojecido
flushing *(v)*	ponerse colorado
foamy *(adj)*	espumoso
foggy *(adj)*	brumoso
footwear *(n)*	calzado
force *(n)*	fuerza
for example	por ejemplo
forgetful *(adj)*	olvidadizo
fracture *(n)*	fractura
frantic *(adj)*	frenético
free (cost) *(adj)*	gratis
frequent *(adj)*	frecuente
frequently *(adv)*	frecuentemente
fresh *(adj)*	fresco
friction *(n)*	fricción

English	Español
frightened *(adj)*	asustado
frostbite *(n)*	congelación de una sección del cuerpo humana
frozen *(adj)*	congelado; helado
full *(adj)*	completo; lleno
fumes *(n)*	humo; vapor
funeral *(n)*	entierro
fungal infection *(n)*	infección de hongos
fungus *(n)*	hongo
funny *(adj)*	gracioso
future *(n)*	futuro
gain (weight) *(v)*	aumentar de peso; engordar
gallon *(n)*	galón
gallstone *(n)*	cálculo biliar
gangrene *(n)*	gangrena
gargle *(v)*	gargarizar; hacer gárgaras
gas, to pass *(v)*	pasar gas
gay (homosexual) *(adj)*	gay; homosexual
gay (mood) *(adj)*	alegre
generic *(adj)*	genérico
genetic *(adj)*	genético
genitals *(n)*	órganos genitales
gentle *(adj)*	apacible; suave
germ *(n)*	germen; microbio
German measles *(n)*	rubeola; sarampión alemán
girl *(n)*	chica; niña
give *(v)*	dar
gland *(n)*	glándula
glass (drinking) *(n)*	vaso
glucose *(n)*	glucosa
go *(v)*	ir
goal *(n)*	objetivo; fin
goiter *(n)*	bocio; buche
good *(adj)*	bueno
gout *(n)*	gota

English	Español
gradient *(n)*	gradiente
gradual *(adj)*	gradual
graft (skin) *(n)*	injerto
grand mal *(n)*	gran mal
grasp *(v)*	agarrar(se)
great *(adj)*	grasoso
greenish *(adj)*	verdoso
grief *(n)*	pena; pesadumbre
grieve *(v)*	afligir
growing (increasing) *(adj)*	creciente
growth *(n)*	crecimiento
guilt *(n)*	culpa
~y feelings	sentimiento de culpabilidad
gum (chewing) *(n)*	chicle; goma de mascar
gum (of mouth) *(n)*	encía
habit (addiction) *(n)*	adicción; hábito
habit (custom) *(n)*	costumbre
habit (vice) *(n)*	vicio
hair *(n)*	pelo
hairy *(adj)*	hirsuto; velludo; peludo
hall *(n)*	pasillo
hallucination *(n)*	alucinación; visión
handicap *(n)*	impedimento; incapacidad
handicapped *(adj)*	incapacitado
hangnail *(n)*	pellejo; pedazo de úna sobresaliente
hangover *(n)*	resaca; cruda; guayabo
happen *(v)*	ocurrir; pasar
happy *(adj)*	feliz; contento
hard (consistency) *(adj)*	duro
hard (difficult) *(adj)*	difícil

English	Español
harm *(v)*	dañar
harmful *(adj)*	dañino
harmless *(adj)*	inocuo; inofensivo
hardware *(n)*	ferretería
have *(v)*	hacer (aux. verb)
have (to possess) *(v)*	tener
~ to (must)	tener que (+ infinitive)
hay fever *(n)*	fiebre del heno
haziness *(n)*	opacidad
heal *(v)*	curar
healer *(n)*	curandero; curador
health (of a person) *(n)*	salud
healthcare *(n)*	atención médica
healthy *(adj)*	saludable
hear *(v)*	oír
hearing *(n)*	audición; sentido
~ aid *(n)*	aparato auditivo
heart *(n)*	corazón
heart attack *(n)*	ataque del corazón; ataque cardíaco
heartbeat *(n)*	latido cardíaco; palpitación
rapid ~	palpitacion rádipa
slow ~	palpitación lenta
heart blockage *(n)*	bloqueo cardíaco
heartburn *(n)*	acidez estomacal; acedía
heart bypass *(n)*	derivación del flujo coronario
heart defect, congenital *(n)*	defecto congénito del corazón
heart disease *(n)*	enfermedad del corazón
heart failure, congestive *(n)*	insuficiencia cardíaca congestiva
heart-lung *(adj)*	cardiorespiratorio
heart rate *(n)*	frecuencia cardíaca

English	Español
heart valve *(n)*	válvula del corazón
heat (warmth) *(n)*	calor
dry ~	calor seco
~ exhaustion	agotamiento por calor; cansancio excesivo debido al calor
~stroke	insolación
heating pad, electric *(n)*	almohadilla eléctrica; almohadilla térmica
heaviness *(n)*	pesadez
height (person's) *(n)*	altura; estatura
help *(n)*	ayuda; asistencia
help *(v)*	ayudar
hemodialysis *(n)*	hemodiálisis
hemoglobin *(n)*	hemoglobina
hemophilia *(n)*	hemofilia
hemorrhage *(n)*	desangramiento; hemorragia
hemorrhoids *(n)*	hemorroides
herb *(n)*	hierba; baqueña
herbal *(adj)*	herbario
herbalist *(n)*	herbolario; experto en hierbas
hernia *(n)*	hernia
heroin *(n)*	heroina
herpes *(n)*	herpes
heterosexual *(adj/n)*	heterosexual
hex *(n)*	mal de ojo
hiccup *(n)*	hipo; jipar; hipar
high *(adj)*	alto
high (on drugs) *(adj)*	drogado
hit (strike) *(v)*	golpear
HIV/human immunodeficiency virus *(n)*	VIH/virus de inmunodeficiencia humana

English	*Español*
hives *(n)*	ronchas; granos
hoarse *(adj)*	afónico; ronco
hoarseness *(n)*	carraspera; ronquera
hobby *(v)*	pasatiempo
hold (an object) *(v)*	tener
~ onto	agarrar
~ one's breath	aguantar la respiración
~ up (lift up)	levantar
hole *(n)*	orificio
home *(n)*	casa; domicilio
homeless *(adj)*	sin hogar; sin casa; sin hogar; destituido; guacho
homosexual *(adj/n)*	homosexual
hookworm *(n)*	anquilostoma
hop *(v)*	saltar
hope *(n)*	esperanza
hope *(v)*	esperar
hopeless *(adj)*	desperado; sin esperanza
hormonal *(adj)*	hormonal
hormone *(n)*	hormona
~ treatment	tratamiento hormonal
horn *(n)*	cuerno; tarro
hose (stockings) *(n)*	medias
hospice *(n)*	hospicio
hospital *(n)*	hospital
county ~	hospital del condado
mental ~	hospital psiquiátrico
private ~	hospital privado
public ~	hospital público
Veterans Administration~	hospital para veteranos
hospitalization *(n)*	hospitalización

English	*Español*
hospitalized *(adj)*	hospitalizado; internado
hot (spicy) *(adj)*	picante
hot (temperature; sexuality) *(adj)*	caliente; ardiente
~ flashes	olas de color
to be ~ (weather)	sofocado/a
to feel ~	caliente; caluroso/a
hour *(n)*	hora
office ~s	horas de consulta
visiting ~s	horas de vista
house *(n)*	horas de visita de casa
HPV/human papillomavirus *(n)*	virus de papiloma humano
hug *(n)*	abrazo
humid *(adj)*	húmedo
humidified *(adj)*	humedecido
humidity *(n)*	humedad
hunger *(n)*	hambre
hungover *(adj)*	resaca; cruda; guayabo
hungry *(adj)*	hambriento
to be ~	tener hambre
hurry *(v)*	apresurarse; darse prisa
hurt (to ache) *(v)*	doler(ue)
hydrocephalus *(n)*	agua en los sesos; hidrocéfalo
hydrocortisone *(n)*	hidrocortisona
hygiene *(n)*	higiene
hymen *(n)*	himen
hyperactive *(adj)*	hiperactivo
hyperglycemia *(n)*	hiperglicemia
hyperpara-thyroidism *(n)*	hiperparatiroidismo
hypertension *(n)*	alta presión
hyperthyroidism *(n)*	hipertiroidismo

English	Español
hypnosis *(n)*	hipnosis
hypoglycemia *(n)*	hipoglicemia
hypothyroidism *(n)*	hipotiroidismo
hysterectomy *(n)*	histerectomia
total ~	histerectomia total
partial ~	histerectomia parcial
ice *(n)*	hielo
~ bag	bolsa de hielo
~ chips	pedacitos de hielo
~ cream	helado
~ pack	bolsa de hielo
idea *(n)*	idea; noción
ideal *(adj)*	ideal
identical *(adj)*	idéntico
idle *(adj)*	desocupado; inactivo; inerte; haragán; vagabundear; haronear; ocroso
ill *(adj)*	enfermo; malo
seriously ~	grave
illiterate *(adj)*	analfabeto
illness *(n)*	enfermedad
imbalance *(n)*	desequilibrio
immediate *(adj)*	inmediato
immediately *(adv)*	inmediatamente
immobile *(adj)*	inmóvil
immobilize *(v)*	inmovilizar
immodest *(adj)*	inmodesto
immune *(adj)*	inmune
immunity *(n)*	inmunidad
immunization *(n)*	inmunización; vacuna
immunize *(v)*	vacunar
impacted *(adj)*	impactado
~ tooth	diente incluido
impatient *(adj)*	impaciente

English	Español
impediment *(n)*	impedimento
speech ~	defecto del habla
imperative *(adj)*	imperativo; de gran importancia; muy urgente
impetigo *(n)*	erupción cutánea
implant *(n)*	implatación; injerto
important *(adj)*	importante
impotence *(n)*	impotencia
improbable *(adj)*	improbable
improve *(v)*	mejorar
impulse *(n)*	impulso
impulsive *(adj)*	impulsivo
inaccurate (not accurate) *(adj)*	inexacto; errático
inaccurate (not correct) *(adj)*	incorrecto
inactive *(adj)*	inactivo
incapable*(adj)*	incapaz
incest *(n)*	incesto
inch *(n)*	pulgada
incident *(n)*	incidente
include *(v)*	incluir
incoherent *(adj)*	incoherencia
income *(n)*	ingresos
incompetent *(adj)*	incompetente
incontinence *(n)*	incontinencia
fecal ~	incontinencia fecal
urinary ~	incontinencia urinaria
incontinent *(adj)*	incontinente
increase *(v)*	aumentar
increase *(n)*	aumento
incubator *(n)*	incubadora
incurable *(adj)*	incurable
indecisive *(adj)*	indeciso; irresoluto
indigestion *(n)*	indigestión; dispepsia
acid ~	acidez

English	Español
infant *(n)*	infante
infect *(v)*	contagiar; infectar
infected *(adj)*	infectado
infection *(n)*	infección
infectious *(adj)*	infeccioso
infertile *(adj)*	infértil; estéril; infecundo; machio; yermo
influenza *(n)*	gripe; influenza
ingrown toenail *(n)*	uña encarnada; uñero
inhale *(v)*	inspirar; inhalar
inhaler *(n)*	inhalador; aerosol
metered-dose ~	aerosol dosificante
inherited *(adj)*	heredado; ancestral
initial *(adj)*	inicial
inject (oneself) *(v)*	inyectar(se)
injection *(n)*	inyección; jeringazo
injure *(v)*	injuriar; causar daño; damnificar; lesionar
injured *(adj)*	herido
injury *(n)*	herida
inner ear *(n)*	oído interno
innocent murmur *(n)*	soplo cardíaco inocente; soplo cardíaco inofensivo
inoperable *(adj)*	inoperable
inpatient *(n)*	hospitalizado
insane *(adj)*	demente; loco
insect bite *(n)*	picadura de insecto
insecticide *(n)*	insecticida
insect repellent *(n)*	loción contra los insectos
insemination *(n)*	inseminación
artificial ~	inseminación artificial
inside *(adv)*	adentro

English	Español
inside *(adj/n)*	interior
insight *(n)*	entendimiento; perspicacia; lucidez; conocimiento profunda
insole (shoes) *(n)*	plantilla
insomnia *(n)*	insomnio
instability *(n)*	inestabilidad
instep (foot) *(n)*	empeine
instinct *(n)*	instinto
instruction *(n)*	instrucción
insufficiency *(n)*	insuficiencia
insufficient *(adj)*	insuficiente
insulin *(n)*	insulina
insurance *(n)*	seguro medico
intelligent *(adj)*	inteligente
intense *(adj)*	intenso
intensify *(v)*	intensificar
intensive care *(n)*	cuidado intensivo
intentional *(adj)*	intencional
intercourse, sexual *(n)*	relaciónes sexuales
interest *(n)*	interés
interested *(adj)*	interesado
intermediate *(adj)*	intermediario
intermittent *(adj)*	intermitente
intern *(n)*	interno; médico interno
internal *(adj)*	interno
internist *(n)*	internista
interpret *(v)*	interpretar
interpretation *(n)*	interpretación
interpreter *(n)*	intérprete
interrupted *(adj)*	interrumpido
interval *(n)*	intervalo
interview *(n)*	entrevista
intestinal *(adj)*	intestinal

English	Español
intestine *(n)*	intestino
large ~	intestino grueso
small ~	intestino delgado
intimacy *(n)*	intimidad
intoxicated *(adj)*	intoxicado; embriagado; ebrio; borracho
intrauterine device (IUD) *(n)*	DIU (dispositivo Intrauterino)
intravenous *(adj)*	intravenoso
intubate *(v)*	intubar
invalid *(adj)*	inválido
invasive *(adj)*	invasor
involuntary *(adj)*	involuntario
IQ *(n)*	cociente de inteligencia
iron (metal) *(n)*	hierro
~ deficiency	ferropenia; insuficiencia ferrica; Bajo en nierro
irradiate *(v)*	irradiar
irregular *(adj)*	irregular
irreversible *(adj)*	irreversible; irrevocable
irrigate *(v)*	irrigar
irritable *(adj)*	irritable
irritant *(n)*	irritante
irritate *(v)*	irritar
irritating *(adj)*	irritante
irritation *(n)*	irritación
ischemia *(n)*	isquemia
ischemic *(adj)*	isquémico
isolation *(n)*	aislamiento
itch *(n)*	picazón; comezón; picor; prurito
ivy, poison *(n)*	hiedra venenosa
jar *(n)*	frasco; bote
jaundice *(n)*	piel amarilla
jaundiced *(adj)*	ictérico
jealous *(adj)*	celoso
jellyfish *(n)*	medusa; aguamala; aguamar
job *(n)*	trabajo
jock itch *(n)*	tinea cruris; tiña inguinal
jockstrap *(n)*	suspensorio
jog *(v)*	trotar
jump *(v)*	saltar
juvenile *(adj)*	juvenil
Kaposi's sarcoma *(n)*	sarcoma de Kaposi
keep *(v)*	guardar; mantener
~ alive	mantener con vida
keloid *(n)*	queloide
kilogram *(n)*	kilogramo
kind *(adj)*	amable
kit *(n)*	equipo; juego de . . .; accesorios
kitten *(n)*	gatito
Kleenex *(n)*	kleenex
kleptomania *(n)*	cleptomanía
kneel *(v)*	arrodillar
knife *(n)*	cuchillo
knot (tissue swelling) *(n)*	nudo; hinchazón
know (facts, how to) *(v)*	saber
know (people, places) *(v)*	conocer
label *(n)*	etiqueta
labor *(n)*	labor; parto
false ~	parto falso
~ pains	dolores de parto
~ room	sala de parto
laboratory *(n)*	laboratorio
laceration *(n)*	cortada; herida; laceración
lack *(n)*	falta; deficiencia
lack *(v)*	faltar

English	Español
lactose *(n)*	lactosa
lancet *(n)*	sangradera; lanceta
lapse *(n)*	lapso
large *(adj)*	grande
laryngitis *(n)*	laringitis
laser *(n)*	láser
last *(adj)*	último
~ name	apellido
~ rites	santos óleos; extremaunción; ultimos ritos
~ week	la semana pasada
late *(adj)*	tarde
later *(adv)*	más tarde
latex *(n)*	látex
lather *(n)*	espuma
lavender *(n)*	espliego; lavanda; lavándula
law *(n)*	ley
lawsuit *(n)*	pleito
lawyer *(n)*	abogado
laxative *(n)*	laxante
layer *(n)*	capa
LDL/low-density lipoprotein *(n)*	lipoproteína de baja densidad
lead (metal) *(n)*	plomo
~ poisoning	envenenamiento de plomo; intoxicación de plomo
leak *(v)*	gotear; escape; fuga; chorreo
learn *(v)*	aprender
leather *(n)*	cuero
leathery (skin) *(adj)*	curtido
leave *(v)*	salir
leech (parasite) *(n)*	sanguijuela
left *(adj)*	izquierdo
leftovers *(n)*	sobras
leggings (surgical) *(n)*	medias compresivas

English	Español
lens *(n)*	lente
lens (of eye) *(n)*	Lente del ojo
contact ~	lente de contacto
hard contact ~	lente de contacto duro
soft contact ~	lente de contacto blando
Lent *(n)*	Cuaresma
leprosy *(n)*	lepra
lesbian *(adj/n)*	lesbiana
less *(adj)*	menos
lessen *(v)*	reducir; atenuar; disminuir; rebajar
lethal *(adj)*	letal
lethargic *(adj)*	aletargado; letárgico
leukemia *(n)*	leucemia; cancer de la sangre
libido *(n)*	libido
lice *(n)*	piojos
license *(n)*	licencia
lidocaine *(n)*	lidocaína
lie down *(v)*	acostarse
life *(n)*	vida
~ expectancy	expectativa de vida; longevidad esperada
~ insurance	seguro de vida
~ support device	sustenimiento de vida aparato para prolongar la vida
ligament *(n)*	ligamento
light *(n)*	luz
~ therapy	fototerapia
light-headed *(adj)*	mareado
light-headedness *(n)*	sensación de desmayo; temperamento ligero

English	Español
lightning *(n)*	relámpago
like *(v)*	gustar
like this	así
limb *(n)*	miembro
phantom ~	miembro fantasma
limber *(adj)*	agíl; flexible
limit *(n)*	límite
limitation *(n)*	limitación
limited *(adj)*	limitado
~ activity	actividad limitada
limp *(v)*	cojear
line *(n)*	línea
lingering (illness) *(adj)*	enfermedad crónica
lining *(n)*	forro
lipid *(n)*	lípido
lipoma *(n)*	lipoma
liposuction *(n)*	liposucción
liquid *(adj/n)*	líquido
list *(n)*	lista
listen *(v)*	escuchar
listless *(adj)*	decaído
liter *(n)*	litro
little (amount) *(adj)*	poco
little (size) *(adj)*	pequeño
live *(adj)*	vivo
live *(v)*	vivir
loading dose *(n)*	dosis inicial alta
loan *(n)*	préstamo
lobby *(n)*	salón principal
local anesthesia *(n)*	anestesia local
localize *(v)*	localizar
lockjaw *(n)*	pasmo seco; tétano; espasmo masticatorio
long *(adj)*	largo; prolongado
~ acting	de acción prolongada
loose *(adj)*	suelto
~ fitting	ajustado; acoplado
lose *(v)*	suelto
~ consciousness	perder la conciencia perder(ie) conocimiento
loss *(n)*	pérdida
lotion *(n)*	loción
loud *(adj)*	ruidoso
lozenge *(n)*	pastilla para chuipar
lubricant *(n)*	lubricante
lubricate *(v)*	lubricar
lukewarm *(adj)*	templado; tibio
lump *(n)*	bulto; masa; chichón
lumpectomy *(n)*	lumpectomía
lunch *(n)*	almuerzo
lupus *(n)*	lupus
systemic ~ erythematosus	lupus eritematoso generalizado
lymph *(n)*	linfa
~ glands	glándulas linfáticas
~ node	nódulo linfático
machine *(n)*	máquina; aparato
mad (angry) *(adj)*	enojado
made *(adj)*	hecho
magnesia, milk of *(n)*	leche de magnesia
magnesium *(n)*	magnesio
magnet *(n)*	imán
maid *(n)*	criada; camerara; doncella; sirvienta muchacha del servicio
maiden name *(n)*	nombre de soltera/o

English	Español
mail *(n)*	correo
main *(adj)*	principal; esencial
maintenance dose *(n)*	dosis de mantenimiento
majority *(n)*	mayoría
make (brand) *(n)*	marca
make *(v)*	hacer
makeup (cosmetics) *(n)*	cosméticos
malabsorption *(n)*	malabsorción
maladjusted *(adj)*	inadaptado
malaise *(n)*	malestar
malaria *(n)*	malaria
male *(adj/n)*	varón
malignant *(adj)*	maligno
malnourished *(adj)*	desnutrido
malpractice *(n)*	negligencia médica
man *(n)*	hombre
manage *(v)*	dirigir; administar
mania *(n)*	manía
manic depression *(n)*	manía co-depresivo
manicure *(n)*	manicura
manifestation *(n)*	manifestación
manual *(adj)*	manual
margin *(n)*	borde
married *(adj)*	casado/a
masculine *(adj)*	masculino
mask *(n)*	máscara
oxygen ~	mascarilla de oxígeno
massage *(n)*	masaje
massive *(adj)*	masivo
mastectomy *(n)*	mastectomía
masturbate *(v)*	masturbar
masturbation *(n)*	masturbación
mattress *(n)*	colchón; colchoneta
mature *(adj)*	maduro
meal *(n)*	comida
Meals On Wheels *(n)*	comidas a domicilio

English	Español
measles *(n)*	sarampión
measure *(n)*	medida
measure *(v)*	estimar
Medicaid *(n)*	Medicaid
medical *(adj)*	médico
~ attention	atención medica
~ examiner	médico forense
~ records	registros médicos; archivos médicos
~ student	estudiante de medicina
Medicare *(n)*	Medicare
medicated *(adj)*	medicado
medication *(n)*	medicamento; medicina
medicine *(n)*	droga; medicamento; medicina
~ dropper	cuentagotas; gotero
meditate *(v)*	meditar; reunirse; tener una reunión; encontrarse
medium *(adj)*	mediano
meet *(v)*	encontrar
meeting *(n)*	encuentro
melanoma *(n)*	melanoma
memorize *(v)*	memorizar
memory *(n)*	memoria
long-term ~	memoria remota
short-term ~	memoria de cortio plazo; memoria de corto término
menarche *(n)*	menarca
mend *(v)*	reparar
Ménière's disease *(n)*	enfermedad de Ménière's;
meningitis *(n)*	meningitis

English	Español
menopausal *(adj)*	menopáusico
menopause *(n)*	menopausia; cambio de vida
menses *(n)*	menstruación
mental *(adj)*	mental
~ illness	enfermedad mental
menu *(n)*	menú
merciful *(adj)*	misericordioso
mesh *(n)*	malla
~ graft	injerto en malla
message *(n)*	mensaje
metabolism *(n)*	metabolismo
metal *(n)*	metal
metallic *(adj)*	metálico
metastasis *(n)*	metástasis
meter *(n)*	metro
methadone *(n)*	metadona
method *(n)*	método
microwave *(n)*	microonda
middle *(adj)*	medio
~ age	edad madura; edad media
~ name	segundo nombre
midget *(n)*	enano
midwife *(n)*	partera
migraine *(n)*	migraña
mild *(adj)*	leve
mild (medicine) *(adj)*	suave
~ sedative	sedante ligero; sedante suave; colmante suave
milky *(adj)*	lácteo; lechoso
mind *(n)*	mente
mineral oil *(n)*	aceite mineral
minimum *(n)*	mínimo
minister *(n)*	pastor

English	Español
misbehave *(v)*	portarse mal; comportarse mal; manejarse mal
miscarriage *(n)*	aborto
misinformed *(adj)*	mal informado
mistake *(n)*	error
misunderstanding *(n)*	equivocación
misuse *(n)*	abuso
mite (insect) *(n)*	ácaro
mitral *(adj)*	mitral
mixture *(n)*	mezcla; mixtura
mobility *(n)*	movilidad
moderate *(adj)*	moderado
moderation *(n)*	moderación
moist *(adj)*	húmedo
moment *(n)*	momento
money *(n)*	dinero
monitor *(v)*	monitorizar
mood *(n)*	humor
more *(adj)*	más
~ or less	más o menos
morgue *(n)*	cuarto de deposito de cadaveres; morgue; necronomio
morning sickness *(n)*	nauseas matutinas; nauseas del embazo; mareos matutinos
mortality *(n)*	mortalidad
~ rate	indice de mortalidad
mortuary *(n)*	depósito de cadáveres
mosquito *(n)*	mosquito
motion *(n)*	movimiento

English	Español
motor *(n)*	motor
mountain sickness *(n)*	puna; mal de montaña
mourning *(n)*	luto
mouthpiece *(n)*	bocal; boquilla
movement *(n)*	movimiento
mucus *(n)*	flema
muggy (weather) *(adj)*	clima bochornoso
multiple *(adj)*	múltiple
~ birth	parto mútiple
~ myeloma	mieloma múltiple
~ sclerosis	esclerosis mútiple
mumps *(n)*	paperas
murmur *(n)*	soplo
muscle bundle *(n)*	fascículo muscular
musculoskeletal *(adj)*	musculoesquelético
myasthenia gravis *(n)*	miestenia grave; miastenia aguda
myocardial *(adj)*	miocárdico
nail (metal) *(n)*	clavo
nail (finger/toe) *(n)*	uña
naked *(adj)*	desnudo
name *(n)*	nombre
nap *(n)*	siesta
narcolepsy *(n)*	narcolepsia
narcotic *(adj)*	narcótico
narrowing *(n)*	estrechez
nasal *(adj)*	nasal
~ drip	goteo nasal
native *(adj)*	nativo
natural *(adj)*	natural
nature*(n)*	naturaleza
~ of the illness	naturaleza de la enfermedad
nausea *(n)*	nausea
navel *(n)*	ombligo
near *(adj)*	cerca

English	Español
nearsighted *(adj)*	miope; corto de vista
nebulizer *(n)*	nebulizador; atomizador
necessity *(n)*	necesidad
necessary *(adj)*	necesario
need *(v)*	necesitar
needle (hypodermic) *(n)*	aguja
negative *(adj)*	negativo
neglect *(n)*	negligenica
neighborhood *(n)*	barrio
nerve *(n)*	nervio
~ block	bloqueo del nervio
pinched ~	nervio atrapado; nervio pinzado
~ root	raíz nerviosa
nervous *(adj)*	nervioso
nervousness *(n)*	nerviosidad
neurologic *(adj)*	neurológico
neurologist *(n)*	neurólogo
neuropathy *(n)*	neuropatía
neurosurgeon *(n)*	neurocirujano
neurosyphillis *(n)*	neurosífilis
never *(adv)*	nunca
new *(adj)*	nuevo
newborn *(n)*	recién nacido
newlywed *(n)*	recién casado
news *(n)*	noticias
newspaper *(n)*	periódico
next *(adj)*	próximo
niacin *(n)*	niacina
nicotine *(n)*	nicotina
night *(adj)*	noche; anochecido
~ blindness	ceguera nocturna
~ sweats	sudor nocturno
~ terrors	terrores nocturnos
nightmare *(n)*	pesadilla

English	Español
nitroglycerin *(n)*	nitroglicerina
nobody *(pron)*	nadie
node *(n)*	nodo; nódulo
nodule *(n)*	nódulo
noise *(n)*	ruido
noisy *(adj)*	ruidoso
none *(adj)*	ninguno
nonflammable *(adj)*	no inflamable
noninfectious *(adj)*	no infeccioso
noninvasive *(adj)*	no invasivo
nonspecific *(adj)*	inespecífico
nonsteroidal anti-inflammatory *(n)*	antiinflamatorio no esteroide
nontoxic *(adj)*	atóxico
normal *(adj)*	normal
nosebleed *(n)*	sangralo por la nariz
nothing *(pron)*	nada
~ by mouth	nada por boca
notice *(v)*	notar
noticeable *(adj)*	perceptible
nourishing *(adj)*	nutritivo
nourishment *(n)*	alimentación
novocaine *(n)*	novocaína
now *(adv)*	ahora
right ~	ahora mismo
nude *(adj)*	desnudo
numb *(adj)*	entumecido; insensible
numb *(v)*	entumecer
numbness *(n)*	entumecimiento
nun *(n)*	monja
nurse *(n)*	enfermera
nurse's aide	auxiliar de enfermeras
charge nurse	enfermera de cargo
head nurse	jefa de enfermeras
visiting nurse	enfermera visitadora

English	Español
nursery *(n)*	cuarto para niños; guardería
nutrient *(n)*	nutritivo
nutrition *(n)*	nutrición
nutritious *(adj)*	nutritivo
nylon *(n)*	nilón
obese*(adj)*	obeso
object *(n)*	objeto
objection *(n)*	objeción
objective *(adj)*	objetivo
obligation *(n)*	obligación
observation *(n)*	observación
obsession *(n)*	obsesión
obsessive-compulsive *(adj)*	obsesivo-compulsivo
obsolete *(adj)*	obsoleto
obstacle *(n)*	obstáculo
obstetrician *(n)*	obstétrico
obstruction *(n)*	bloqueo; obstrucción
obvious *(adj)*	obvio
occasionally *(adv)*	a veces
occluding *(adj)*	oclusante
occupation *(n)*	ocupación
occupational *(adj)*	ocupacional
~ therapist	terapeuta ocupacional
~ therapy	terapia ocupacional
occupied *(adj)*	ocupado
occur *(v)*	ocurir
odd (strange) *(adj)*	chocante
odor *(n)*	olor
odorless *(adj)*	inodoro; sin olor
of *(prep)*	de
office *(n)*	oficina
~ hours	horas de consulta
official *(adj)*	oficial
often *(adv)*	a menudo; frecuentemente

English	Español
ointment *(n)*	pomada
old *(adj)*	viejo
older *(adj)*	mayor
on *(prep)*	en
oncologist *(n)*	oncólogo
only *(adv)*	solo; solamente
only *(adj)*	único
onset *(n)*	comienzo
ooze *(v)*	superar
opacity *(n)*	opacidad
open *(adj)*	abierto
operable *(adj)*	operable
operate *(v)*	operar
operating room *(n)*	sala de cirugía
operation *(n)*	operación
ophthalmologist *(n)*	oftalmólogo
opinion *(n)*	opinión
opportunity *(n)*	oportunidad
opposite *(adj)*	opuesto
optical *(adj)*	óptico
optician *(n)*	óptico
orally *(adv)*	vía oral
order *(n)*	orden
order *(v)*	ordenar
organ *(n)*	órgano
orgasm *(n)*	orgasmo
original *(adj)*	original
orthodontist *(n)*	ortodontista
orthopedist *(n)*	ortopédico
osteoporosis *(n)*	osteoporosis
other *(adj)*	otro
otorhinolaryngologist *(n)*	otorrinolaringólogo
outbreak (of disease) *(n)*	epidemia
outbreak (rash) *(n)*	erupción
outcome *(n)*	resultado
outdated *(adj)*	anticuado
outer *(adj)*	exterior; externo

English	Español
outpatient *(n)*	paciente ambulatorio
outside *(adv)*	afuera
outside *(adj/n)*	exterior
overcrowded *(adj)*	atestado
overdose *(n)*	dosis excesiva
overdue (pregnancy) *(adj)*	tardío; atrasado; retrasado
over-the-counter *(adj)*	sin receta médica sobre el mostrador
overweight *(adj)*	exceso de peso
ovulate *(v)*	ovular
ovulation *(n)*	ovulación
owe *(v)*	deber
own *(v)*	tener
oxygen *(n)*	oxígeno
~ tank	tanque de oxígeno
pacemaker *(n)*	marcapaso
pacifier *(n)*	chupete; tete
pack (cigarettes) *(n)*	cajetilla
package *(n)*	paquete
pad *(n)*	almohadilla
heating ~	almohadilla caliente eléctrica
pain *(n)*	dolor
painful *(adj)*	doloroso
painless *(adj)*	sin dolor
paint *(n)*	pintura
lead-based ~	pintura con plomo
pale *(adj)*	pálido
palpitation *(n)*	palpitación
pamphlet *(n)*	folleto
Pap smear *(n)*	Papanicolaou; citologia vaginal
paper *(n)*	papel
paralysis *(n)*	parálisis
paralyzed *(adj)*	paralítico

English	Español
paramedic *(n)*	paramédico
paranoia *(n)*	paranoia
paranoid *(adj)*	paranoico
Parkinson's disease *(n)*	enfermedad de Parkinson
parotid gland *(n)*	glándula parótida
part *(n)*	parte
part-time *(adv)*	tiempo parcial
pass *(v)*	pasar
pathologist *(n)*	patólogo
patience *(n)*	paciencia
patient *(n)*	paciente
pay *(v)*	pagar
payment *(n)*	pago
peace *(n)*	paz
peak *(n)*	punto máximo
pediatrician *(n)*	pediátra
pedicure *(n)*	pedicura
pelvic *(adj)*	pelvico
pen *(n)*	pluma
pencil *(n)*	lápiz
pending *(adj)*	pendiente
penetrating *(adj)*	penetrante
penetration *(n)*	penetración
penicillin *(n)*	penicilina
per *(adv/prep)*	por
perfect *(adj)*	perfecto
perforated *(adj)*	perforado
~ eardrum	tímpano perforado
perhaps *(adv)*	tal vez
period *(n)*	período
periodontist *(n)*	periodontista
permanent *(adj)*	permanente
permission *(n)*	permiso
permit *(n)*	permiso
peroxide, hydrogen *(n)*	peróxido de hidrógeno
person *(n)*	persona
personal *(adj)*	personal
personal hygiene *(n)*	higiene personal
personality *(n)*	personalidad
~ change	cambio de personalidad
~ disorder	trastorno de personalidad; desorden de personalidad
perspiration *(n)*	sudor; transpiración
pessary *(n)*	pesario
pesticide *(n)*	pesticida
petit mal *(n)*	tipo de epilepsia
pharmacist *(n)*	farmacéutico
phencyclidine/PCP *(n)*	fenciclidina
phlegm *(n)*	flema
phobia *(n)*	fobia
photosensitive *(adj)*	fotosensible
physical *(adj)*	físico
physical therapist *(n)*	terapista físico
physically *(adv)*	físicamente
physician *(n)*	doctor; médico
pick (scratch) *(v)*	rascar; arañar; rasguñar
pigment *(n)*	pigmento
pill (capsule) *(n)*	cápsula
pill (solid) *(n)*	pastilla; píldora
pillbox *(n)*	cajita de pastillas
pillow *(n)*	almohada
pimple *(n)*	grano
pinched nerve *(n)*	nervio pinzado
pinworm *(n)*	oxiuro; lumbriz intestinal
pipe (tobacco) *(n)*	pipa
please *(adv)*	por favor
plenty *(adv)*	bastante
pneumonia *(n)*	neumonía
podiatrist *(n)*	podiatra; podiatrista

English	Español
point *(n)*	apuntar
point *(v)*	señalar
poison *(n)*	veneno
poisoning *(n)*	envenenamiento
poisonous *(adj)*	venenoso
police *(n)*	policía
polio *(n)*	parálisis infantil; poliomielitis
pollution, air *(n)*	contaminación del aire
polyp *(n)*	pólipo
pore *(n)*	poro
portion (food) *(n)*	ración
position *(n)*	posición
positive *(adj)*	positivo
possible *(adj)*	posible
postnasal drip *(n)*	escurrimiento posnasal
postoperative *(adj)*	posoperatorio
~ pain	dolor posoperatorio
potassium *(n)*	potasio
potency *(n)*	potencia; fuerza
pound *(n)*	libra
powder *(n)*	polvo
powerful *(adj)*	potente; poderoso
precaution *(n)*	precaución
precise *(adj)*	preciso
predict *(v)*	predicir
prednisone *(n)*	prednisona
preferable *(adj)*	preferible
pregnancy *(n)*	embarazo
pregnant *(adj)*	embarazada
prejudiced *(adj)*	predispuesto
preliminary *(adj/n)*	preliminar
premature *(adj)*	prematuro
prenatal *(adj)*	prenatal
preoperative *(adj)*	preoperatorio
preparation *(n)*	preparación

English	Español
prepare *(v)*	preparar
prescribe *(v)*	prescribir; recetar
prescription *(n)*	receta
present *(adj)*	presente
present (gift) *(n)*	regalo
pressure *(n)*	presión
prevention *(n)*	prevención
preventive *(adj)*	preventivo
previous *(adj)*	previo
prick (needle) *(n)*	pinchazo; puntura
prick (insect) *(n)*	picadura
priest *(n)*	sacerdote; cura; párroco; padre
primary *(adj)*	primario
procedure *(n)*	procedimiento
proceed *(v)*	proceder
progesterone *(n)*	progesterona
prognosis *(n)*	prognóstica
program *(n)*	programa
progressive *(adj)*	progresivo
prolonged *(adj)*	prolongado
promise *(n)*	promesa
prosthesis *(n)*	miembro artificial; prótesis
prostitute *(n)*	prostituta
protection *(n)*	protección
protective *(adj)*	proteccionista; protector
protein *(n)*	proteína
psychiatrist *(n)*	siquiatra
psychosis *(n)*	sicosis
psychotherapy *(n)*	sicoterapia
psychotic *(adj)*	sicótico
puberty *(n)*	pubertad
pubic *(adj)*	púbico
pulse *(n)*	pulso
pump *(n)*	bomba
puncture *(n)*	pinchazo; perforar
pus *(n)*	pus

English	Español
quackery *(n)*	charlatanismo; curanderia
quality *(n)*	calidad
quandary *(n)*	dilema; incertidumbre; aprieto; duda
quantity *(n)*	cantidad
quarantine *(n)*	cuarentena
quart *(n)*	cuarto
quarter *(n)*	cuarto
question *(n)*	pregunta
quick *(adj)*	rápido
quickly *(adv)*	rápidamente
quiet (no noise) *(adj)*	silencioso
rabies *(n)*	rabia
radiating *(adj)*	radiandose
radiation *(n)*	radiación
radioactive *(adj)*	radioactivo
radiologist *(n)*	radiólogo
rage *(n)*	furor
raise *(v)*	levantar
rancid *(adj)*	rancio
random *(adj)*	al azar
rape *(v)*	violar
rapid *(adj)*	rápido
rarely *(adv)*	raras veces
rash (skin) *(n)*	salpullido
diaper ~	salpullido de pañal
rat bite *(n)*	mordedura de rata
rattlesnake *(n)*	serpiente de cascabel
ravenous *(adj)*	hambriento
raw (food) *(adj)*	crudo
razor *(n)*	navaja/hoja/maquinilla/cuchilla de afeitar
reach *(v)*	alcanzar
reaction *(n)*	reacción
adverse ~	reacción adversa
allergic ~	reacción alérgica
read *(v)*	leer
ready *(adj)*	listo
reason *(n)*	razón
rebound *(n)*	rebote
receipt *(n)*	recibo
receive *(v)*	recibir
recent *(adj)*	reciente
receptionist *(n)*	recepcionista
recommend *(v)*	recomendar
record (patient's chart) *(n)*	historial médico; archivo médico
recover *(v)*	recuperar
recovery *(n)*	recuperación
~ room	sala de recuperación
rectal *(adj)*	rectal
recuperate *(v)*	recuperar
recurrence *(n)*	reaparición
reduction *(n)*	reducción
refer *(v)*	enviar
refill *(n)*	recargo; recarga; repuesto; renovación de receta
reflex *(n)*	reflejo
reflux *(n)*	reflujo
register *(v)*	registrar
regular *(adj)*	regular
regularly *(adv)*	con regularidad
rehabilitation *(n)*	rehabilitación
reinfection *(n)*	reinfección
rejection *(n)*	rechazo
relapse *(n)*	recaida; reincidar
related *(adj)*	relacionado; de la misma familia; emparentado

English	Español
relaxant *(n)*	relajante
muscle ~	relajante muscular
relaxation *(n)*	descanso
relief *(n)*	alivio
remember *(v)*	recordar
remission *(n)*	remisión
remnant *(n)*	residuo
removal *(n)*	ablación; extirpación
remove *(v)*	extirpar
renal *(adj)*	renal
~ failure	insuficiencia renal
repellent *(n)*	repelente
insect ~	repelente contra insectos
replacement *(n)*	reemplazo
knee ~	reemplazo de rodilla
total hip ~	reemplazo total de la cadera
research *(n)*	investigación
residence *(n)*	residencia
resist *(v)*	resistir
resistance *(n)*	resistencia
resource *(n)*	recurso
respiration *(n)*	respiración
response *(n)*	respuesta; contestacion
responsibility *(n)*	responsibilidad
rest *(n)*	descanso; reposo
rest *(v)*	descansar
restless *(adj)*	inquieto
restraints *(n)*	ataduras
restrictive *(adj)*	restringido
result *(n)*	resultado
resuscitation *(n)*	resuscitación
retinopathy *(n)*	retinopatía
retired *(adj)*	jubilado
reusable *(adj)*	reusable

English	Español
reversal *(n)*	inversión
rheumatic *(adj)*	reumático
~ fever	fiebre reumática
rheumatoid *(adj)*	reumatoide
~ arthritis	artritis reumatoide
rheumatologist *(n)*	reumatólogo
rhythm *(n)*	ritmo
right *(adj/n)*	derecho
rigid *(adj)*	rígido
ringworm *(n)*	tiña; tinea; dermatofitosis
rinse *(n)*	enjuague
risk *(n)*	riesgo
~ factor	factor de riesgo
high ~	alto riesgo
room *(n)*	cuarto; sala
roseola *(n)*	roséola
roundworm *(n)*	ascáride
rule *(n)*	regla
run *(v)*	correr
ruptured *(adj)*	perforado
sad *(adj)*	triste
safety *(n)*	seguridad
salary *(n)*	salario
saline *(n)*	salino
~ solution	solución salina
saliva *(n)*	saliva
salmonella *(n)*	salmonela
salty *(adj)*	salado
same as	así como
sample *(n)*	muestra
sand *(n)*	arena
say *(v)*	decir
scab *(n)*	costra
scab *(v)*	formar costra
scabies *(n)*	sarna
scald *(n)*	escaldadura; quemadura

English	Español
scalding *(adj)*	hirviendo
scar *(n)*	cicatriz
scarlet fever *(n)*	fiebre escarlatina
scarred *(adj)*	cicatrizado
schedule *(n)*	programa
schizophrenia *(n)*	esquizofrénia
school *(n)*	escuela
school (university) *(n)*	universidad
sciatica *(n)*	ciática
scratch *(v)*	rascar
scream *(n)*	grito
scream *(v)*	gritar
screening *(n)*	servicio de análisis; rastreo; exploración
seasickness *(n)*	mal de mar; mareo
seat *(n)*	asiento
secretion *(n)*	secreción
sedative *(n)*	sedante
see *(v)*	ver
seizure *(n)*	convulsión
seldom *(adv)*	pocas veces
self-control *(n)*	autocontrol
semen *(n)*	semen
sensation *(n)*	sensación
sensitive *(adj)*	sensible
separated *(adj)*	separado
serious *(adj)*	serio; grave
setback *(n)*	recaída
several *(adj)*	varios
severe *(adj)*	severo
sex *(n)*	sexo
sexual *(adj)*	sexual
~ activity	actividad sexual
shaky *(adj)*	tembloroso
shave *(v)*	afeitar
sheet *(n)*	sábana
shelter (homeless) *(n)*	centro de acogida; casa de acogida refugio para desamparados; albergue para desamparados
shock *(n)*	choque
short *(adj)*	bajo; pequeño; corto; breve; achicado; escaso; falto
shortage *(n)*	escasez
shortness of breath *(n)*	falta de aire; falta de respiración
short-term *(adj)*	corto plazo
shot (beverage) *(n)*	trago
shot (injection) *(n)*	inyección
shower *(n)*	ducha
shower *(v)*	duchar
sick *(adj)*	enfermo; malo
side *(n)*	lado
~ effect	efecto secundario
sidewalk *(n)*	acera
SIDS/sudden infant death syndrome *(n)*	síndrome de muerte infantil repentina
sight *(n)*	visión; vista
sign *(n)*	signo
signature *(n)*	firma
silver *(n)*	plata
similar *(adj)*	semejante
simple *(adj)*	sencillo
single (marital status) *(adj)*	soltero
sinus *(n)*	seno nasal; cavidad nasal
sinusitis *(n)*	sinusitis
sip *(n)*	sorbo; traguito
sit *(v)*	sentar
sitz bath *(n)*	baño de asiento; polibán

English	Español
size *(n)*	tamaño
skinny *(adj)*	flaco; delgado
sleep *(n)*	sueño
~ apnea	apnea del sueño; apnea durante el sueño
sleep *(v)*	dormir
sleepy *(adj)*	soñoliento; adormecido; con sueño
slice *(n)*	raja; rebanada; lasca
slice (bread) *(n)*	rebanada de pan
slipped disc *(n)*	disco desplazado
slow *(adj)*	lento
slowly *(adv)*	despacio
slurred speech	pronuciación inarticulada
small *(adj)*	pequeño
smallpox *(n)*	viruelas
smart *(adj)*	inteligente
smell *(n)*	olfato; olor
smell *(v)*	oler
smoke *(v)*	fumar
snake *(n)*	serpiente; culebra
sneeze *(n)*	estornudo
sneeze *(v)*	estornudar
snore *(v)*	roncar
snow *(n)*	nieve
soak *(v)*	remojar
soap *(n)*	jabón
soapy *(adj)*	jabonoso; lleno de jabón
sober *(adj)*	sobrio
social *(adj)*	social
~ security	seguro social
~ worker	trabajador social
sodium *(n)*	sodio
soft *(adj)*	suave
sole (foot) *(n)*	planta del pie
solid *(adj/n)*	sólido
sometimes *(adv)*	a veces; de vez en cuando; algunas veces
soon *(adv)*	pronto
sound *(n)*	sonido
spanking *(n)*	zurra; paliza; tunda; zumba regañina
speak *(v)*	hablar
specialist *(n)*	especialista
speech *(n)*	lenguaje
~ therapy	terapeuta del haba
spell *(v)*	deletrear
sperm *(n)*	esperma
sphincter *(n)*	esfínter
spina bifida *(n)*	espina bífida
spinal *(adj)*	espinal
~ tap	punción lumbar
spirometer *(n)*	espirómetro
spirometry *(n)*	espirometría
spit *(n)*	saliva; esputo
spit *(v)*	escupir
splint *(n)*	tablilla
spoon *(n)*	cuchara
spoonful *(n)*	cucharada
sprain *(v)*	torcer
sprain *(n)*	esguince; torcedura
spray *(n)*	rociada; aerosol; atomizador; vaporizador
spread *(v)*	prapagar
spread (disease) *(v)*	propagar la enfermedad; regar la enfermedad
sputum *(n)*	esputo; flema
stable *(adj)*	estable
stage *(n)*	fase
stair *(n)*	escalera

English	Español
stairs, flight of *(n)*	tramo de escalera
stand *(v)*	estar de pies; estar parado
~ up	levantarse; ponarse de pie
start *(v)*	empezar(ie); comenzar(ie)
starvation *(n)*	inanición; hambre
state *(n)*	estado
station *(n)*	estación
STD/sexually transmitted disease *(n)*	ETS (enfermedad de transmisión sexual)
steady (constant) *(adj)*	constante
steam *(n)*	vapor
sterile *(adj)*	estéril; aséptico
steroid *(n)*	esteroide
sticky *(adj)*	pegajoso; viscoso
stiff (joint) *(adj)*	rigido; tieso; agarrotado
stillbirth *(n)*	mortinato; natimuerto
stimulant *(n)*	estimulante
sting (insect) *(n)*	picadura; picada
stinging *(adj)*	causado por una picadura; capaz de causan picazón
stocking (elastic) *(n)*	calceta elástica; medias elasticas; calcetin elastico
stocking (knee-length) *(n)*	calceta; medias hasta la rodilla; calcetines hasta la radilla
stocking (surgical) *(n)*	calceta compresiva; medias compresivas calcetines compresivos
stone *(n)*	cálculo; piedra
gall~	cálculo biliar; piedra biliar
kidney ~	cálculo renal; piedra renal
stool *(n)*	excremento; heces
stop *(v)*	parar; pare de caminar
stop *(n)*	alto; pare; parada
strain (muscle) *(v)*	torcedura de musculo
strain (voice) *(v)*	forzar su voz; afanarse
strange *(adj)*	extraño
straw (drinking) *(n)*	paja; popote; paja para beber pajilla; pitillo; sorbeto
stream *(n)*	chorro; corriente; raudal
street *(n)*	calle
strength *(n)*	fuerza
strenuous *(adj)*	estrenuo
strep throat	faringitis
stress *(n)*	estrés; tensión
~ test	prueba de tolerancia al esfuerzo; prueba de cinta rodante
stretch marks *(n)*	estrias
stretcher *(n)*	camilla
stricture *(n)*	constricción
stroke *(n)*	embolia cerebral; derrame cerebral; accidente cerebrovascular; apoplegia
strong *(adj)*	fuerte
student *(n)*	estudiante; alumno

English	Español
stuffy (nose) *(adj)*	nariz tapada
stump (amputation) *(n)*	munón por amputación
stuttering *(n)*	tartamudez
sty *(n)*	orzuelo
success *(n)*	éxito
sudden *(adj)*	repentino
suddenly *(adv)*	de repente
sue *(v)*	demandar entablar una demanda; poner pleito
suffer *(v)*	sufrir
sufficient *(adj)*	bastante; suficiente
suicide *(n)*	suicidio
sulfa drug *(n)*	sulfamida
sun *(n)*	sol
~ therapy	terapia por medio de luz
sunbathing *(n)*	tomar el sol; asolearse
sunburn *(n)*	quemadura de sol
sunburned *(adj)*	quemado del sol
sunglasses *(n)*	gafas de sol; anteojos de sol; lentes de sol
sunlight *(n)*	luz del sol
sunscreen *(n)*	filtro solar
sunstroke *(n)*	insolación
suntanned *(adj)*	bronceado
superficial *(adj)*	superficial
supermarket *(n)*	supermercado
supervision *(n)*	supervisión
supplement *(n)*	suplemento
supplies *(n)*	provisiones
support *(n)*	apoyo
support *(v)*	apoyar
suppository *(n)*	supositorio
vaginal ~	supositorio vaginal
surgeon *(n)*	cirujano

English	Español
surgery *(n)*	cirugía
surname *(n)*	apellido
survive *(v)*	sobrevivir
susceptible *(adj)*	susceptible
suture *(n)*	sutura
swallow *(n)*	trago
swallow *(v)*	tragar
sweat *(n)*	sudor
sweat *(v)*	sudar
swell *(v)*	hinchar
swelling *(n)*	hinchazón
swim *(v)*	nadar
swollen *(adj)*	hinchado
symmetrical *(adj)*	simétrico
sympathy *(n)*	simpatía
symptom *(n)*	síntoma
syphilis *(n)*	sifilis
syringe *(n)*	jeringa
system *(n)*	sistema
systemic *(adj)*	sistemático
table *(n)*	mesa
tablet *(n)*	pastilla
take *(v)*	tomar
tall *(adj)*	alto
tampon *(n)*	tampón
tan *(adj)*	bronceado
tangled *(adj)*	enredado
tantrum (temper) *(n)*	pataletas; rabieta, berrinche
tap *(n)*	punción; golpe ligero; polmadita
~ water	agua del grifo; agua de la llave
tape (medical) *(n)*	cinta medica
taper *(v)*	disminuir; reducir
tapeworm *(n)*	tenia; solitaria; lombriz solitaria
tar *(n)*	alquitrán

English	Español
taste *(n)*	gusto; sabor
tasteless *(adj)*	desabrido; sin sabor
tattoo *(n)*	tatuaje
teach *(v)*	enseñar
team *(n)*	equipo
tear (eyes) *(n)*	lágrima
technology *(n)*	tecnología
teethe *(v)*	dentar
telephone *(n)*	teléfono
television *(n)*	televisión
tell (say) *(v)*	decir
temper *(n)*	disposición; humor
temperature *(n)*	temperatura
temporary *(adj)*	temporal
tempting *(adj)*	tentador
tendency *(n)*	tendencia
tender *(adj)*	sensible; doloroso
test *(n)*	análisis, examen; prueba
testosterone *(n)*	testosterona
tetanus *(n)*	tétano
therapist *(n)*	terapeuta
therapy *(n)*	terapia; tratamiento
thermometer *(n)*	termómetro
thick (consistency) *(adj)*	espeso
thin *(adj)*	flaco; delgado; fino
think *(v)*	pensar
thinner, blood *(n)*	anticoagulante
thirst *(n)*	sed
throbbing (pain) *(adj)*	punzante
thrombophlebitis *(n)*	tromboflebitis
thyroidectomy *(n)*	amputación de las tiroides
tick (insect) *(n)*	garrapata
tickle *(n)*	cosquilleo
tight *(adj)*	apretado
tightness *(n)*	estrechez; tensión; opresión
tingling *(n)*	hormigueo
tip *(n)*	punta
tired *(adj)*	cansado
tiredness *(n)*	cansancio
tobacco *(n)*	tabaco
chewing ~	tabaco de mascar
toilet *(n)*	inodoro; excusado; retrete
tolerance *(n)*	tolerencia
tolerate *(v)*	tolerar
tone *(n)*	tono
tonsilitis *(n)*	tonsilitis
tonsillectomy *(n)*	tonsilotomía
tooth *(n)*	diente
toothbrush *(n)*	cepillo de dientes
topical *(adj)*	tópico
torn *(adj)*	desgarrado
total *(adj)*	total
touch *(v)*	tocar
Tourette's disease *(n)*	enfermedad de Tourette
tourniquet *(n)*	torniquete
towel *(n)*	toalla
toxic *(adj)*	tóxico
transfusion *(n)*	transfusión
blood ~	transfusión sanguínea
translator *(n)*	intérprete; traductor
transplant *(n)*	trasplante
transportation *(n)*	transporte
transsexual *(n)*	transexual
transvestite *(n)*	transvestista; travestí
traumatic *(adj)*	traumático
tray *(n)*	bandeja
treatment *(n)*	tratamiento
tremor *(n)*	temblor
Trichomonas *(n)*	tricomonas

English	Español
trimester *(n)*	trimestre
trip (on/over) *(v)*	tropezar; caerse
triplets *(n)*	tripletos
trust *(n)*	confianza
trust *(v)*	confiar en
try *(v)*	probar
tub *(n)*	bañera
tubal *(adj)*	tubal; tubárico
~ ligation *(n)*	ligadura de trompas
~ pregnancy *(n)*	embarazo tubárico; embarazo ectopico
tuberculosis *(n)*	tuberculosis
tumor *(n)*	tumor
benign ~	tumor benigno
fibroid ~	tumor fibroideo
twins *(n)*	gemelos
fraternal ~	gemelos fraternos
identical ~	gemelos idénticos
type *(n)*	tipo
blood ~	grupo sanguíneo; tipo de sangre
typhoid *(n)*	tifoidea
typical *(adj)*	típico
ulcer *(n)*	úlcera
ultrasound *(n)*	ultrasonido
umbilical *(adj)*	umbilical
~ cord *(n)*	cordón umbilical
unbutton *(v)*	desabotonar
unconscious *(adj)*	inconsciente
undernourished *(adj)*	desnutrido
understand *(v)*	comprender; entender
underweight *(adj)*	falta de peso; bajo en peso
unemployed *(adj)*	desempleado
unhappy *(adj)*	infeliz

English	Español
unhealthy *(adj)*	enfermizo
unit *(n)*	unidad
unknown *(adj)*	desconocido
unpleasant *(adj)*	desagradable; antipatico; ingrato
unpredictable *(adj)*	imprevisible
unstable *(adj)*	inestable
unusual *(adj)*	atípico; no usual
upper *(adj)*	superior
urge *(n)*	impulso
urgency *(n)*	urgencia
urgent *(adj)*	urgente
urinalysis *(n)*	análisis de la orina
urinate *(v)*	orinar
urination *(n)*	urinación
urine *(n)*	orina
urologist *(n)*	urólogo
use *(v)*	usar
useful *(adj)*	útil
usual *(adj)*	usual
VA/Veteran's Administration *(n)*	Administración de Veteranos
vaccinate *(v)*	vacunar
vaccination *(n)*	inoculación; vacuna
vaccine *(n)*	vacuna
vaginal *(adj)*	vaginal
vague *(adj)*	vago
valuable *(adj)*	valioso
valve *(n)*	válvula
vaporizer *(n)*	vaporizador
variable *(adj)*	variable
variation *(n)*	variación
varicose *(adj)*	varicoso
~ veins *(n)*	várices; venas varicosas
varied *(adj)*	variado
variety *(n)*	variedad

English	Español
vary *(v)*	variar
Vaseline *(n)*	vaselina
vegetarian *(adj)*	vegetariano
vending machine *(n)*	distribuidor automático
ventilator *(n)*	ventilador
vibration *(n)*	vibración
victim *(n)*	víctima
view *(n)*	vista
viewpoint *(n)*	punto de vista
vigorous *(adj)*	enérgico; vigoroso
violate (rape) *(v)*	violar
violence *(n)*	violencia
violent *(adj)*	violento
viral *(adj)*	viral
virgin *(n)*	virgen
virus *(n)*	virus
visible *(adj)*	visible
vision *(n)*	visión
visit *(n)*	visita
visit *(v)*	visitar
visiting hours *(n)*	horas de vista
visiting nurse *(n)*	enfermera visitante
visitor *(n)*	visita
vitamin *(n)*	vitamina
vocal *(adj)*	vocal
~ cord *(n)*	cuerda vocal
voice *(n)*	voz
voluntary *(adj)*	voluntario
volunteer *(n)*	voluntario
vomit *(n)*	vómito
vomit *(v)*	vomitar
vomiting *(n)*	vómito
voucher *(n)*	vale; cupón
vulnerable *(adj)*	vulnerable
wait *(n)*	espera
wait *(v)*	esperar
waiting *(n)*	espera
~ list	lista de espera
~ room	sala de espera
wake *(v)*	despertar
walk *(v)*	caminar
wall *(n)*	pared
want (love) *(v)*	desear; querer
warm *(adj)*	caliente; cálido afectuoso; amoroso
warmer *(adj)*	más caliente
warmth *(n)*	calor
warning *(n)*	aviso
wart *(n)*	verruga
wash *(v)*	lavar
wasp *(n)*	avispa
watch *(n)*	reloj
watch (look after) *(v)*	cuidar
watch (look at) *(v)*	mirar
water *(n)*	agua
watery *(adj)*	aguoso; aquoso; lagrimoso; diluido
wax (ear) *(n)*	cera; cerumen
weak *(adj)*	débil
weakened *(adj)*	debilitado
weakness *(n)*	debilidad
weekend *(n)*	fin de semana
weeping (crying) *(n)*	lloroso
weeping (oozing) *(n)*	supurante; exudante; rezumante
weigh *(v)*	pesar
weight *(n)*	peso
to gain ~	aumentar de peso
to lose ~	bajar de peso
welfare (social program) *(n)*	asistencia social

English	Español
well *(adv)*	bien
wet *(adj)*	mojado
what *(pron)*	qué
wheeze *(n)*	resollo
wheeze *(v)*	resollar
whisper *(v)*	murmurar; hablar en voz baja; hablar entre dientes
white (of eggs) *(n)*	clara
whole *(adj)*	entero; todo
whole *(n)*	completo; totalidad
whooping cough *(n)*	tosferina
why *(adv/conj)*	por qué; para qué
wide *(adj)*	amplio
widespread *(adj)*	difuso
widow *(n)*	viuda
widower *(n)*	viudo
wig *(n)*	peluca
will (legal) *(n)*	testamento
will (volition) *(n)*	voluntad
wind (air) *(n)*	viento
window *(n)*	ventana
wipe (clean) *(v)*	limpiar
wipe (dry) *(v)*	pasar un paño; enjugar
wire *(n)*	alambre

English	Español
witch hazel *(n)*	agua de hamamelis
withdrawal *(n)*	retirada
witness *(n)*	testigo
woman *(n)*	mujer
wood *(n)*	madera
work *(n)*	trabajo
work *(v)*	trabajar
world *(n)*	mundo
worm *(n)*	lombriz
worried *(adj)*	preocupado
worrisome *(adj)*	preocupante
worse *(adj/adv)*	peor
worsening *(n)*	empeoramiento
wound *(n)*	herida
wrinkle *(n)*	arruga
write *(v)*	escribir
x-ray *(n)*	radiografía; rayos equis
yawn *(n)*	bostezo
yell *(v)*	gritar
yes *(adv/n)*	sí
yesterday *(adv/n)*	ayer
yoga *(n)*	yoga
young *(adj)*	joven
zoster *(n)*	zoster

Español	English
abajo	below *(adj)*
abeja	bee *(n)*
abierto	open *(adj)*
ablación	removal *(n)*
abnormalidad	abnormality *(n)*
abogado	lawyer *(n)*
aborto	miscarriage ; abortion *(n)*
abrasión	abrasion *(n)*
abrazo	hug *(n)*
absorber	absorb *(v)*
abstener	abstain *(v)*
abuso	misuse *(n)*
ácaro	mite *(n)*
accidente	accident *(n)*
aceite mineral	mineral oil *(n)*
aceptar	accept *(v)*
acera	sidewalk *(n)*
acidez estomacal	heartburn *(n)*
ácido	acid *(n)*
aclarar	bleach *(n)*
acné	acne *(n)*
acostarse	lie down *(v)*
actividad	activity *(n)*
actividad limitada	limited activity *(n)*
actividad sexual	sexual activity *(n)*
acupuntura	acupuncture *(n)*
adentro	inside *(adv)*
adherencia	adhesion *(n)*
adhesivo	adhesive *(n)*
adicción	addiction *(n)*; habit (addiction) *(n)*
adictivo	addictive *(adj)*
adicto	addicted *(adj)*
administar	manage *(v)*
Administración de Veteranos	VA/Veteran's Administration *(n)*
admisión	admission *(n)*
adolescencia	adolescence *(n)*

Español	English
adolescente	adolescent *(n)*
adopción	adoption *(n)*
adoptar	adopt *(v)*
adrenalina	adrenaline *(n)*
adverso	adverse *(adj)*
aeróbicos	aerobics *(n)*
aerosol	inhaler *(n)*
aerosol dosificador	metered-dose inhaler *(n)*
afectar	affect *(v)*
afeitar	shave *(v)*
afeminado	effeminate *(adj)*
afligir	afflict *(v)*; grieve *(v)*
afónico	hoarse *(adj)*
afuera	outside *(adv)*
agarrar	hold on to *(v)*
agarrar(se)	grasp *(v)*
agencia	agency *(n)*
agente	agent *(n)*
àgíl	limber *(adj)*
ágil	agile *(adj)*
agnóstico	agnostic *(n)*
agotado	exhausted *(adj)*
agotamiento por calor; cansancio excesivo debido al calor	heat exhaustion *(n)*
agraviar; causar daño; lesionar; damnificar	injure *(v)*
agresivo	aggressive *(adj)*
agrietado	chapped *(adj)*
agua	water *(n)*
agua de hamamelis	witch hazel *(n)*
agua del grifo	tap water *(n)*
agua en los sesos	hydrocephalus *(n)*
aguantar la respiración	hold one's breath *(v)*
aguja	needle (hypodermic) *(n)*

Español	English
aguoso; aquoso	watery *(adj)*
ahogar	choke (fumes) *(v)*
ahogo	choking *(adj)*
ahora	now *(adv)*
ahora mismo	right now *(adv)*
aire	air *(n)*
aire acondicionado	air conditioning *(n)*
aislamiento	isolation *(n)*
ajustado; acoplado	loose fitting *(adj)*
ajustar	adjust *(v)*
alambre	wire *(n)*
alarma	alarm *(n)*
al azar	random *(adj)*
alcanzar	reach *(v)*
alcohólico	alcoholic *(n)*
alegre	gay (mood) *(adj)*
alergia	allergy *(n)*
alérgico	allergic *(adj)*
alerta	alert *(adj)*
aletargado	lethargic *(adj)*
alfombra	carpet *(n)*
algún	any *(adj)*
algunas veces	sometimes *(adv)*
alguna vez	ever *(adv)*
aliento	breath *(n)*
alimentación	nourishment *(n)*
alinear	align *(v)*
alivio	relief *(n)*
almohadilla	pad *(n)*
almohadilla caliente eléctrica	heating pad, electric *(n)*
almohada	pillow *(n)*
almuerzo	lunch *(n)*
al lado	beside *(adv)*
alquitrán	tar *(n)*
alrededor	around *(adv)*
alta presión	hypertension *(n)*
alternativa	alternative *(adj)*
altitud	altitude *(n)*

Español	English
alto	high *(adj)*; tall *(adj)*; stop *(n)*
alto riesgo	high risk *(adj)*
altura	height (person's) *(n)*
alucinación	hallucination *(n)*
alumno	student *(n)*
amable	amiable *(adj)*; kind *(adj)*
amargo	bitter *(adj)*
ambas	both *(adj)*
ambiental	environmental *(adj)*
ambiente	environment *(n)*
ambiguo	ambiguous *(adj)*
ambulancia	ambulance *(n)*
ambulatorio	ambulatory *(adj)*
a menudo	often *(adv)*
amnesia	amnesia *(n)*
amniocentesis	amniocentesis *(n)*
amplio	wide *(adj)*
amputación	amputation *(n)*
amputar	amputate *(v)*
analfabeto	illiterate *(adj)*
analgesía	analgesia *(n)*
analgésico	analgesic *(n)*
análisis	test *(n)*
análisis de la orina	urinalysis *(n)*
anestesia	anesthesia *(n)*
anestesia local	local anesthesia *(n)*
anestesiólogo	anesthesiologist *(n)*
anestético	anesthetic *(n)*
anfetamina	amphetamine *(n)*
angina	angina *(n)*
angiograma	angiogram *(n)*
angioplastia	angioplasty *(n)*
ángulo	angle *(n)*
animal	animal *(n)*
aniversario	anniversary *(n)*
anquidostoma	hookworm *(n)*
ansiedad	anxiety *(n)*

Español	English
ansioso	anxious *(adj)*
antiácido	antacid *(n)*
antibiótico	antibiotic *(n)*
anticoagulante	anticoagulant *(n)*; blood thinner *(n)*
anticuado	outdated *(adj)*
anticuerpo	antibody *(n)*
antidepresivo	antidepressant *(n)*
antiespasmódico	antispasmodic *(adj)*
antihistamina	antihistamine *(n)*
antiinflamatorio	anti-inflammatory *(adj)*
antiinflamatorio no esteroide	nonsteroidal anti-inflammatory *(n)*
antipsicotico	antipsychotic *(adj)*
antojo	craving *(n)*
ántrax	anthrax *(n)*
anual	annual *(adj)*
apacible	gentle *(adj)*
apaleado; moler a golpes; aporreado	beaten up *(adj)*
aparato	apparatus *(n)*; device *(n)*; equipment *(n)*; machine *(n)*
aparato auditivo	hearing aid *(n)*
aparato intrauterino	intrauterine device (IUD) *(n)*
aparato para prolongar la vida	life support device *(n)*
aparatos ortodónticos	braces (dental) *(n)*
aparatos ortopédicos	braces (orthopedic) *(n)*
apellido	surname *(n)*
apendicéctomia	appendectomy *(n)*
apendicitis	appendicitis *(n)*
apetito	appetite *(n)*

Español	English
aplastante	crushing *(adj)*
a plazo corto; corto plazo	short-term *(adj)*
aplicar	apply *(v)*
apnea del sueño; apnea durante el sueño	sleep apnea *(n)*
apoyar	support *(v)*
apoyo	support *(n)*
aprender	learn *(v)*
apresurarse	hurry *(v)*
apretado	tight *(adj)*
apretar	clench (fist) *(v)*
apropiado	appropriate *(adj)*
aproximadamente	approximately *(adv)*
a prueba de niños	childproof *(adj)*
archivo	file (archive) *(n)*
área	area *(n)*
arena	sand *(n)*
arrodillar	kneel *(v)*
arrollador	devastating *(adj)*
arruga	wrinkle *(n)*
arteria	artery *(n)*
artificial	artificial *(adj)*
artritis	arthritis *(n)*
artritis reumatoide	rheumatoid arthritis *(n)*
ascáride	roundworm *(n)*
aséptico	sterile *(adj)*
así	like this *(adv)*; same as *(adj)*
asiento	seat *(n)*
asiento de coche	car seat *(n)*
asiento de coche para niños	car seat *(n)*
asistencia	help *(n)*
asistencia médica	medical attention *(n)*
asistencia social	welfare (social program) *(n)*

Español	English
áspero	coarse *(adj)*
aspirar	aspirate *(v)*
aspirina	aspirin *(n)*
asustado	frightened *(adj)*
ataduras	restraints *(n)*
ataque	attack *(n)*
ataque cardíaco	heart attack *(n)*
ataque del corazón	heart attack *(n)*
atención	attention *(n)*; care *(n)*
atención médica	health care *(n)*
ateo	atheist *(n)*
atestado	overcrowded *(adj)*
atípico	unusual *(adj)*
atomizador	nebulizer *(n)*
atóxico	nontoxic *(adj)*
atragantar	choke (on food) *(v)*
atrás	behind *(adv)*
atrasado	relapse *(n)*
aturdido	dazed *(adj)*
audición	hearing *(n)*
aumentar de peso	gain (weight) *(v)*; increase *(v)*
aumentar de peso; engordar	to gain weight *(v)*
aumento	increase *(n)*
autocontrol	self-control *(n)*
autoizar	authorize *(v)*
autorización	authorization *(n)*
auxiliar de enfermeras	nurse's aide *(n)*
avanzado	advanced *(adj)*
a veces	occasionally *(adv)*; sometimes *(adv)*
avión	airplane *(n)*
aviso	warning *(n)*
avispa	wasp *(n)*
ayer	yesterday *(adv/n)*
ayuda	aid *(n)*; help *(n)*

Español	English
ayudar	assist *(v)*; help *(v)*
ayunar	fast *(v)*
ayuno	fasting *(adj)*
babeandose	drooling *(n)*
bacinilla	bedpan *(n)*
bacteriano	bacterial *(adj)*
bajar de peso	to lose weight *(v)*
bajo	short *(adj)*
balance	equilibrium *(n)*
balbucear	babble (baby) *(n)*
balón; pelota	ball *(n)*
bandeja	tray *(n)*
bañar	bathe *(v)*
bañera	bathtub *(n)*; tub *(n)*
baño de asiento	sitz bath *(n)*
baños de sol	sunbathing *(n)*
baqueña	herb *(n)*
barandal	bedrail *(n)*
barato	cheap *(adj)*
barrio	neighborhood *(n)*
básico	basic *(adj)*
bastante	plenty *(adv)*; sufficient *(adj)*
bastón	cane *(n)*
bateria	battery *(n)*
bebé	baby *(n)*
bella	beautiful *(adj)*
beneficioso	beneficial *(adj)*
benificio	benefit *(n)*
bien	well *(adv)*
biliar	bile *(n)*
biopsía	biopsy *(n)*
bioretroalimentación	biofeedback *(n)*
bizco	cross-eyed *(adj)*
blanco	fair (complexion) *(adj)*
blanquear	bleach *(v)*
bloqueo	obstruction *(n)*
bloqueo cardíaco	heart blockage *(n)*

Español	English
bloqueo del nervio	nerve block *(n)*
bocal; boquilla	mouthpiece *(n)*
bocio	goiter *(n)*
bolas	knot (tissue swelling) *(n)*
bolsa de hielo	ice bag *(n)*; ice pack *(n)*
bomba	pump *(n)*
bomba para el seno	breast pump *(n)*
boquilla	mouthpiece *(n)*
borde	edge *(n)*; margin *(n)*
borracho	intoxicated *(adj)*
borroso	blurred *(adj)*
bostezo	yawn *(n)*
botánico	herbalist *(n)*
bote	can *(n)*; jar *(n)*
botella	bottle *(n)*
botulismo	botulism *(n)*
breve	brief *(adj)*
bronceado	suntanned *(adj)*; tan *(adj)*
bronquitis	bronchitis *(n)*
brumoso	foggy *(adj)*
buche	goiter *(n)*
bueno	good *(adj)*
bueno salud	fitness (good health) *(n)*
bulimia	bulimia *(n)*
bulto; masa; chichón	lump *(n)*
bursitis	bursitis *(n)*
cada	every *(adj)*
caer	fall *(v)*
caerse (usted se cayo)	trip (on/over) *(v)*
caída	fall *(n)*
cajero	cashier *(n)*
cajetilla	pack (cigarettes) *(n)*
cajita de pastillas	pillbox *(n)*
calambre	cramp *(n)*
calamina	calamine *(n)*
calceta; medias; calcetin	stocking (knee-length) *(n)*
calceta compresiva; medias compresivas; calcetin compresivo	stocking (surgical) *(n)*
calceta elástica; medias elasticas; calcetines elasticos	stocking (elastic) *(n)*
calcio	calcium *(n)*
cálculo	estimate *(n)*; stone *(n)*
cálculo biliar	gallstone *(n)*
cálculo renal	kidney stone *(n)*
calidad	quality *(n)*
caliente	hot (temperature; sexuality) *(adj)*
calmar	calm *(v)*
calor	heat (warmth) *(n)*; warm *(adj)*; warmth *(n)*
calor seco	dry heat *(n)*
caluroso	hot (weather) *(adj)*
calvo	bald *(adj)*
calzado	footwear *(n)*
calle	street *(n)*
callo	callus *(n)*
cama	bed *(n)*
cambiar	change *(v)*
cambio	change *(n)*
cambio de personalidad	personality change *(n)*
cambio de vida	change of life *(n)*; menopause *(n)*
camilla	stretcher *(n)*
caminar	walk *(v)*
cancancio	fatigue *(n)*
cancelar	cancel *(v)*

Español	English
cancer de la sangre	leukemia *(n)*
canceroso	cancerous *(adj)*
candidato	candidate *(n)*
canguro; niñera	babysitter *(n)*
cansado	tired *(adj)*
cansancio	tiredness *(n)*
cansar	fatigue *(v)*
cantidad	amount *(n)*; quantity *(n)*
capa	layer *(n)*
capacidad	capacity *(n)*
capaz	capable *(adj)*
capón	infertile *(adj)*
característico	characteristic *(adj)*
cardenal	bruise *(n)*
cardíaco	cardiac *(adj)*
cardiólogo	cardiologist *(n)*
cardiomiopatía	cardiomyopathy *(n)*
cardiorespiratorio	heart-lung *(adj)*
carie	cavity (dental) *(n)*
carraspera	hoarseness *(n)*
carro	car *(n)*
cartílago	cartilage *(n)*
casa	house *(n)*; home *(n)*
casado	married *(adj)*
casi	almost *(adv)*
caspa	dandruff *(n)*
castración	castration *(n)*
castrar	castrate *(v)*
catarata	cataract *(n)*
catarro	cold (illness) *(n)*
cateter	catheter *(n)*
cateterismo	catheterization *(n)*
cateterizar	catheterize *(v)*
causado por una picadura; capaz de causar picazón	stinging *(adj)*
causar	cause *(v)*

Español	English
cavidad	cavity (dental) *(n)*
celoso	jealous *(adj)*
celulitis	cellulitis *(n)*
centímetro	centimeter *(n)*
central	central *(adj)*
centro	center *(n)*
centro de acogida; refugio para desamparados	shelter (homeless) *(n)*
cepillo de dientes	toothbrush *(n)*
cequera nocturna	night blindness *(n)*
cera	wax (ear) *(n)*
cera del oído	cerumen *(n)*
cerca	near *(adj)*
cercano	close *(adj)*; close (proximity) *(adj)*
cerrado	closed *(adj)*
cerrar	close *(v)*
certificación	certification *(n)*
certificado	certificate *(n)*
certificado de defunción	death certificate *(n)*
certificado del nacimiento	birth certificate *(n)*
cerumen	wax (ear) *(n)*
cesación	cessation *(n)*
cesárea	cesaerean section *(n)*
cianuro	cyanide *(n)*
cíatica	sciatica *(n)*
cicatriz	scar *(n)*
cicatrizado	scarred *(adj)*
ciclo	cycle *(n)*
cicuncidar	circumcise *(v)*
ciego	blind *(adj)*
cierto	certain *(adj)*
cigarillo	cigarette *(n)*
cigarro	cigar *(n)*
cinta	tape (medical) *(n)*
circulación	circulation *(n)*

Español	English
círculo	circle *(n)*
circumcisión	circumcision *(n)*
cirrosis	cirrhosis *(n)*
cirugía	surgery *(n)*
cirujano	surgeon *(n)*
cita	appointment *(n)*
citrato	citrate *(n)*
ciudad	city *(n)*
ciudadano	citizen *(n)*
clamidia	chlamydia *(n)*
clara	white (of eggs) *(n)*
claro	clear *(adj)*
clase	class *(n)*
claustrofopia	claustrophobia *(n)*
clavo	nail (metal) *(n)*
cleptomanía	kleptomania *(n)*
clero	clergy *(n)*
clic	click *(n)*
clima bochornoso	muggy (weather) *(adj)*
clínica	clinic *(n)*
cloro	chlorine *(n)*
coagulación	coagulation *(n)*
coagulante	coagulant *(n)*
coagular	coagulate *(v)*
coágulo	clot *(n)*
cobija	blanket *(n)*
cobrar	charge *(v)*
cobro	charge *(n)*
cocaina	cocaine *(n)*
cociente de inteligencia	IQ *(n)*
cohabitar	cohabit *(v)*
cojear	limp *(v)*
colcha	blanket *(n)*
colchón	mattress *(n)*
colectomía	colectomy *(n)*
cólera	cholera *(n)*
cólico	colic *(n)*

Español	English
colitis ulcerosa	colitis, ulcerative *(n)*
color	color *(n)*
colorante	dye *(n)*
comatoso	comatose *(adj)*
combinación	combination *(n)*
comenzar	begin *(v)*; start *(v)*
comer	eat *(v)*
comida	lunch *(n)*; meal *(n)*
comidas llevadas al domicilio	Meals On Wheels *(n)*
comienzo	onset *(n)*
comité	committee *(n)*
como	as *(adv)*; same as *(adj)*
cómoda	commode *(n)*
cómodo	comfortable *(adj)*
compañero	companion *(n)*
compasión	compassion *(n)*
competente	competent *(adj)*
complejo	complex *(adj)*
completo	complete *(adj)*
completo	full *(adj)*; whole *(n)*
complicación	complication *(n)*
complicado	complicated *(adj)*
componente	component *(n)*
comprar	buy *(v)*
comprender	understand *(v)*
compresa	compress *(n)*
compresión	compression *(n)*
comprimido	lozenge *(n)*
compulsión	compulsion *(n)*
compulsivo	compulsive *(adj)*
común	common *(adj)*
comunidad	community *(n)*
con el tiempo	eventually *(adv)*
con regularidad	regularly *(adv)*
con soltura	fluently *(adv)*
concentración	concentration *(n)*
concentrar	concentrate *(v)*

Español	English
concepción	conception *(n)*
concubinato	common-law marriage *(n)*
concusión	concussion *(n)*
condado	county *(n)*
condición	condition *(n)*
condicionado	conditioned *(adj)*
condón	condom *(n)*
confianza	faith *(n)*; trust *(n)*
confiar en	trust *(v)*
conflicto	conflict *(n)*
confundido	confused *(adj)*
confusión	confusion *(n)*
confuso	confused *(adj)*
congelación	frostbite *(n)*
congelado	frozen *(adj)*
congénito	congenital *(adj)*
congestión	congestion *(n)*
congestionado	congested *(adj)*
congestivo	congestive *(adj)*
coniforme	cone-shaped *(adj)*
conocer	know (people, places) *(v)*
conocido	familiar *(adj)*
consciente	conscious *(adj)*
consejero	counselor *(n)*
consejo	advice *(n)*
constante	constant *(adj)*; steady (constant) *(adj)*
constipación	constipation *(n)*
constricción	stricture *(n)*
consulta	advice *(n)*
consultar	consult *(v)*
contacto	contact *(n)*
contagiar	infect *(v)*
contagioso	contagious *(adj)*
contaminación del aire	pollution, air *(n)*

Español	English
contaminar	contaminate *(v)*
contener	contain *(v)*
contenido	content *(n)*
contento	content *(adj)*; happy *(adj)*
contestar	answer *(v)*
continuado	continuous *(adj)*
continuamente	continuously *(adv)*
contra	against *(prep)*
contracción	contraction (labor) *(n)*
contraceptivo	contraceptive *(n)*
contradictorio	conflicting *(adj)*
control	control *(n)*
controlar	control *(v)*
convaleciente	convalescent *(n)*
conveniente	convenient *(adj)*
convulsión	seizure *(n)*
coodinar	coordinate *(v)*
cooperativo	cooperative *(adj)*
coordinación	coordination *(n)*
copa	cup (drinking) *(n)*
copioso	copious *(adj)*
corazón	heart *(n)*
cordón	cord *(n)*
cordón umbilical	umbilical cord *(n)*
corona	crown *(n)*
correctamente	correctly *(adv)*
correcto	correct *(adj)*
correo	mail *(n)*
correr	run *(v)*
cortada	laceration *(n)*
cortar	cut *(v)*
cortisona	cortisone *(n)*
corto de vista	nearsighted *(adj)*
cosmético	cosmetic *(adj)*
cosméticos	makeup (cosmetics) *(n)*
cosquilleo	tickle *(n)*

Español	English
coste; costo	cost *(n)*
costoso	expensive *(adj)*
costra	crust *(n)*; scab *(n)*
costumbre	habit (custom) *(n)*
creciente	growing (increasing) *(adj)*
crecimiento	growth *(n)*
crema	lotion *(n)*
criada	maid *(n)*
cristalino	lens (of eye) *(n)*
critiano	Christian *(n)*
crítico	critical *(adj)*
crónico	chronic *(adj)*
crónico	lingering (illness) *(adj)*
crudo	hungover *(adj)*; raw (food) *(adj)*
crup	croup *(n)*
cuajar	clot *(v)*
cuarentena	quarantine *(n)*
Cuaresma	Lent *(n)*
cuarto	bedroom *(n)*; quart *(n)*; quarter *(n)*; room *(n)*
cuarto de depósito de cadaveres	morgue *(n)*
cubierto	coated *(adj)*
cubrir	cover *(v)*
cuchara	spoon *(n)*
cucharada	spoonful *(n)*
cuchilla de afeitar	razor *(n)*
cuchillo	knife *(n)*
cuentagotas	medicine dropper *(n)*
cuerda vocal	vocal cord *(n)*
cuerno	horn *(n)*
cuero	leather *(n)*
cuerpo	body *(n)*
cuidado	care *(n)*
cuidado intensivo	intensive care *(n)*

Español	English
cuidador	caregiver *(n)*
cuidadoso	careful *(adj)*
cuidar	care (for) *(v)*; watch (look after) *(v)*
culebra	snake *(n)*
culpa	guilt *(n)*
cumpleaños	birthday *(n)*
cuna	crib (baby's) *(n)*
cuna de mimbre; bacinete	bassinet *(n)*
cupón	voucher *(n)*
cura	priest *(n)*; cure *(n)*; dressing (bandage) *(n)*
curador	healer *(n)*
curanderia	quackery *(n)*
curandero	healer *(n)*
curar	cure *(v)*; heal *(v)*
curtido	leathery (skin) *(adj)*
champu de alquitrán	tar shampoo *(n)*
charlatanismo	quackery *(n)*
chequeo	check-up *(n)*
chica; niña	girl *(n)*
chicle	gum (chewing) *(n)*
chico	boy *(n)*
chocante	odd (strange) *(adj)*
choque	bump *(n)*; shock *(n)*
chorro	stream *(n)*
chupete; tete	pacifier *(n)*
daltónico	color-blind *(adj)*
dañar	harm *(v)*
dañino	harmful *(adj)*
dar	give *(v)*
dar de alta	discharge *(v)*
dar de pecho	breast-feed *(v)*
de	of *(prep)*
de acción prolongada	long acting *(adj)*
deber	owe *(v)*

Español	*English*
débil	weak *(adj)*
debilidad	weakness *(n)*
debilitado	weakened *(adj)*
decaído	listless *(adj)*
decir	say *(v)*; tell (say) *(v)*
decongestivo	decongestant *(adj/n)*
defecar	defecate *(v)*
defecto	defect *(n)*
defecto congénito del corazón	heart defect, congenital *(n)*
defecto del habla	speech defect *(n)*
defecto de nacimiento	birth defect *(n)*
defectuoso	defective *(adj)*
defensa	defense *(n)*
deficiencia	lack *(n)*
deficiente	deficient *(adj)*
definitivo	definite *(adj)*
deforme	deformed *(adj)*
deformidad	deformity *(n)*
defunción	death *(n)*
deletrear	spell *(v)*
delicado	delicate *(adj)*
delirio	delirium *(n)*
delusorio	delusional *(adj)*
demencia	dementia *(n)*
dementado	demented *(adj)*
demente	demented *(adj)*; insane *(adj)*
demora	delay *(n)*
densidad	density *(n)*
dentadura	denture *(n)*
dentar	teethe *(v)*
dentista	dentist *(n)*
despacio	slowly *(adv)*
dependencia	dependence *(n)*
dependiente	clerk *(n)*; dependent *(adj)*
despertar	wake *(v)*
depósito de cadáveres	mortuary *(n)*
deprimido	depressed *(adj)*
derecho	right *(n/adj)*
de repente	suddenly *(adv)*
derivación del flujo coronario	heart bypass *(n)*
derramar	leak *(v)*
desabotonar	unbutton *(v)*
desabrido	tasteless *(adj)*
desagradable	unpleasant *(adj)*
desangramiento	hemorrhage *(n)*
desanimado	despondent *(adj)*
desarrollo	development *(n)*
desbridar	debride *(v)*
descalzo	barefoot *(adj/adv)*
descansar	rest *(v)*
descanso	relaxation *(n)*; rest *(n)*
desconocido	unknown *(adj)*
describir	describe *(v)*
desear	want (love) *(v)*
desempleado	unemployed *(adj)*
desensibilizar	desensitize *(v)*
deseo	desire *(n)*
desesperado	desperate *(adj)*
desequilibrio	imbalance *(n)*
desgarrado	torn *(adj)*
desgaste; desgaste por fricción	chafing *(n)*
deshidratado	dehydrated *(adj)*
desmayo	blackout *(n)*; faint *(adj)*
desnudo	bare *(adj)*; naked *(adj)*; nude *(adj)*
desnutrido	malnourished *(adj)*; undernourished *(adj)*
desocupado	idle *(adj)*

Español	English
desodorante	deodorant *(n)*
desperado	hopeless *(adj)*
despertar	arouse *(v)*
despierto	awake *(adj)*
después	after *(adv)*
desviación	deviation *(n)*
determinación	determination *(n)*
detoxicación	detoxication *(n)*
de vez en cuando	sometimes *(adv)*
diagnosticar	diagnose *(v)*
diagnóstico	diagnostic *(adj)*
diente	tooth *(n)*
diente incluido	impacted tooth *(n)*
dieta	diet *(n)*
dietético	dietician *(n)*
difícil	hard (difficult) *(adj)*
difunto	deceased *(adj/n)*
difuso	widespread *(adj)*
digerir	digest *(v)*
dilema	quandary *(n)*
diluir	dilute *(v)*
dinero	money *(n)*
dinero en efectivo	cash *(n)*
dirección	address *(n)*
dirigir	manage *(v)*
disco	disc *(n)*
disco desplazado	slipped disc *(n)*
disentería	dysentery *(n)*
dislocado	dislocated *(adj)*
disminución	decrease *(n)*
disminuir	decrease *(v)*; taper *(v)*
disolver	dissolve *(v)*
dispepsia	indigestion *(n)*
disponible	available *(adj)*; disposable *(adj)*
disposición	temper *(n)*
distender	strain (muscle) *(v)*
distribuidor automático	vending machine *(n)*
diván; sofa; canape; camilla	couch *(n)*
doblar	bend *(v)*
doble	double *(adj)*
doctor	physician *(n)*
doler	ache *(v)*; hurt *(v)*; ache *(n)*; pain *(n)*
dolor de espalda	backache *(n)*
dolores de parto	labor pains *(n)*
dolor posoperatorio	postoperative pain *(n)*
dolorido	aching *(adj)*
doloroso	painful *(adj)*
domicilio	home *(n)*
dominante	dominant *(adj)*
donar	donate *(v)*
dormido	asleep *(adj)*
dormir	sleep *(v)*
dorso	back (of a hand) *(n)*
dosis	dose *(n)*
dosis de mantenimiento	maintenance dose *(n)*
dosis excesiva	overdose *(n)*
dosis inicial alta	loading dose *(n)*
dren	drain *(n)*
drenaje	drain *(n)*; drainage *(n)*
drenante	draining *(adj)*
drenar	drain *(v)*
droga	medicine *(n)*
drogado	high (on drugs) *(adj)*
ducha	douche *(n)*; shower *(n)*
duchar	shower *(v)*
dudar	doubt *(v)*

Español	*English*
duro	hard (consistency) *(adj)*
ebrio	intoxicated *(adj)*
eccema	eczema *(n)*
ecocardiograma	echocardiogram *(n)*
edad	age *(n)*
edad madura; edad media	middle age *(n)*
educación	education *(n)*
efectivo	effective *(adj)*
efecto	effect *(n)*
efecto secundario	side effect *(n)*
ejercicio	exercise *(n)*
elasticidad	elasticity *(n)*
electivo	elective *(adj)*
electrocardiograma	ECG/electro-cardiogram *(n)*
electroence-falograma	EEG/electroen-cephalogram *(n)*
elegir	choose *(v)*
elevado	elevated *(adj)*
elevar	elevate *(v)*
eliminar	eliminate *(v)*
embarazada	pregnant *(adj)*
embarazo	pregnancy *(n)*
embarazo tubárico; embarazo ectopico	tubal pregnancy *(n)*
embolia cerebral; derrame cerebral; accidente cardiomuscular; apoplegia	stroke *(n)*
embolio	stroke *(n)*
emborrachado; tomado ebrio; bebido; embriagado	drunk *(adj)*
embriagado	intoxicated *(adj)*
empaste	filling (tooth) *(n)*
empeine	instep (foot) *(n)*
empeoramiento	worsening *(n)*
empeorar	deteriorate *(v)*
empezar	begin *(v)*; start *(v)*
empleador; emplezario; patrón	employer *(n)*
empleo	employment *(n)*
en	on *(prep)*
enano	dwarf *(n)*; midget *(n)*
encía	gum (of mouth) *(n)*
en cinta; en estado; esperando un bebe	expecting (pregnant) *(adj)*
encontrar	meet *(v)*
en cualquier momento	anytime *(adv)*
encuentro	meeting *(n)*
enema	enema *(n)*
energía	energy *(n)*
enérgico	vigorous *(adj)*
enfadado	angry *(adj)*
enfermedad	disease *(n)*; illness *(n)*
enfermedad del corazón	heart disease *(n)*
enfermedad de Ménière's	Ménière's disease *(n)*
enfermedad de Parkinson	Parkinson's disease *(n)*
enfermedad de Tourette	Tourette's disease *(n)*
enfermedad de transmisión sexual (ETS)	sexually transmitted disease (STD) *(n)*
enfermedad mental	mental illness *(n)*
enfermera	nurse *(n)*
enfermera de cargo	charge nurse *(n)*

Español	English
enfermera visitadora	visiting nurse *(n)*
enfermera visitante	visiting nurse *(n)*
enfermizo	unhealthy *(adj)*
enfermo	ill *(adj)*; sick *(adj)*
enfermo hospitalizado	inpatient *(n)*
enjuague	rinse *(n)*
enjugar; pasar un paño	wipe (dry) *(v)*
en medio	in between *(adv)*
enojado	mad (angry) *(adj)*
enredado	tangled *(adj)*
enrojecido	flushed *(adj)*
enseñar	teach *(v)*
entendimiento; perspicacia; lucidez	insight *(n)*
entero	entire *(adj)*; whole *(adj)*
entierro	funeral *(n)*
en todas partes	everywhere *(adv)*
entrada	entrance *(n)*
entre	between *(prep)*
entrepierna	crotch *(n)*
entrevista	interview *(n)*
entumecer	numb *(v)*
entumecido	numb *(adj)*
entumecimiento	numbness *(n)*
envenenamiento	poisoning *(n)*
enviar	refer *(v)*
enzima	enzyme *(n)*
epidemia	outbreak (of disease) *(n)*
epidémico	epidemic *(adj)*
epilepsia	epilepsy *(n)*
episodio	episode *(n)*; event *(n)*
equilibrio	balance (physical) *(n)*; equilibrium *(n)*
equipo	equipment *(n)*; team *(n)*
equipo; juego de . . . accesorios	kit *(n)*
equivocación	misunderstanding *(n)*
erección	erection *(n)*
erosión	erosion *(n)*
erosionar	erode *(v)*
errático	erratic *(adj)*
error	mistake *(n)*
eructo	burp *(v)*
erupción	eruption *(n)*; outbreak (rash) *(n)*
erupción cutánea	impetigo *(n)*
escabiosis	scabies *(n)*
escalar	climb *(v)*
escaldadura; quemadura	scald *(n)*
escalera	stair *(n)*
escalera mecánica	escalator *(n)*
escalofrios	chills *(n)*
escamoso	flaky *(adj)*
escasez	shortage *(n)*
esclerosis mútiple	multiple sclerosis *(n)*
escoger	choose *(v)*
escribir	write *(v)*
escuchar	listen *(v)*
escuela	school *(n)*
escupir	spit *(v)*
escurrimiento postnasal; secreción; cronica mucosa postnasal	postnasal drip *(n)*
esfínter	sphincter *(n)*
esfuerzo	effort *(n)*
esguince; torcer	sprain *(n)*
esmalte	enamel *(n)*

Español	*English*
espalda	back (of a person) *(n)*
espasmo masticatorio	lockjaw *(n)*
especialista	specialist *(n)*
espera	wait *(n)*; waiting *(n)*
esperanza	hope *(n)*
esperanza de vida	life expectancy *(n)*
esperar	expect *(v)*; wait *(v)*
esperma	sperm *(n)*
espeso	thick (consistency) *(adj)*
espina bífida	spina bifida *(n)*
espinal	spinal *(adj)*
espinilla	blackhead *(n)*
espirometría	spirometry *(n)*
espirómetro	spirometer *(n)*
espliego; lavanda; lavándula	lavender *(n)*
espuma	lather *(n)*
espumoso	foamy *(adj)*
esputo	spit *(n)*; sputum *(n)*
esquizofrénica	schizophrenia *(n)*
estable	stable *(adj)*
establecido	established *(adj)*
estación	station *(n)*
estado	state *(n)*
estar de pies; estar de panado	stand *(v)*
estatura	height (person's) *(n)*
estéril	sterile *(adj)*
estéril; infecundo; yermo machio	pill (capsule) *(n)*
esteroide	steroid *(n)*
estimar; medir	measure *(v)*
estimulante	exciting *(adj)*; stimulant *(n)*
estornudar	sneeze *(v)*
estornudo	sneeze *(n)*

Español	*English*
estrechez; tension; opresión	narrowing *(n)*; tightness *(n)*
estrellita	floater (eye) *(n)*
estrenuo	strenuous *(adj)*
estreñido	constipated *(adj)*
estrés	stress *(n)*
estrias	stretch marks *(n)*
estrógeno	estrogen *(n)*
estudiante	student *(n)*
estudiente de medicina	medical student *(n)*
ética	ethics *(n)*
ética medica	medical ethics *(n)*
ético	ethical *(adj)*
etiqueta	label *(n)*
étnico	ethnic *(adj)*
ETS (enfermedad de transmisión sexual)	STD (sexually transmitted disease) *(n)*
evaluación	evaluation *(n)*
evaluar	evaluate *(v)*
evidencia	evidence *(n)*
evidente	evident *(adj)*
evitar	avoid *(v)*
exacerbación	exacerbation *(n)*
examen; prueba	examination *(n)*; test *(n)*
examinar	examine *(v)*
excesivo	excessive *(adj)*
exceso de peso	overweight *(adj)*
excitación	excitement *(n)*
excitar	arouse sexually *(v)*
excremento	feces *(n)*; stool *(n)*
excusa	excuse *(n)*
excusado; retrete	bathroom *(n)*; toilet *(n)*
exhalar	exhale *(v)*
éxito	success *(n)*
expansivo	expanding *(adj)*

Español	English
expectorante	expectorant *(n)*
experiencia	experience *(n)*
experimental	experimental *(adj)*
experimentar	experience *(v)*
experto	experienced *(adj)*
explicación	explanation *(n)*
explicar	explain *(v)*
exploración	screening *(n)*
explorar	explore *(v)*
exponer	expose *(v)*
éxtasis	ecstasy *(n)*
extender	spread *(v)*
extenso	extensive *(adj)*
exterior	outside *(adj/n)*; outer *(adj)*
externo	outer *(adj)*
extirpación	removal *(n)*
extirpar	remove *(v)*
extraño	strange *(adj)*
extremidad	extremity *(n)*
extremo	extreme *(adj)*
eyacular	ejaculate *(v)*
fácil	easy *(adj)*
fácilmente	easily *(adv)*
factor de riesgo	risk factor *(n)*
facultad; universidad	school (university) *(n)*
falta	lack *(n)*
falta de aire	shortness of breath *(n)*
falta de peso	underweight *(adj)*
faltar	lack *(v)*
farmacéutico	pharmacist *(n)*
fascículo muscular	muscle bundle *(n)*
fase	stage *(n)*
fatal	fatal *(adj)*
fatiga	fatigue *(n)*
fatiga sin causa	unexplained fatigue *(n)*
felicitaciónes	congratulations *(n)*
feliz	happy *(adj)*
feliz cumpleaños	happy birthday
fenciclidina	phencyclidine/ PCP *(n)*
ferretería	hardware *(n)*
ferropenia	iron deficiency *(n)*
fértil	fertile *(adj)*
feto	fetus *(n)*
fibra	fiber *(n)*
fibrocístico	fibrocystic *(adj)*
fibroide	fibroid *(n)*
fiebre	fever *(n)*
fiebre del heno	hay fever *(n)*
fiebre escarlatina	scarlet fever *(n)*
fiebre reumática	rheumatic fever *(n)*
fíjador	fixative *(n)*
filtro solar	sunscreen *(n)*
fin	goal *(n)*
fin de semana	weekend *(n)*
firma	signature *(n)*
físicamente	physically *(adv)*
físico	physical *(adj)*
fisura	fissure *(n)*
flacido	flaccid *(adj)*
flaco; delgado	skinny *(adj)*; thin *(adj)*
flatulencia	flatulence *(n)*
flebitis	thrombophlebitis *(n)*
flema	mucus *(n)*; phlegm *(n)*; sputum *(n)*
flexible	flexible *(adj)*
flor	flower *(n)*
fluido	fluid *(n)*
fobia	phobia *(n)*
folleto	pamphlet *(n)*
forma de admisión	admission form *(n)*
formar costra	scab *(v)*

Español	English
formulario de admisión	admission form *(n)*
forro	lining *(n)*
forzar	strain (voice) *(v)*
fotosensible	photosensitive *(adj)*
fototerapia	light therapy *(n)*
fractura	fracture *(n)*
fracturado	broken *(adj)*
fracturar	break (bone) *(v)*
fragil	brittle *(adj)*
frágil	delicate*(adj)*
frasco	jar *(n)*
frecuencia cardíaca	heart rate *(n)*
frecuente	frequent *(adj)*
frecuentemente	frequently *(adv)*; often *(adv)*
frenético	frantic *(adj)*
fresco	cool *(adj)*; fresh *(adj)*
fricción	friction *(n)*
frío	cold (temperature) *(adj)*
fuego	fire *(n)*
fuerte	strong *(adj)*
fuerza	force *(n)*; potency *(n)*; strength *(n)*
fugaz	fleeting *(adj)*
fumar	smoke *(v)*
furor	rage *(n)*
furunculo	boil *(n)*
futuro	future *(n)*
gafas de sol	sunglasses *(n)*
galón	gallon *(n)*
gangrena	gangrene *(n)*
gargarizar	gargle *(v)*
garrapata	tick *(n)*
gatear	crawl *(v)*
gatito	kitten *(n)*
gay	gay (homosexual) *(adj)*

Español	English
gemelos	twins *(n)*
gemelos fraternos	fraternal twins *(n)*
gemelos idénticos	identical twins *(n)*
genérico	generic *(adj)*
genético	genetic *(adj)*
germen	germ *(n)*
glándula	gland *(n)*
glándula parótida	parotid gland *(n)*
glándulas linfáticas	lymph glands *(n)*
glucosa	glucose *(n)*
glucosa en aynunas	fasting glucose *(n)*
golpe	bump *(n)*
golpeado	beaten *(adj)*
golpear	hit (strike) *(v)*
golpe ligero; palmadita	tap *(n)*
gordo	fat (obese) *(adj)*
gota	gout *(n)*
gotear	dribble *(v)*
goteo nasal	nasal drip *(n)*
gracioso	funny *(adj)*
gradiente	gradient *(n)*
gradual	gradual *(adj)*
grande	big *(adj)*; large *(adj)*
gran mal	grand mal *(n)*
grano	pimple *(n)*
granos	hives *(n)*
grasoso	fatty *(adj)*; great *(adj)*
gratis	free (cost) *(adj)*
grave	serious *(adj)*; seriously ill *(adj)*
gripa	flu *(n)*
gripe	flu *(n)*; influenza *(n)*
gritar	scream *(v)*; yell *(v)*
grito	scream *(n)*
grupo sanguíneo; tipo de sangre	blood type *(n)*
guardar	keep *(v)*

Español	English
guardería	nursery *(n)*
gustar	like *(v)*
gusto	taste *(n)*
hábito	habit (addiction) *(n)*
hablar	speak *(v)*
hacer	make *(v)*
hacer *(aux. verb)*	have *(v)*
hacer ejercicio	exercise *(v)*
hambre	hunger *(n)*
hambriento	hungry *(adj)*; ravenous *(adj)*
heces depigmentadas; excreta color barró	clay-colored stools *(n)*
hecho	made *(adj)*
helado	frozen *(adj)*; ice cream *(n)*
hembra	female *(n)*
hemodiálisis	hemodialysis *(n)*
hemofilia	hemophilia *(n)*
hemoglobina	hemoglobin *(n)*
hemograma	blood count *(n)*
hemorragia	hemorrhage *(n)*
hemorragia nasal	nosebleed *(n)*
hemorroides	hemorrhoids *(n)*
hendidura palatina	cleft palate *(n)*
herbario	herbal *(adj)*
herbolario; experto en hierbas	herbalist *(n)*
heredado; ancestral	inherited *(adj)*
herida	injury *(n)*; wound *(n)*
herido	injured *(adj)*
hernia	hernia *(n)*
heroína	heroin *(n)*
herpes	herpes *(n)*
heterosexual	heterosexual *(adj/n)*
hidrocéfalo	hydrocephalus *(n)*

Español	English
hidrocortisona	hydrocortisone *(n)*
hiedra venenosas	poison ivy *(n)*
hielo	ice *(n)*
hierba	herb *(n)*
hierro	iron (metal) *(n)*
higiene	hygiene *(n)*
higiene personal	personal hygiene *(n)*
himen	hymen *(n)*
hinchado	swollen *(adj)*
hinchar	swell *(v)*
hinchazón	swelling *(n)*
hiperactivo	hyperactive *(adj)*
hiperglicemia; alto de azucar	hyperglycemia *(n)*
hipermetrope	farsighted *(adj)*
hiperparatiroidismo	hyperparathyroidism *(n)*
hipertiroidismo; tiroides altas	hyperthyroidism *(n)*
hipnosis	hypnosis *(n)*
hipo	hiccup *(n)*
hipoglicemia; bajo de azucar	hypoglycemia *(n)*
hipotiroidismo; tiroides bajas	hypothyroidism *(n)*
hirsuto; peludo	hairy *(adj)*
hirviendo	scalding *(adj)*
histerectomia	hysterectomy *(n)*
histerectomia parcial	partial hysterectomy *(n)*
histerectomia total	total hysterectomy *(n)*
historial médico	record (patient's chart) *(n)*
hoja de afeitar	razor *(n)*
hombre	man *(n)*
homosexual	homosexual *(n/adj)*
hongo	fungus *(n)*
honorrios; tarifa cargo; cuota; factura	fee *(n)*

Español	*English*
hopitalizado	hospitalized *(adj)*
hora	hour *(n)*
horas de consulta	office hours *(n)*
horas de vista	visiting hours *(n)*
hormiga	ant *(n)*
hormigueo	tingling *(n)*
hormón; hormona	hormone *(n)*
hormonal	hormonal *(adj)*
hospicio	hospice *(n)*
hospital	hospital *(n)*
hospital del condado	county hospital *(n)*
hospitalización	hospitalization *(n)*
hospital para veteranos	Veteran's Administration hospital *(n)*
hospital privado	private hospital *(n)*
hospital psiquiátrico	mental hospital *(n)*
hospital público	public hospital *(n)*
humedad	humidity *(n)*
humedecido	humidified *(adj)*
húmedo	damp *(adj)*; humid *(adj)*; moist *(adj)*
humo	fumes *(n)*
humor	mood *(n)*; temper *(n)*
ictérico	jaundiced *(adj)*
idea	idea *(n)*
ideal	ideal *(adj)*
idéntico	identical *(adj)*
imán	magnet *(n)*
impaciente	impatient *(adj)*
impactado	impacted *(adj)*
impedimento	handicap *(n)*
impedimento	impediment *(n)*
imperativo; de gran importancia; muy urgente	imperative *(adj)*

Español	*English*
implatación	implant *(n)*
importante	important *(adj)*
impotencia	impotence *(n)*
impreso de admisión	admission form *(n)*
imprevisible	unpredictable *(adj)*
improbable	improbable *(adj)*
impulsivo	impulsive *(adj)*
impulso	drive (impulse) *(n)*; impulse *(n)*; urge *(n)*
inactivo	inactive *(adj)*
inadaptado	maladjusted *(adj)*
inanición; hambre	starvation *(n)*
incapacidad	handicap *(n)*
incapacitado	disabled *(adj)*; handicapped *(adj)*
incapaz	incapable *(adj)*
incendio	fire *(n)*
incesto	incest *(n)*
incidente	incident *(n)*
incluir	include *(v)*
incoherencia	incoherent *(adj)*
incómodo	bothersome *(adj)*
incompetente	incompetent *(adj)*
inconsciente	unconscious *(adj)*
incontinencia	incontinence *(n)*
incontinencia fecal	fecal incontinence *(n)*
incontinencia urinaria	urinary incontinence *(n)*
incontinente	incontinent *(adj)*
incorrecto	inaccurate (not correct) *(adj)*
incubadora	incubator *(n)*
incurable	incurable *(adj)*
indeciso; irresoluto	indecisive *(adj)*
indice de mortalidad	mortality rate *(n)*

Español	English
indigestión	indigestion *(n)*
indigestión acída	acid indigestion *(n)*
inespecífico	nonspecific *(adj)*
inestabilidad	instability *(n)*
inestable	unstable *(adj)*
inexacto	inaccurate (not accurate) *(adj)*
infante	infant *(n)*
infección	infection *(n)*
infección de hongos	fungal infection *(n)*
infeccioso	infectious *(adj)*
infectado	infected *(adj)*
infectar	infect *(v)*
infeliz	unhappy *(adj)*
infértil	infertile *(adj)*
inflamable	flammable *(adj)*
inflamación séptica de garganta	strep throat *(n)*
ingresar	admit (to hospital) *(v)*
ingresos	income *(n)*
inhalador	inhaler *(n)*
inhalar	inhale *(v)*
inicial	initial *(adj)*
injerto	graft (skin) *(n)*; implant *(n)*
injerto en malla	mesh graft *(n)*
inmediatamente	immediately *(adv)*
inmediato	immediate *(adj)*
inmodesto	immodest *(adj)*
inmóvil	immobile *(adj)*
inmovilizar	immobilize *(v)*
inmune	immune *(adj)*
inmunidad	immunity *(n)*
inmunización	immunization *(n)*
inoculación	vaccination *(n)*
inocuo	harmless *(adj)*
inodoro; desodorizado	odorless *(adj)*

Español	English
inoperable	inoperable *(adj)*
inquieto	restless *(adj)*
insecticida	insecticide *(n)*
inseminación	insemination *(n)*
inseminación artificial	artificial insemination *(n)*
insensible	numb *(adj)*
insolación	sunstroke *(n)*
insomnio	insomnia *(n)*
inspirar	inhale *(v)*
instinto	instinct *(n)*
instrucción	instruction *(n)*
insuficiencia	failure (organ) *(n)*; insufficiency *(n)*
insuficiencia cardíaca congestiva	heart failure, congestive *(n)*
insuficiencia renal	renal failure *(n)*
insuficiente	insufficient *(adj)*
insulina	insulin *(n)*
inteligente	intelligent *(adj)*; smart *(adj)*
intencional	intentional *(adj)*
intensificar	intensify *(v)*
intenso	intense *(adj)*
intercambiable	exchangeable *(adj)*
interés	interest *(n)*
interesado	interested *(adj)*
interior	inside *(adj/n)*
intermediario	intermediate *(adj)*
intermitente	intermittent *(adj)*
internado	hospitalized *(adj)*
internista	internist *(n)*
interno	intern *(n)*; internal *(adj)*
interpretación	interpretation *(n)*
interpretar	interpret *(v)*
intérprete; traductor	interpreter *(n)*; translator *(n)*

Español	English
interrumpido	interrupted *(adj)*
intervalo	interval *(n)*
intestinal	intestinal *(adj)*
intestino	bowel *(n)*; intestine *(n)*
intestino delgado	small bowel *(n)*
intestino grueso	large bowel *(n)*
intimidad	intimacy *(n)*
intoxicación de plomo; envenenamiento de plomo	lead poisoning *(n)*
intoxicado	intoxicated *(adj)*
intravenoso	intravenous *(adj)*
intubar	intubate *(v)*
inválido	invalid *(adj)*
invasor	invasive *(adj)*
inversión	reversal *(n)*
investigación	research *(n)*
involuntario	involuntary *(adj)*
inyección	injection *(n)*; shot (injection) *(n)*
inyectar(se)	inject (oneself) *(v)*
ir	go *(v)*
irradiar	irradiate *(v)*
irratador	irritating *(adj)*
irregular	irregular *(adj)*
irreversible	irreversible *(adj)*
irrigar	irrigate *(v)*
irritable	irritable *(adj)*
irritación	irritation *(n)*
irritante	irritant *(n)*; irritating *(adj)*
irritar	irritate *(v)*
isquemia	ischemia *(n)*
isquémico	ischemic *(adj)*
izquierdo	left *(adj)*
jabón	soap *(n)*
jabonoso; lleno de jabón	soapy *(adj)*
jadeante; falto de aire; sin aliento; sin resuello	breathless *(adj)*
jefa de enfermeras	head nurse *(n)*
jeringa	syringe *(n)*
jipar	hiccup *(n)*
joven	young *(adj)*
jubilado	retired *(adj)*
juvenil	juvenile *(adj)*
kilogramo	kilogram *(n)*
kleenex	Kleenex *(n)*
labio leporino	cleft lip *(n)*
labor	labor *(n)*
laboratorio	laboratory *(n)*
lácteo	dairy *(adj)*; milky *(adj)*
lactosa	lactose *(n)*
lado	side *(n)*
lágrima	tear (eyes) *(n)*
lápiz	pencil *(n)*
lapso	lapse *(n)*
largo	long *(adj)*
laringitis	laryngitis *(n)*
la semana pasada	last week
láser	laser *(n)*
látex	latex *(n)*
latido cardíaco	heartbeat *(n)*
lavar	wash *(v)*
laxante	laxative *(n)*
leche de magnesia	milk of magnesia *(n)*
lechoso	milky *(adj)*
leer	read *(v)*
lenguaje	speech *(n)*
lente	lens *(n)*
lente de contacto	contact lens *(n)*
lente de contacto blando	soft contact lens *(n)*
lente de contacto duro	hard contact lens *(n)*

Español	English
lentes	eyeglasses *(n)*
lento	slow *(adj)*
lepra	leprosy *(n)*
lesbiana	lesbian *(n/adj)*
lesionar; causar daño; damnificar	injure *(v)*
letal	lethal *(adj)*
letárgico; aletargado	lethargic *(adj)*
leucemia	leukemia *(n)*
levantar	hold up (lift up) *(v)*; raise *(v)*
levantarse	stand up *(v)*
leve	mild *(adj)*
ley	law *(n)*
libido	libido *(n)*
libra	pound *(n)*
licencia	license *(n)*
lidocaína	lidocaine *(n)*
ligadura de los tubos	tubal ligation *(n)*
ligamento	ligament *(n)*
limitación	limitation *(n)*
limitado	limited *(adj)*
límite	limit *(n)*
limpiar	clean *(v)*; wipe (clean) *(v)*
limpio	clean *(adj)*
línea	line *(n)*
linfa	lymph *(n)*
lípido	lipid *(n)*
lipoma	lipoma *(n)*
lipoproteína de baja densidad	LDL/low density lipoprotein *(n)*
liposucción	liposuction *(n)*
líquido	liquid *(n/adj)*
lisiado	crippled *(adj)*
lista	list *(n)*
lista de espera	waiting list *(n)*

Español	English
listo	ready *(adj)*
litro	liter *(n)*
llaga de cama	bedsore *(n)*
llamar	call *(v)*
llano	flat *(adj)*
llegar	arrive *(v)*
llenar	fill *(v)*
lleno	full *(adj)*
llevar	carry *(v)*
llorar	cry *(v)*
lloroso	weeping (crying) *(n)*
localizar	localize *(v)*
loción	lotion *(n)*
loción contra los insectos	insect repellent *(n)*
loco	insane *(adj)*
lombriz	worm *(n)*
lubricante	lubricant *(n)*
lubricar	lubricate *(v)*
lucha	fight *(n)*
lumpectomía	lumpectomy *(n)*
lupus	lupus *(n)*
lupus eritematoso generalizado	systemic lupus erythematosus *(n)*
luto	mourning *(n)*
luz	light *(n)*
luz del sol	sunlight *(n)*
machacar	crush (pulverize) *(v)*
madera	wood *(n)*
maduro	mature *(adj)*
magnesito	magnesium *(n)*
mal	badly *(adv)*
malabsorción	malabsorption *(n)*
mal aliento	bad breath *(n)*
malaria	malaria *(n)*
mal de mar; mareo	seasickness *(n)*
mal de ojo	hex *(n)*
malestar	malaise *(n)*

Español	*English*
mal informado	misinformed *(adj)*
maligno	malignant *(adj)*
malo	bad *(adj)*; ill *(adj)*; sick *(adj)*
maltrato infantil	child abuse *(n)*
malla	mesh *(n)*
manejar; guiar	drive *(v)*
manía	mania *(n)*
manía depresiva	manic depression *(n)*
manicura	manicure *(n)*
manifestación	manifestation *(n)*
manta	blanket *(n)*
mantener	keep *(v)*
mantener con vida	keep alive *(v)*
manual	manual *(adj)*
máquina	machine *(n)*
maquinilla de afeitar	razor *(n)*
marca	make (brand) *(n)*
marca de nacimiento	birthmark *(n)*
marcapaso	pacemaker *(n)*
mareado	dizzy *(adj)*; light-headed *(adj)*
mareado; mareo del aire; mal de vuelo	airsick *(adj)*
mareo	dizziness *(n)*
mareo de coche/carro	car sickness *(n)*
margen	edge *(n)*
más	more *(adj)*
masaje	massage *(n)*
más caliente	warmer *(adj)*
mascar	chew *(v)*
máscara	mask *(n)*
mascarilla de oxígeno	oxygen mask *(n)*
masculino	masculine *(adj)*
masivo	massive *(adj)*

Español	*English*
más o menos	more or less *(adv)*
más tarde	later *(adv)*
mastectomía	mastectomy *(n)*
masturbación	masturbation *(n)*
masturbar	masturbate *(v)*
mate	flat *(adj)*
matrimonio consuetudinario; union libre; matrimonio de hecho; union consensual	common-law marriage *(n)*
mayor	older *(adj)*
mayoría	majority *(n)*
media compresiva	stocking (surgical) *(n)*
mediano	medium *(adj)*
medias	hose (stockings) *(n)*
medias compresivas	leggings (surgical) *(n)*
medicado	medicated *(adj)*
Medicaid	Medicaid *(n)*
medicamento	medication *(n)*; medicine *(n)*
Medicare	Medicare *(n)*
medicina	medication *(n)*; medicine *(n)*
médico	medical *(adj)*; physician *(n)*
médico forense	coroner *(n)*; medical examiner *(n)*
médico interno	intern *(n)*
medida	measure *(n)*
medio; promedio	average *(adj)*; middle *(adj)*
meditar	meditate *(v)*
medula osea	bone marrow *(n)*
medusa	jellyfish *(n)*
mejor	better *(adj)*
mejorar	improve *(v)*

Español	English
melanoma	melanoma *(n)*
memoria	memory *(n)*
memoria a corte termino	short-term memory *(n)*
memoria remota	long-term memory *(n)*
memorizar	memorize *(v)*
menarca	menarche *(n)*
meningitis	meningitis *(n)*
menopausia	menopause *(n)*
menopáusico	menopausal *(adj)*
menos	less *(adj)*
mensaje	message *(n)*
menstruación	menses *(n)*
mental	mental *(adj)*
mente	mind *(n)*
menú	menu *(n)*
mesa	table *(n)*
metabolismo	metabolism *(n)*
metadona	methadone *(n)*
metal	metal *(n)*
metálico	metallic *(adj)*
metástasis	metastasis *(n)*
método	method *(n)*
metro	meter *(n)*
mezcla	mixture *(n)*
microbio	germ *(n)*
microonda	microwave *(n)*
miedo	fear *(n)*
mieloma múltiple	multiple myeloma *(n)*
miembro	limb *(n)*
miembro artificial	prosthesis *(n)*
miembro fantasma	phantom limb *(n)*
miestenia grave	myasthenia gravis *(n)*
migraña	migraine *(n)*
mínimo	minimum *(n)*
miocárdico	myocardial *(adj)*
miope	nearsighted *(adj)*
mirar	watch (look at) *(v)*
misericordioso	merciful *(adj)*
mitral	mitral *(adj)*
mixtura	mixture *(n)*
moderación	moderation *(n)*
moderado	moderate *(adj)*
mojado	wet *(adj)*
molestar	bother *(v)*
momento	moment *(n)*
mongolismo	Down syndrome *(n)*
monitor de presión arterial	blood pressure monitor *(n)*
monitor de presión sanguínea	blood pressure monitor *(n)*
monitorizar	monitor *(v)*
monja	nun *(n)*
morado	bruise *(n)*; bruised *(adj)*
moratón	bruised *(adj)*
mordedura	bite (animal) *(n)*
mordedura de ratas	rat bite *(n)*
moretón	bruise *(n)*
morgue vivero	nursery *(n)*
morir	die *(v)*
mortal	fatal *(adj)*
mortalidad	mortality *(n)*
mosquito	mosquito *(n)*
motor	motor *(n)*
movilidad	mobility *(n)*
movimiento	motion *(n)*; movement *(n)*
muerte	death *(n)*
muerto	dead *(adj)*
muestra	sample *(n)*
mujer	woman *(n)*
muleta	crutch *(n)*
múltiple	multiple *(adj)*
mundo	world *(n)*

Español	*English*
muñon	stump (amputation) *(n)*
murmurar; hablar en voz baja	whisper *(v)*
musculoesquelético	musculoskeletal *(adj)*
nacido muerto; parto de un niño muerto; mortinato	stillbirth *(n)*
nacimiento	birth *(n)*
nada	nothing *(pron)*
nada por boca	nothing by mouth
nadar	swim *(v)*
nadie	nobody *(pron)*
narcolepsia	narcolepsy *(n)*
narcótico	narcotic *(adj)*
nariz sangrienta	bloody nose *(n)*
nariz tapada	stuffed (nose) *(adj)*
nasal	nasal *(adj)*
natimuerto	stillbirth *(n)*
nativo	native *(adj)*
natural	natural *(adj)*
naturaleza	nature *(n)*
naturaleza de la enfermedad	nature of the illness
nausea	nausea *(n)*
nauseas del embrazo	morning sickness *(n)*
nauseas matutinas; mareos matutinos	morning sickness *(n)*
navaja de afeitar	razor *(n)*
navidad	Christmas *(n)*
nebulizador	nebulizer *(n)*
necesario	necessary *(adj)*
necesidad	necessity *(n)*
necesitar	need *(v)*
negativo	negative *(adj)*

Español	*English*
negligencia	neglect *(n)*
negligencia médica	malpractice *(n)*
nervio	nerve *(n)*
nervio atrapado	pinched nerve *(n)*
nervio pinzado	pinched nerve *(n)*
nerviosidad	nervousness *(n)*
nervioso	anxious *(adj)*; nervous *(adj)*
neumonía	pneumonia *(n)*
neurocirujano	neurosurgeon *(n)*
neurológico	neurologic *(adj)*
neurólogo	neurologist *(n)*
neuropatía	neuropathy *(n)*
neurosífilis	neurosyphillis *(n)*
niacina	niacin *(n)*
nicotina	nicotine *(n)*
nieve	snow *(n)*
nigua (in Guatemala, a nigua is also a crybaby or coward); garrapata	chigger *(n)*
nilón	nylon *(n)*
ninguno	none *(adj)*
niño	boy *(n)*
nitroglicerina	nitroglycerin *(n)*
noción	idea *(n)*
nocturno	night *(n)*
nodo	node *(n)*
nódulo	nodule *(n)*
nódulo linfático	lymph node *(n)*
no infeccioso	noninfectious *(adj)*
no inflamable	nonflammable *(adj)*
no invasor	noninvasive *(adj)*
nombre	name *(n)*
nombre de soltera	maiden name *(n)*
normal	normal *(adj)*
notar	notice *(v)*

Español	English
noticias	news *(n)*
novocaína	novocaine *(n)*
nudo	bag *(n)*; bursa *(n)*
nuevo	new *(adj)*
nunca	never *(adv)*
nutrición	nutrition *(n)*
nutritivo	nourishing *(adj)*; nutrient *(n)*; nutritious *(adj)*
obeso	obese *(adj)*
objeción	objection *(n)*
objetivo	objective *(adj)*; goal *(n)*
objeto	object *(n)*
obligación	obligation *(n)*
observación	observation *(n)*
obsesión	obsession *(n)*
obsesivo-compulsivo	obsessive-compulsive *(adj)*
obsoleto	obsolete *(adj)*
obstáculo	obstacle *(n)*
obstétrico	obstetrician *(n)*
obstrucción	blockage *(n)*; obstruction *(n)*
obvio	obvious *(adj)*
oclusante	occluding *(adj)*
ocupación	occupation *(n)*
ocupacional	occupational *(adj)*
ocupado	busy *(adj)*; occupied *(adj)*
ocurrir	happen *(v)*
oficial	official *(adj)*
oficina	office *(n)*
oftalmólogo	ophthalmologist *(n)*
oído interno	inner ear *(n)*
oír	hear *(v)*
ojo negro	black eye *(n)*
olas de calor	hot flashes *(n)*
oler(ue)	smell *(v)*

Español	English
olfato	smell *(n)*
olor	odor *(n)*; smell *(n)*
olvidadizo	forgetful *(adj)*
ombligo	navel *(n)*
oncólogo	oncologist *(n)*
onsentimiento	consent *(n)*
opacidad	haziness *(adj)*; opacity *(n)*
opción	choice *(n)*
operable	operable *(adj)*
operación	operation *(n)*
operar	operate *(v)*
opinión	opinion *(n)*
oportunidad	opportunity *(n)*
opresivo	crushing *(adj)*
oprimir	click *(n)*
óptico	optical *(adj)*; optician *(n)*
opuesto	opposite *(adj)*
orden	order *(n)*
ordenar	order *(v)*
órgano	organ *(n)*
órganos genitales	genitals *(n)*
orgasmo	climax (sexual) *(n)*; orgasm *(n)*
orificio	hole *(n)*
original	original *(adj)*
orina	urine *(n)*
orinal	bedpan *(n)*
orinar	urinate *(v)*
ortodontista	orthodontist *(n)*
ortopédico	orthopedist *(n)*
orzuelo	sty *(n)*
oscuro	dim *(adj)*
osteoporosis	osteoporosis *(n)*
otorinolaringólogo	otorhinolaryngologist *(n)*
otro	another *(adj)*; other *(adj)*

Español	*English*
otro véz	again *(adv)*
ovulación	ovulation *(n)*
ovular	ovulate *(v)*
oxígeno	oxygen *(n)*
oxiuro; lombriz intestinal	pinworm *(n)*
paciencia	patience *(n)*
paciente	patient *(n)*
paciente ambulatorio	outpatient *(n)*
padre	priest *(n)*
pagar	pay *(v)*
pago	payment *(n)*
país	country *(n)*
paja; papete; pajilla sorbeto	straw (drinking) *(n)*
pálido	pale *(adj)*
palpitación	heartbeat *(n)*; palpitation *(n)*
palpitación lenta	slow heartbeat *(n)*
palpitacion rádipa	rapid heartbeat *(n)*
Papanicolaou; citologia vaginal	Pap smear *(n)*
papel	paper *(n)*
paperas	mumps *(n)*
paquete	package *(n)*
parada	stop *(n)*
parálisis	paralysis *(n)*
parálisis facial	Bell's palsy *(n)*
parálisis infantil	polio *(n)*
paralítico	paralyzed *(adj)*
paramédico	paramedic *(n)*
paranoia	paranoia *(n)*
paranoico	paranoid *(adj)*
para qué	why *(adv/conj)*
parar	stop *(v)*
pare	stop *(n)*; stop *(v)*
pared	wall *(n)*
pare de caminar	stop *(v)*

Español	*English*
parpadear	blink *(v)*
párroco	priest *(n)*
parte	part *(n)*
partera	midwife *(n)*
parto	childbirth *(n)*; delivery (parturition) *(n)*; labor *(n)*
parto falso	false labor *(n)*
parto mútiple	multiple birth *(n)*
pasajero; de corta duración; transitorio	fleeting *(adj)*
pasar	happen *(v)*; pass *(v)*
pasar gas	gas, to pass *(v)*
pasatiempo	hobby *(n)*
pase usted	come in *(v)*
pasillo	hall *(n)*
pasmo seco	lockjaw *(n)*
pastilla	tablet *(n)*; pill (solid) *(n)*
pastor	minister *(n)*
pataletas	tantrum (temper) *(n)*
patiestevado	bowlegged *(adj)*
patio trasero; jardin posterior; traspatio	backyard *(n)*
patizambo	bowlegged *(adj)*
patólogo	pathologist *(n)*
paz	peace *(n)*
pedacitos de hielo	ice chips *(n)*
pedazo de una sobresaliente	hangnail *(n)*
pedir	ask *(v)*
pedíatra	pediatrician *(n)*
pedicura	pedicure *(n)*
pegajoso	sticky *(adj)*
peligroso	dangerous *(adj)*
pélivo	pelvic *(adj)*

Español	English
pelo	hair *(n)*
pelota	ball *(n)*
peluca	wig *(n)*
pellejo de una sobresaliente	hangnail *(n)*
pena	grief *(n)*
pendiente	pending *(adj)*
penetración	penetration *(n)*
penetrante	penetrating *(adj)*
penicilina	penicillin *(n)*
pensar(ie)	think *(v)*
peor	worse *(adj/adv)*
pequeño	little (size) *(adj)*; small *(adj)*
perceptible	detectable *(adj)*; noticeable *(adj)*
perder(ie)	lose *(v)*
perder(ie) conocimiento	lose consciousness *(v)*
pérdida	loss *(n)*
perdida de conocimiento	blackout *(n)*
perdón	excuse *(n)*
perfecto	perfect *(adj)*
perforado	perforated *(adj)*; ruptured *(adj)*
perforar	puncture *(n)*
periódico	newspaper *(n)*
período	period *(n)*
periodontista	periodontist *(n)*
permanente	permanent *(adj)*
permiso	permission *(n)*; permit *(n)*
peróxido de hidrógeno	peroxide, hydrogen *(n)*
perro	dog *(n)*
persona	person *(n)*
personal	personal *(adj)*
personalidad	personality *(n)*

Español	English
pesadez	heaviness *(n)*
pesadilla	nightmare *(n)*
pesadumbre	grief *(n)*
pesar	weigh *(v)*
pesario	pessary *(n)*
peso	weight *(n)*
pesticida	pesticide *(n)*
picadura	bite (insect) *(n)*; prick (insect) *(n)*; sting (insect) *(n)*
picadura de insecto	insect bite *(n)*
picante	hot (spicy) *(adj)*
picazón	itch *(n)*
pie deforme	clubfoot *(n)*
piel amarilla	jaundice *(n)*
pigmento	pigment *(n)*
píldora	pill (solid) *(n)*
pinchazo	prick (needle) *(n)*; puncture *(n)*
pintura	paint *(n)*
pintura con plomo	lead-based paint *(n)*
piojos	lice *(n)*
pipa	pipe (tobacco) *(n)*
piso	floor (of building) *(n)*
placenta	afterbirth *(n)*
planta del pie	sole (foot) *(n)*
plantilla	insole (shoes) *(n)*
plata	silver *(n)*
playa	beach *(n)*
pleito	lawsuit *(n)*
plomo	lead (metal) *(n)*
pluma	pen *(n)*
pocas veces	seldom *(adv)*
poco	little (amount) *(adj)*
poder	can *(v)*
podiatra	podiatrist *(n)*
podiatrista	podiatrist *(n)*

Español	English
policía	police *(n)*
poliomielitis	polio *(n)*
pólipo	polyp *(n)*
polvo	dust *(n)*; powder *(n)*
polvo de ángel	angel dust/PCP *(n)*
pomada	ointment *(n)*
poner pleito; demandar; entablar una demanda	sue *(v)*
ponerse colorado	flushing *(v)*
ponerse de pie	stand up *(v)*
por	by *(prep)*; per *(prep/adv)*
por día	daily *(adj)*
por ejemplo	for example
por favor	please *(adv)*
poro	pore *(n)*
por qué	why *(adv/conj)*
porque	because *(conj)*
portador	carrier (of disease) *(n)*
portarse mal; comportarse mal; manejarse mal	misbehave *(v)*
posible	possible *(adj)*
posición	position *(n)*
positivo	positive *(adj)*
posoperatorio	postoperative *(adj)*
potasio	potassium *(n)*
potencia	potency *(n)*
potente; poderoso	powerful *(adj)*
precaución	precaution *(n)*
preciso	precise *(adj)*
predicir	predict *(v)*
predispuesto	prejudiced *(adj)*
prednisona	prednisone *(n)*
preferible	preferable *(adj)*
pregunta	question *(n)*

Español	English
preguntar	ask (question) *(v)*
preliminar	preliminary *(n/adj)*
prematuro	premature *(adj)*
prenatal	prenatal *(adj)*
preocupado	concerned *(adj)*; worried *(adj)*
preocupante	worrisome *(adj)*
preoperatorio	preoperative *(adj)*
preparación	preparation *(n)*
preparar	prepare *(v)*
prescribir	prescribe *(v)*
presentación de nalgas	breech (birth) *(n)*
presente	present *(adj)*
presión	pressure *(n)*
presionar	click *(n)*
presión sanguínea	blood pressure *(n)*
préstamo	loan *(n)*
prevención	prevention *(n)*
preventivo	preventive *(adj)*
previo	previous *(adj)*
primario	primary *(adj)*
principal; esencial	main *(adj)*
probabilidad	chance (probability) *(n)*
probar(ue)	try *(v)*
proceder	proceed *(v)*
procedimiento	procedure *(n)*
profundo	deep *(adj)*
progesterona	progesterone *(n)*
prognóstica	prognosis *(n)*
programa	program *(n)*; schedule *(n)*
progresivo	progressive *(adj)*
prolongado	long *(adj)*; prolonged *(adj)*
promesa	promise *(n)*
pronto	soon *(adv)*

Español	English
pronunciación inarticulada	slurred speech *(n)*
propagar	spread (disease) *(v)*
prostituta	prostitute *(n)*
protección	protection *(n)*
proteccionista; protector	protective *(adj)*
proteína	protein *(n)*
prótesis	prosthesis *(n)*
proturberante	bulging *(adj)*
provisiones	supplies *(n)*
próximo	next *(adj)*
prueba de tolerancia al estuerzo; prueba de cinta rodante	stress test *(n)*
pubertad	puberty *(n)*
púbico	pubic *(adj)*
pujo	contraction (labor) *(n)*
pulga	flea *(n)*
pulgada	inch *(n)*
pulso	pulse *(n)*
pulverizador; aereosol; rociada	spray *(n)*
puna; mal de montaña	mountain sickness *(n)*
punción	tap *(n)*
punción lumbar	spinal tap *(n)*
punta	point *(n)*; tip *(n)*
punto de vista	viewpoint *(n)*
punto máximo	peak *(n)*
puntura; pinchazo	prick (needle) *(n)*
punzante	throbbing (pain) *(adj)*
puño	fist *(n)*
pus	pus *(n)*
qué	what *(prep)*
queja	complaint *(n)*
quejar	complain *(v)*

Español	English
queloide	keloid *(n)*
quemado del sol	sunburned *(adj)*
quemadura	burn *(n)*
quemadura de sol	sunburn *(n)*
quemante	burning *(adj)*
quemar	burn *(v)*
querer(ie)	want (love) *(v)*
quimoterápia	chemotherapy *(n)*
rabia	rabies *(n)*
ración	portion (food) *(n)*
radiación	radiation *(n)*
radiar; resplandecer, irradiar luz	radiating *(adj)*
radioactivo	radioactive *(adj)*
radiografía	x-ray *(n)*
radiólogo	radiologist *(n)*
raíz nerviosa	nerve root *(n)*
raja	slice *(n)*
rancio	rancid *(adj)*
rápidamente	quickly *(adv)*
rápido	fast *(adj)*; quick *(adj)*
raras veces	rarely *(adv)*
rascar; arañar; rasguñar	pick (scratch) *(v)*; scratch *(v)*
rastreo	screening *(n)*
rayos equis	x-ray *(n)*
razón	reason *(n)*
reacción	reaction *(n)*
reacción adversa	adverse reaction
reacción alérgica	allergic reaction *(n)*
reaparición	recurrence *(n)*
rebanada	slice (bread) *(n)*
rebote	rebound *(n)*
recaída	setback *(n)*
recargo; renovación de receta; renovación	refill *(n)*
recepcionista	receptionist *(n)*

Español	*English*
receta	prescription *(n)*
recetar	prescribe *(v)*
recibir	receive *(v)*
recibo	receipt *(n)*
recién casado	newlywed *(n)*
recién nacido	newborn *(n)*
reciente	recent *(adj)*
recomendar	recommend *(v)*
recordar(ue)	remember *(v)*
rectal	rectal *(adj)*
recuento de globulos	blood count *(n)*
recuperación	recovery *(n)*
recuperar	recover *(v)*; recuperate *(v)*
recurso	resource *(n)*
rechazo	rejection *(n)*
reducción	reduction *(n)*
reducir	lessen *(v)*
reemplazo	replacement *(n)*
reemplazo de la rodilla	knee replacement *(n)*
reemplazo total de la cadera	total hip replacement *(n)*
reflejo	reflex *(n)*; response *(n)*
reflujo	reflux *(n)*
regalo	present (gift) *(n)*
registrar	register *(v)*
registros médicos	medical records *(n)*
regla	rule *(n)*
regular	regular *(adj)*
regusto	aftertaste *(n)*
rehabilitación	rehabilitation *(n)*
reinfección	reinfection *(n)*
relacionado	related *(adj)*
relaciónes sexuales	sexual intercourse *(n)*
relajante	relaxant *(n)*
relajante muscular	muscle relaxant *(n)*
relámpago	lightning *(n)*
reloj	clock *(n)*; watch *(n)*
remedio	cure *(n)*
remisión	remission *(n)*
remojar	soak *(v)*
renal	renal *(adj)*
reparar	mend *(v)*
repelente	repellent *(n)*
repelente contra insectos	insect repellent *(n)*
repentino	sudden *(adj)*
reposo	rest *(n)*
resaca	hangover *(n)*
residencia	residence *(n)*
residuo	remnant *(n)*
resistencia	resistence *(n)*
resistir	resist *(v)*
resollar	wheeze *(v)*
resollo	wheeze *(n)*
respiración	respiration *(n)*
respirar	breathe *(v)*
responsibilidad	responsibility *(n)*
respuesta; contestación	answer *(n)*; response *(n)*
restringido	restrictive *(adj)*
resultado	outcome *(n)*; result *(n)*
resuscitación	resuscitation *(n)*
retina desprendida	detached retina *(n)*
retinopatía	retinopathy *(n)*
retirada	withdrawl *(n)*
reumático	rheumatic *(adj)*
reumatoide	rheumatoid *(adj)*
reumatólogo	rheumatologist *(n)*
reusable	reusable *(adj)*
revisar	check *(v)*
riesgo	risk *(n)*

Español	English
rígido	rigid *(adj)*
rigido; tieso; agarrotamiento	stiff (joint) *(adj)*
ritmo	rhythm *(n)*
roncar	snore *(v)*
ronco	hoarse *(adj)*
ronchas	hives *(n)*
ronquera	hoarseness *(n)*
roséola	roseola *(n)*
rubeola	German measles *(n)*
ruido	noise *(n)*
ruidoso	loud *(adj)*; noisy *(adj)*
sábana	sheet *(n)*
saber	know (facts, how to) *(v)*
sabor	flavor *(n)*; taste *(n)*
sacerdote	priest *(n)*
sala	room *(n)*
sala de cirugía	operating room *(n)*
sala de clase; salón de clase	classroom *(n)*
sala de espera	waiting room *(n)*
sala de parto	labor room *(n)*
sala de recuperación	recovery room *(n)*
salado	salty *(adj)*
salario	salary *(n)*
sal de epsom	Epsom salt *(n)*
salida	exit *(n)*
salino	saline *(n)*
salir	leave *(v)*
saliva	saliva *(n)*; spit *(n)*
salmonela	salmonella *(n)*
salón principal	lobby *(n)*
salpullido	fleabite *(n)*; rash (skin) *(n)*
salpullido de pañal	diaper rash *(n)*
saltar	hop *(v)*; jump *(v)*
salud	health (of a person) *(n)*
saludable	healthy *(adj)*
sangradera; lanceta	lancet *(n)*
sangrando	bleeding *(n)*
sangrar	bleed *(v)*
sangre	blood *(n)*
sangriento	bloody *(adj)*
sanguijuela	leech (parasite) *(n)*
santos óleos; ùltimos titos; extremaunción	last rites *(n)*
sarampión	measles *(n)*
sarampión alemán	German measles *(n)*
sarcoma de Kaposi	Kaposi's sarcoma *(n)*
sarpullido	eruption (skin) *(n)*
seco	dry *(adj)*
secreción	secretion *(n)*
sed	thirst *(n)*
sedante	sedative *(n)*
sedante ligero	mild sedative *(n)*
segundo nombre	middle name *(n)*
seguridad	safety *(n)*
seguro	insurance *(n)*
seguro de vida	life insurance *(n)*
seguro social	Social Security *(n)*
semejante	similar *(adj)*
semen	semen *(n)*
sencillo	simple *(adj)*
seno nasal; cavidad nasal	sinus *(n)*
sensación	feeling (sensation) *(n)*; sensation *(n)*
sensación de desmayo	light-headedness *(n)*
sensible	sensitive *(adj)*
sensible; doloroso	tender *(adj)*
sentar	sit *(v)*
sentido	hearing *(n)*

Spanish	*English*
sentir	feel *(v)*
señalar	point *(v)*
senimiento de culpabilidad	guilty feelings *(n)*
sentirse cadiente	to feel *(v)*
separado	separated *(adj)*
sequedad	dryness *(n)*
serio	serious *(adj)*
serpiente	snake *(n)*
serpiente de cascabel	rattlesnake *(n)*
servicio de análisis	screening *(n)*
severo	severe *(adj)*
sexo	sex *(n)*
sexual	sexual *(adj)*
sí	yes *(adv/n)*
sicosis	psychosis *(n)*
sicoterapia	psychotherapy *(n)*
sicótico	psychotic *(adj)*
siempre	always *(adv)*
siesta	nap *(n)*
sifilis	syphilis *(n)*
signo	sign *(n)*
silencioso	quiet (no noise) *(adj)*
silla	chair *(n)*
simétrico	symmetrical *(adj)*
simpatía	sympathy *(n)*
sin dolor	painless *(adj)*
sindrome de Down	Down syndrome *(n)*
síndrome de muerte infantil repentina	SIDS/sudden infant death syndrome *(n)*
sin esperanza	hopeless *(adj)*
sin olor	odorless *(adj)*
sin receta medica; sobre el mostrador	over-the-counter *(adj)*
sin techo	homeless *(adj)*

Español	*English*
síntoma	symptom *(n)*
sinusitis	sinusitis *(n)*
siquiatra	psychiatrist *(n)*
sistema	system *(n)*
sistema nervioso central	central nervous system *(n)*
sistemático	systemic *(adj)*
sobras	leftovers *(n)*
sobrevivir	survive *(v)*
sobrio	sober *(adj)*
social	social *(adj)*
sodio	sodium *(n)*
sofocado	to be hot (weather) *(adj)*
sol	sun *(n)*
solamente	only *(adv)*
sólido	solid *(n/adj)*
solo	alone *(adj)*; only *(adv)*
soltero	single (marital status) *(adj)*
solución salina	saline solution *(n)*
somnoliento; adormecido	drowsy *(adj)*
sonar	blow *(v)*
sonido	sound *(n)*
soñoliento; con sueño	sleepy *(adj)*
soplar	blow (breathe out) *(v)*
soplo cardiaco	murmur *(n)*
soplo funcional	innocent murmur *(n)*
sopor; soñera; amodorramiento	drowsiness *(n)*
sorbo	sip *(n)*
sordo	deaf *(adj)*
sótano	basement *(n)*

Español	English
suave	gentle *(adj)*; mild (medicine) *(adj)*; soft *(adj)*
suave (comida suave)	bland *(adj)*
suciedad; basura; mugre	dirt *(n)*
sudar	sweat *(v)*
sudor	perspiration *(n)*; sweat *(n)*
sudor nocturno	night sweats *(n)*
suelo	floor (flooring) *(n)*
suelto	loose *(adj)*
sueño	dream *(n)*; sleep *(n)*
suficiente	enough *(adj)*; sufficient *(adj)*
sufrir	suffer *(v)*
sufrir un colapso	collapse *(v)*
suicidio	suicide *(n)*
sulfamida	sulfa drug *(n)*
superar	ooze *(v)*
superficial	superficial *(adj)*
superior	upper *(adj)*
supermercado	supermarket *(n)*
supervisión	supervision *(n)*
suplemento	supplement *(n)*
supositorio	suppository *(n)*
supositorio vaginal	vaginal suppository *(n)*
supuración	drainage *(n)*
supurante	weeping (oozing) *(n)*
susceptible	susceptible *(adj)*
suspensorio	jockstrap *(n)*
sutura	suture *(n)*
tabaco	tobacco *(n)*
tabaco de mascar	chewing tobacco *(n)*
tablilla	splint *(n)*
talipédico	clubfooted *(adj)*
tal vez	perhaps *(adv)*
tamaño	size *(n)*
tambien	also *(adv)*
tampón	tampon *(n)*
tan	as *(adv)*
tanque de oxígeno	oxygen tank *(n)*
tanto	as much *(adv)*
tarde	afternoon *(n)*; late *(adj)*
tardío; atrasado; rotrasado	overdue (pregnancy) *(adj)*
tartamudez	stuttering *(n)*
tatuaje	tattoo *(n)*
taza de medir	measuring cup *(n)*
tecnología	technology *(n)*
teléfono	telephone *(n)*
televisión	television *(n)*
temblor	tremor *(n)*
tembloroso	shaky *(adj)*
temperatura	temperature *(n)*
templado	lukewarm *(adj)*; warm *(adj)*
temporal	temporary *(adj)*
tendencia	tendency *(n)*
tener	have (to possess) *(v)*; hold (an object) *(v)*; own *(v)*
tener frío	to be cold *(v)*
tener hambre	to be hungry *(v)*
tener miedo	to be afraid *(v)*
tener que (+ infinitive)	have to (must) *(v)*
tenia	tapeworm *(n)*
tensión	stress *(n)*
tentador	tempting *(adj)*
terapeuta	therapist *(n)*
terapeuta del habla	speech therapy *(n)*
terapeuta ocupacional	occupational therapist *(n)*

Español	*English*
terapia	therapy *(n)*
terapia electroconvulsiva	ECT/electroconvulsive therapy *(n)*
terapia electrochoque	ECT/electroconvulsive therapy *(n)*
terapia ocupacional	occupational therapy *(n)*
terapia por medio de luz	sun therapy *(n)*
terapista físico	physical therapist *(n)*
termómetro	thermometer *(n)*
terrores nocturnos	night terrors *(n)*
testamento	will (legal) *(n)*
testigo	witness *(n)*
testosterona	testosterone *(n)*
tétano	lockjaw *(n)*; tetanus *(n)*
tez; cutis	complexion *(n)*
tiempo parcial	part-time *(adv)*
tifoidea	typhoid *(n)*
tímpano perforado	perforated eardrum *(n)*
tiña	ringworm *(n)*
tinea cruris; tiña inguinal	jock itch *(n)*
típico	typical *(adj)*
tipo	type *(n)*
tipo de epilepsia	petit mal *(n)*
tiroidectomía	thyroidectomy *(n)*
toalla	towel *(n)*
tocar	touch *(v)*
todo	all *(adj)*; whole *(adj)*
tolerar	tolerate *(v)*
tolerencia	tolerance *(n)*
tomar	take *(v)*
tono	tone *(n)*
tonsilitis	tonsilitis *(n)*
tonsilotomía	tonsillectomy *(n)*
tópico	topical *(adj)*
toque	dab *(n)*
torcedura	sprain *(v)*
torcedura de musculo	strain (muscle) *(v)*
torniquete	tourniquet *(n)*
torpe	clumsy *(adj)*
tos	cough *(n)*
toser	cough *(v)*
tosferina	whooping cough *(n)*
total	total *(adj)*
totalidad	whole *(n)*
tóxico	toxic *(adj)*
trabajador social	social worker *(n)*
trabajar	work *(v)*
trabajo	employment*(n)* ; job *(n)*; work *(n)*
traer	bring *(v)*
tragar	swallow *(v)*
trago	shot (beverage) *(n)*; swallow *(n)*
tramo de escalera	flight of stairs *(n)*
tranquilo	calm *(adj)*
transexual	transsexual *(n)*
transfusión	transfusion *(n)*
transfusión sanguínea	blood transfusion *(n)*
transpiración	perspiration *(n)*
transporte	transportation *(n)*
transvestido	transvestite *(n)*
trasplante	transplant *(n)*
trastorno de la personalidad	personality disorder *(n)*
tratamiento	therapy *(n)*
tratamiento hormonal	hormone treatment *(n)*
tratamiento	treatment *(n)*
traumático	traumatic *(adj)*
tricomonas	Trichomonas *(n)*

Español	English
trimestre	trimester *(n)*
tripletos	triplets *(n)*
triste	sad *(adj)*
tropezar (usted se tropezó)	trip (on/over) *(v)*
trotar	jog *(v)*
tubárico	tubal *(adj)*
tubario	tubal *(adj)*
tuberculosis	tuberculosis *(n)*
tumor	tumor *(n)*
tumor benigno	benign tumor *(n)*
tumor fibroideo	fibroid tumor *(n)*
turbio	cloudy (liquid) *(adj)*
úlcera	ulcer *(n)*
último	last *(adj)*
ultrasonido	ultrasound *(n)*
umbilical	umbilical *(adj)*
anquilostoma	hookworm *(n)*
único	only *(adj)*
unidad	unit *(n)*
union consensual	common-law marriage *(n)*
uña	nail (finger/toe) *(n)*
uña encarnada	ingrown toenail *(n)*
uñero	ingrown toenail *(n)*
urgencia	urgency *(n)*
urgente	urgent *(adj)*
urinación	urination *(n)*
urólogo	urologist *(n)*
usar	use *(v)*
usual	usual *(adj)*
útil	useful *(adj)*
vaciar	empty *(v)*
vacío	empty *(adj)*
vacuna	immunization *(n)*; vaccination *(n)*; vaccine *(n)*

Español	English
vacunar	immunize *(v)*; vaccinate *(v)*
vaginal	vaginal *(adj)*
vago	vague *(adj)*
vale	voucher *(n)*
valioso	valuable *(adj)*
válvula	valve *(n)*
válvula del corazón	heart valve *(n)*
vapor	fumes *(n)*; steam *(n)*
vaporizador	vaporizer *(n)*
variable	variable *(adj)*
variación	variation *(n)*
variado	varied *(adj)*
variar	vary *(v)*
varicela	chicken pox *(n)*
várices	varicose veins *(n)*
varicoso	varicose *(adj)*
variedad	variety *(n)*
varios	several *(adj)*
varón	male *(adj/n)*
vaselina	Vaseline *(n)*
vaso	glass (drinking) *(n)*
vegetariano	vegetarian *(adj)*
venas varicosas	varicose veins *(n)*
vendaje	bandage *(n)*
vendar	bandage *(v)*
veneno	poison *(n)*
venenoso	poisonous *(adj)*
venida	coming *(n)*
venir	come *(v)*
ventana	window *(n)*
ventilador	ventilator *(n)*
ver	see *(v)*
verdoso	greenish *(adj)*
verruga	wart *(n)*
vértigo	Ménière's disease *(n)*
vestir	dress *(v)*

Español	*English*
vestirse	dress oneself *(v)*
vestuario	changing room *(n)*
vía oral	orally *(adv)*
vía respiratoria	airway *(n)*
vibración	vibration *(n)*
vicio	habit (vice) *(n)*
víctima	victim *(n)*
vida	life *(n)*
viejo	old *(adj)*
viento	wind (air) *(n)*
vigoroso	vigorous *(adj)*
VIH/virus de inmunodeficiencia humana	HIV/human immunodeficiency virus *(n)*
violar	rape *(v)*; violate *(v)*
violencia	violence *(n)*
violento	aggressive *(adj)*; violent *(adj)*
viral	viral *(adj)*
virgen	virgin *(n)*
viruelas	smallpox *(n)*
virus	virus *(n)*
virus de papiloma humano	HPV/human papillomavirus *(n)*
viscoso; pegajoso	sticky *(adj)*
visible	visible *(adj)*
visión	hallucination *(n)*; vision *(n)*; sight *(n)*

Español	*English*
visita	visitor *(n)*
visitar	visit *(v)*
vista	sight *(n)*; view *(n)*; visit *(n)*
vitamina	vitamin *(n)*
viuda	widow *(n)*
viudo	widower *(n)*
vivir	live *(v)*
vivo	alive *(adj)*; live *(adj)*
vocal	vocal *(adj)*
voluntad	will (volition) *(n)*
voluntario	voluntary *(adj)*; volunteer *(n)*
vomitar	vomit *(v)*
vómito	vomit *(n)*; vomiting *(n)*
voz	voice *(n)*
vulnerable	vulnerable *(adj)*
y	and *(conj)*
ya	already *(adv)*
yeso	cast *(n)*
yoga	yoga *(n)*
zambo	bowlegged *(adj)*
zoster	herpes*(n)* ; zoster *(n)*
zumaque venenosa	poison ivy *(n)*
zumbido	buzz *(n)*
zurra	spanking *(n)*

Index

F

G

H

K

L

M

N

Q

R

S

Y